Dr. Roger De Lange, Jr., D.V.M.

January 23, 1992

OVERDENTURES

OVERDENTURES

ALLEN A. BREWER, D.D.S., F.A.C.D.

Chairman, Department of Prosthodontics, Eastman Dental Center, Rochester,
New York; Associate Professor of Clinical Dentistry and Dental Research,
University of Rochester School of Medicine and Dentistry, Rochester, New York;
Clinical Professor of Prosthodontics, State University of New York School of
Dentistry, Buffalo, New York

ROBERT M. MORROW, D.D.S., F.A.C.D., F.I.C.D.

Colonel, United States Air Force Dental Corps; Chief, Prosthodontics,
USAF Clinic, Honolulu, Hawaii; formerly Clinical Associate Professor,
University of Texas Dental Branch, Houston, Texas, and Assistant Chairman
for Resident Training and Research, Department of Prosthodontics,
Wilford Hall USAF Medical Center, San Antonio, Texas

with 591 *illustrations*

The C. V. Mosby Company

SAINT LOUIS   1975

Copyright © 1975 by The C. V. Mosby Company

All rights reserved. No part of this book may be reproduced in any manner without written permission of the publisher.

Printed in the United States of America

Distributed in Great Britain by Henry Kimpton, London

Library of Congress Cataloging in Publication Data

Brewer, Allen A   1911-
   Overdentures.

  Bibliography: p.
  Includes index.
  1. Overlay dentures. I. Morrow, Robert M., 1931-   joint author. II. Title. [DNLM: 1. Denture, Complete. 2. Denture retention. WU530 B847o]
RK656.B7   617.6'92   74-28500
ISBN 0-8016-3515-2

VH/VH/VH 9 8 7 6 5 4 3 2

CONTRIBUTORS

WILLIAM F. BOURNE, B.S., D.D.S., M.S.,
Colonel USAF DC

Chief, Endodontics Section, USAF Clinic,
Honolulu, Hawaii

ALLEN A. BREWER, D.D.S., F.A.C.D.

Chairman, Department of Prosthodontics,
Eastman Dental Center, Rochester, New York;
Associate Professor of Clinical Dentistry and
Dental Research, University of Rochester
School of Medicine and Dentistry, Rochester,
New York; Clinical Professor of Prosthodontics,
State University of New York School of
Dentistry, Buffalo, New York

ROBERT J. CRONIN, Jr., D.D.S.,
Major USAF DC

Prosthodontic Resident, Wilford Hall USAF
Medical Center, San Antonio, Texas

ROBERT J. CRUM, D.D.S.

Prosthodontics Section Chief, Veterans Administration
Hospital, Hines, Illinois; Clinical Associate Professor,
Prosthodontics, Loyola University School of Dentistry,
Maywood, Illinois; Clinical Associate Professor,
Prosthodontics, University of Illinois College of
Dentistry, Chicago, Illinois

HAMPTON GREEN, Jr., B.S., D.D.S., F.I.C.D.,
Colonel USAF DC

Chief, Dental Services, Dover AFB, Dover, Delaware

LEONARD G. JEWSON, D.D.S., M.S.D.,
Colonel USAF DC

Chairman, Department of Periodontics,
USAF Medical Center, Wright-Patterson AFB,
Dayton, Ohio

JOHN D. LARKIN, D.D.S., F.A.C.D., F.I.C.D.

Clinical Professor, Complete Restorations,
University of Texas Dental Branch, Houston, Texas;
Clinical Professor, Department of Prosthodontics,
University of Texas, Health Science Center
at San Antonio, San Antonio, Texas;
Consultant in Prosthodontics to Veterans
Administration Hospital, Houston, Texas,
Wilford Hall USAF Medical Center, San Antonio,
Texas, and Brooke Army Medical Center,
San Antonio, Texas

MERRILL C. MENSOR, Jr., B.A.,
D.D.S., F.I.C.D.

Formerly Assistant Clinical Professor,
Department of Fixed Prosthodontics,
University of Pacific School of Dentistry,
San Francisco, California

ROBERT M. MORROW, D.D.S., F.A.C.D.,
F.I.C.D.

Colonel, United States Air Force Dental Corps;
Chief, Prosthodontics, USAF Clinic, Honolulu,
Hawaii; formerly Clinical Associate Professor,
University of Texas Dental Branch, Houston, Texas,
and Assistant Chairman for Resident Training
and Research, Department of Prosthodontics,
Wilford Hall USAF Medical Center,
San Antonio, Texas

JOHN W. MYERS, B.S., D.D.S., M.S.

Practice limited to endodontics, San Antonio, Texas

PETER R. REINER, D.D.S., Colonel USAF DC

Chief, Area Dental Laboratory, McChord AFB,
Tacoma, Washington

KENNETH D. RUDD, B.S., D.D.S., F.A.C.D., F.I.C.D., **Colonel USAF DC (Ret.)**

Coordinator for Continuing Education and Professor of Prosthodontics, University of Texas Health Science Center, San Antonio, Texas

IRA L. SHANNON, B.S., D.M.D., M.S.D., F.A.C.D.

Director, Oral Physiology Research Laboratory, Veterans Administration Hospital, Houston, Texas; Professor (Biochemistry), University of Texas Dental Branch, Houston, Texas; Faculty, University of Texas Graduate School of Biomedical Sciences, Houston, Texas

JOHN J. TARSITANO, D.D.S., **Colonel USAF DC**

Director, Dental Services Division, USAF Hospital, Wiesbaden, Germany; Consultant to USAFE Surgeon General

This book is dedicated to the many edentulous patients who have convinced us that one of the worst tragedies that can befall a man is the loss of all his teeth.

FOREWORD

Reference to the dental literature indicates that innumerable techniques have been developed and many textbooks written about complete dentures because of the increasing number of aging and chronically ill patients in need of this type of prosthesis. The majority of the techniques have been rendered obsolete by more advanced procedures.

The present stage of implantology and the retention of teeth for support have led to a close scrutiny and, in some instances, even a reappraisal of previous concepts. This new approach has applied advanced thinking to the anatomic, physiologic, and psychologic aspects of complete denture construction and has not made it necessary to discard established techniques.

Providing additional retentive and stabilizing forces to improve the function of dentures is a worthy goal. Similarly, preventing destruction of the bony foundation deserves every effort because its preservation for support is essential in view of the increased longevity of patients.

The overdenture is a method of meeting these needs, and the authors have oriented their instruction to the dynamic relationship between the tissues and the prosthesis. Their book will serve as a ready reference and a stimulus to research in a new area of investigation. It does not pretend to be encyclopedic, but it includes both basic information and newly accepted techniques that a dentist can apply clinically. Although nothing can take the place of experience, it is of considerable assistance to have available the detailed record of accomplishment of colleagues on which to base one's own work. Fourteen specialists have collaborated to produce this book.

The justification for adding yet another textbook to the shelves of dental literature is to be found in the presentation of the subject matter and the comparative novelty and newness of it. There has been an increasing demand in dentistry for a dependable reference that can be consulted in solving the numerous problems encountered every day in providing an overdenture service. This volume is dedicated to the principles that have been found most reliable in fabricating overdentures. It gives authentic and workable methods that will enable a dentist to treat with a high degree of success those patients who are partially edentulous.

As the authors state, the overdenture concept has been known since 1861; however, it has been used only infrequently. It will be especially gratifying if some of the readers are inspired to apply their ingenuity to develop other applications for the benefit of the patient and the advancement of the dental profession.

Although I am well aware of the faculties and capabilities of the authors, I am amazed at the lengths to which they have gone to present the subject matter so succinctly. Graduates and undergraduates will find this textbook a veritable font of information that will be an extremely valuable reference in the practice of restorative dentistry.

Jerome M. Schweitzer, D.D.S.
New York City

PREFACE

The practicing dentist soon learns that losing all of one's teeth is one of the worst tragedies in a person's life. Frequently, dentists are asked to treat patients in their fifties or sixties who were rendered edentulous between the ages of 16 and 25 years. Generally, they state that their first dentures were excellent, but each subsequent set has been less satisfactory. They find it difficult to accept the fact that continuous resorption of the residual ridges has made them "dental cripples." Many patients retain their teeth until a more advanced age, but the majority of them lack the ability to cope with complete dentures at that time. In other patients, extremely large superstructures placed on teeth with inadequate bony support have literally torn these teeth out of their sockets.

Use of the overdenture allows the patient to retain teeth that are not entrenched in bone firmly enough to support a more conventional prosthesis. Reduction of the coronal height improves the crown-root ratio, thereby permitting mobile teeth to become firm immediately. The life expectancy of these teeth is increased appreciably, the resorption of the residual ridge is retarded, and the stability and retention of the denture are improved.

The overdenture is not a new concept. In 1861 Barker reported on the proceedings of the American Dental Convention in New Haven, Connecticut. Drs. Butler, Roberts, Atkinson, Sutton, and Hayes participated in a symposium entitled "Surgical Preparation of the Mouth for Artificial Dentures: Should the Roots of Broken and Decayed Teeth Always Be Removed?" The consensus was that in many situations retention of the roots or "fangs" would enable the dentist to give the patients with complete dentures treatment superior to that obtained after extraction of all roots. Hayes reported the results of fabricating a complete denture over two roots in the maxillary arch; 12 years later they were still in place, contributing to the comfort of the patient. Since that convention more than a hundred journal articles on the retention of roots or teeth to support a complete denture have appeared. Many authors advocate the use of various attachments to increase retention and stability.

In 1945, Block, of Louisville, Kentucky, provided complete dentures for a 14-year-old girl with a congenital absence of permanent teeth. Four maxillary and four mandibular teeth were retained, and crowns were fitted to the molars. In 1972, 27 years later, the lower deciduous molars were still intact, supporting a complete mandibular denture.

During World War II, many dentists in the military service used overdentures in the treatment of inadequate or mutilated dentitions. Although few of the procedures were documented, Boos reported such a treatment in the July, 1948, issue of the *Dental Digest*. In 1944, the patient had been provided with a complete denture placed over two retained molars after they had been crowned.

An article by Rehn in 1952 advocated the retention of a single "front" tooth for denture support.

Miller reported in the *Journal of Prosthetic Dentistry* in 1958 that retention of a few teeth under complete dentures allowed "weak" teeth to regain healthy status. His foresight was of prime importance in convincing the profession that the overdenture was a superior treatment modality. Lord and Teel, in 1969, reported 7 years of successful treatment with overdentures. The Gerber series of rootcap attachments was developed in 1954. For 20 years, clinically successful hybrid prostheses have been fabricated with the Gerber attachments.

As new materials and products, such as plastic teeth, soft liners, and fluorides, were introduced, the potential for this type of treatment increased materially. Methods that formerly were expensive and time consuming were simplified without sacrificing quality. At present, overdenture treatment can be provided by any adequately oriented dentist at little additional cost beyond that for conventional complete dentures.

In this book we have attempted to present the procedural information that will enable the dental practitioner to use overdenture treatment with a high degree of success. Most of the methods, attachments, and materials currently used are included. In selecting a treatment procedure, we have adopted the premise that it should be as good as or better than any alternative plan and that it is desirable that it be simpler and less costly.

The dentist seldom has time to accomplish all of the procedures required prior to construction of the overdenture. Therefore he relies on those in various other specialties for many of the preliminary procedures. This book contains chapters by recognized authorities in these specialties and by men who have worked with us on overdentures. We greatly appreciate their valuable contributions, for without them this book would not have been possible.

Anyone who has ever written a book knows the myriad details—illustrations, references, acknowledgments, indexing, and general supervision—to which attention must be given. We thank Mrs. Lisa Maves for help in organizing and typing the early sections of the manuscript, and her husband, Bob, for making prints of many illustrations. Later sections of the manuscript were typed by Lynn Allessi, and we thank her too for her excellent help. We are deeply indebted to Jack Oster, Aaron Fenton, Gerald Graser, Edward Plekavich, Henry D. Rohrer, Jr., and William Gray, all graduate students of Dr. Brewer, who worked with him in treating many patients with overdentures. Dr. Gary Rogoff, another of his outstanding graduate students, in addition to treating patients and performing a major portion of the photography, also helped with editing portions of the manuscript, so he deserves a special vote of thanks. Dr. Eugene A. Derricotte and Dr. Frederick D. Birmingham also made significant contributions in planning and completing prerequisite treatment procedures for many of our overdenture patients. We are especially grateful to Rusty and Jamie Bolane, a husband-wife team, for giving unstintingly of their time and efforts to help with the illustrations. We wish to thank particularly Mr. Ralph Montalvo for his superb art work and Mr. George Huffman for his assistance with the photography. Mrs. Kikue K. Townsend has provided the much needed assistance in maintenance of records and schedules that has contributed to the successful completion of the manuscript. We acknowledge the excellent editorial support of Mrs. Gordon Dyer, whose help has been invaluable.

To our wives, Brownie Brewer and Wanita Morrow, whose services have been indispensable, goes credit for their tireless efforts in accomplishing much of the typing and assisting with the organizing of the manuscript. We shall be eternally grateful for their moral support in the completion of an ambitious undertaking.

The views and opinions expressed are those of the authors and do not necessarily reflect those of the United States Air Force.

Allen A. Brewer
Robert M. Morrow

CONTENTS

PART ONE RATIONALE FOR THE OVERDENTURE

1 Rationale for the retention of teeth for overdentures, 3
ROBERT J. CRUM

2 Advantages, disadvantages, indications, and contraindications, 12
ALLEN A. BREWER

PART TWO PRELIMINARY PROCEDURES

3 Special relationship between dentist and prosthodontic patient, 17
JOHN D. LARKIN

4 Examination, diagnosis, treatment planning, and prognosis, 24
ROBERT M. MORROW AND ALLEN A. BREWER

5 Periodontics and the overdenture patient, 37
LEONARD G. JEWSON

6 Endodontic considerations and treatment of overdenture abutments, 52
JOHN W. MYERS AND WILLIAM F. BOURNE

7 Surgical considerations in overdenture therapy, 62
JOHN J. TARSITANO

PART THREE METHODS

8 Overdentures for congenital and acquired defects, 77
ALLEN A. BREWER

9 Transitional overdentures, 88
ALLEN A. BREWER AND ROBERT M. MORROW

- 10 Immediate overdentures, 98
  ROBERT M. MORROW
- 11 Remote overdentures, 119
  ROBERT M. MORROW
- 12 Removable partial overdentures, 156
  ALLEN A. BREWER
- 13 Attachments for the overdenture, 162
  MERRILL C. MENSOR, Jr.
- 14 Laboratory procedures for metal bases, 191
  PETER R. REINER
- 15 Duplicating overdentures, 209
  ROBERT M. MORROW
- 16 Centric check-point procedure for determining the accuracy of jaw relation records, 214
  ROBERT M. MORROW
- 17 Metal occlusal surfaces for overdentures, 220
  ROBERT M. MORROW
- 18 Relining, rebasing, and soft liners, 226
  ALLEN A. BREWER

PART FOUR SPECIAL CONSIDERATIONS

- 19 Chemical protection of tooth surfaces in patients with overdentures, 237
  IRA L. SHANNON AND ROBERT J. CRONIN, Jr.
- 20 Overdenture problems, 248
  ALLEN A. BREWER AND ROBERT M. MORROW
- 21 The future, 256
  ALLEN A. BREWER AND ROBERT M. MORROW

Bibliography, 257

PART ONE
RATIONALE FOR THE OVERDENTURE

1
RATIONALE FOR THE RETENTION OF TEETH FOR OVERDENTURES

ROBERT J. CRUM

Preventive prosthodontics emphasizes the importance of any procedure that can delay or eliminate future prosthodontic problems. The overdenture is a logical method for the dentist to use in preventive prosthodontics. The purpose of this chapter is to present a rationale for retaining teeth, particularly mandibular canines, to support overdentures.

Retention of the roots of one or more canines for overdentures offers the patient several advantages from a functional as well as a biologic standpoint. Overdentures should be considered in the event of loss of alveolar bone support and subsequent development of an unfavorable crown-root ratio. They are considered in every case as an alternative to the extraction of all natural teeth, and they may be used instead of other restorative procedures, such as fixed or removable partial dentures.

Extraction of all natural mandibular dentition and replacement with a complete mandibular denture is not the most desirable treatment. Problems associated with the conventional complete mandibular denture are apparent to every dentist. Many sequelae to the extraction of all mandibular teeth make the complete mandibular denture progressively less effective. Among these sequelae are the loss of discrete tooth proprioception, the progressive loss of alveolar bone, and the transfer of all occlusal forces from the teeth to the oral mucosa.

Although the roots of the mandibular canines are often involved with periodontitis and hypermobility before treatment, it is better to retain them for overdentures than to extract them. Periodontal treatment should always be performed when there is evidence of periodontitis. From the physiologic viewpoint, the roots provide not only a periodontal ligament to support the teeth, but also directional sensitivity, tactile sensitivity to load, dimenional discrimination, and canine response. Sensory innervation is as important to the periodontal ligament as to the other components of mastication.

NEUROMUSCULAR FUNCTION AND SENSORY INPUT

Some definitions should be made to clarify the terminology. *Sensation* is an impression conveyed by an afferent nerve to the higher brain centers. Pure sensation probably only occurs once when a child first experiences that specific sensation. Past experiences, blending, and comparison of one sensation with another transform sensation into perception. *Perception* is the conscious mental registration of a sensory stimulus. *Proprioceptive sensibility* is the unconscious sense that gives knowledge of the position and the state of the parts of the body. *Proprioception,* according to Sherrington's definition (Ramfjord and Ash, 1971), refers to information provided about the position and movements of the body and its parts by receptors. A *receptor* is a sensory nerve terminal that responds to stimuli of various kinds. A *mechanoreceptor* is a receptor that is stimulated by differences of pressure, such as those of touch and hearing. The term mechanoreceptor is currently listed as a subject heading in the Index of Dental Literature (1973) and the Index Medicus (1974). *Proprioceptors* are those receptors located in muscles, tendons, ligaments, joints, and periodontal ligaments which give sensory input regarding movements and position (Posselt, 1968). The periodontal ligament is richly innervated by these receptors, and the tooth is surrounded by a vast array of proprioceptors that can receive mechanical stimulation. These receptors have also been called *pressoreceptors* (Ramfjord and Ash). Receptors are classified into three groups (Ramfjord and Ash): (1) *exteroceptors,* which are affected by changes in the external environment such as stimuli to temperature, vision, hearing, and tactile discrimination, (2) *interoceptors,* which respond to changes in the viscera and are related to perception of hunger, visceral pain, and thirst, and (3) *proprioceptors,* which are concerned with sense of position and movements of the body and its parts.

The receptor population in the periodontal ligament consists of both rapidly and slowly adapting units (Anderson and associates, 1970). The rapidly adapting receptors fire only a few impulses when stimulated, whereas slowly adapting units fire throughout stimulation. Animal studies have shown that slowly adapting receptors in the periodontal ligament maintain spontaneous discharges without any apparent stimualtion of the tooth (Hannam, 1968b). The impulse discharges increase when the tooth is stimulated mechanically, and there may be a silent period in the discharge after the stimulus is removed.

It is probable that receptors other than those of the periodontal ligament are active during mastication. These may be located in the supporting bone, adjacent periosteum, and mucosa. Jerge (1963) observed in animal studies that some periodontal ligament receptors also innervate adjacent soft tissues. When a mandibular tooth is loaded mechanically, receptors in the elevator muscles and the temporomandibular joint may be stimulated. It has also been suggested that auditory receptors may be active in mastication, since tooth contacts may be conducted by vibration through bone (Manly and associates, 1952).

Most of the sensory inputs from the receptors in the periodontal ligament are proprioceptive signals (Sicher and Bhaskar, 1972), since they provide information about the movements and position of the mandible. All of the pressure-sensitive receptors in the periodontal ligament are proprioceptors, and all of their inputs are classed as proprioceptive signals. The majority of the reflex proprioceptive signals from the periodontal ligament are of the subconscious reflex type. However, deliberate conscious mandibular movements that provide occlusal loading of the teeth will result in some proprioceptive signals from the periodontal receptors being received at the higher brain levels as perception. As mentioned previously, perception is the conscious mental registration of a sensory stimulus. During routine mastication, these proprioceptive signals from the periodontal receptors would not be raised to the level of consciousness.

Jerge (1965) said that the periodontal receptors are dually represented in the trigeminal nerve, the cell bodies of these neurons being located in the mesencephalic nucleus and the gasserian ganglion. Ramfjord and Ash also said that proprioception was divided into subconscious and conscious proprioception. In addition, they said that the receptors of the periodontal ligament are called proprioceptors because some of the sensory information goes to the mesencephalic nucleus, the latter having a proprioceptive function. In his research on the mesencephalic nucleus, Jerge (1963) reported two general classes of cells in the nucleus—those which innervated muscle spindles of jaw closing muscles and those which innervated the periodontal ligament of teeth. Corbin and Harrison (1940) observed in animal studies that the mesencephalic nucleus was activated by pressure on teeth from any direction. The mesencephalic nucleus exerts a proprioceptive function in the reflex control of routine masticatory movements.

Kawamura (1964) stated that routine chewing movements of the jaw are performed through the reciprocal relationship of jaw opening and jaw closing muscles; these chewing movements are done rhythmically and unconsciously with only the lower brain center involved. The periodontal receptors are largely responsible for the ability of the mandible to close directly into intercuspal position without interferences (Posselt). Sicher (1956) points out that the proprioceptive signals originating in the periodontal ligaments are unique and of unsurpassed exactness and accuracy. He states that the closing movement in the average patient is automatic and is directed by the engram of the periodontal input. Jerge (1965) said that the activity of specific muscles or parts of muscles attached to the mandible is directed by specific receptors of specific teeth and that the periodontal receptors are important in determining the activity of the trigeminal motor nerves. These statements support the belief that the receptors in the periodontal ligament are proprioceptive and that they function at the subconscious level during routine mastication.

There is general agreement as to the histologic aspects of the neural elements in the periodontal ligament (Anderson and associates). The ligament contains nerve fibers that run from the apical area of the root through the periodontal ligament to the gingival margin. The fibers are joined by small nerve bundles that enter the periodontal ligament laterally from the alveolar bone. The nerves differ in diameter; the larger ones are myelinated, whereas the smaller ones are either myelinated or nonmyelinated. The larger fibers are concerned with touch and the smaller with pain. The manner in which the fibers terminate is not clear. In man, the larger nerve endings have been reported variously as coiled knobs, knoblike, Meissner-like, elongated and spindlelike, and irregular branched.

Numerous studies on the sensory input of the periodontal ligament are cited in support of the rationale for retaining teeth for overdentures. There has been little research on the overdenture and its effect on proprioception. Two studies on the overdenture and sensory perception are cited in this chapter. Every facet of proprioception that is presented here may or may not be used by the overdenture. In view of the paucity of current knowledge, I believe that the sensory input of the periodontal ligament should be preserved for use with overdentures. The use of the overdenture is based on the premise that an attempt should be made to retain every possible sensory input. Two recent reviews (Crum and Loiselle, 1972; Anderson and co-workers), list much of the literature available on proprioception and the sensory input of the masticatory components.

Retention of a root means considerably more than mere physical preservation. In essence, this action preserves an integral component of the sensory feedback system that programs the masticatory system throughout the patient's life.

The neuromuscular function of the masticatory system depends basically on the integration of sensory feedback and motor neuron response at the reflex level. The motor responses are programmed and monitored by the sensory processes of proprioception on the subconscious level and by perception on the conscious level. As these processes relate to oral function, they involve the sensory innervation of the various components, such as the periodontal ligaments, and salivary glands, and the epithelial surface of the oral cavity, the muscles of the tongue and mouth, the muscles of mastication, and the temporomandibular joints. The function of the masticatory system is dependent on the input placed into the system by these components. A defect or nonintegration of the proprioceptive input can result in poor function or pathologic changes to the system. It can result also in proprioceptive inputs that are out of synchronization. A multiplicity of asynchronous sensory inputs can cause disharmony in the function of the system and can result in temporomandibular joint dysfunction.

Retention of any tooth for an overdenture preserves a portion of one of the major sensory inputs, that is; input from periodontal proprioceptors. The afferent input from the periodontal ligament receptors contains information about the magnitude and direction of the occlusal forces as well as about the size and consistency of the food bolus. After this input from the periodontal receptors is integrated with input from the other receptors in the epithelial surface of the mouth, the muscles, and the temporomandibular joints, they contribute to the overall response. The periodontal receptor input is also protective, for it monitors the teeth against occlusal overloading. Extraction of all teeth results in the complete loss of all input from periodontal ligament receptors, whereas use of the overdenture preserves this sensory input.

SENSORY INPUT FROM PERIODONTAL RECEPTORS
Sensitivity of anterior teeth

Sensory input from the periodontal receptors is one of the major determinants of masticatory function, and the roots of the teeth offer more discrete discriminatory input than does the oral mucosa. In studies of human teeth, Manly and associates observed that whereas the mean minimal threshold for detection of load was approximately 1 gm. on the incisal surface of an anterior tooth (natural dentition) in an axial direction, it was 8 to 10 gm. on the occlusal surfaces of first molars. Of eight denture wearers tested for minimal load thresholds to forces applied to the occlusal surfaces of the first premolar of the mandibular denture, five were insensitive to a force of 125 gm., two reacted to 83 gm., and one reacted to 56 gm. The sensitivity of anterior natural teeth was much greater than that achieved with a mandibular denture. The average threshold for denture wearers was more than a hundred times that for anterior natural teeth. The complete denture wearer had considerably less sensitivity than patients who still had natural anterior teeth. Retention of natural teeth for an overdenture preserves some of the sensory input from the periodontal receptors, which is more precise than that able to be obtained from the oral mucosa.

Other investigators corroborated the findings of Manly and associates that the sensitivity of natural anterior teeth was more acute than that of posterior teeth. Kawamura (1964), Grossman (1964a, 1964b), and Grossman and associates (1965) agreed that the sensitivity in the anterior part of the mouth, particularly the periodontal ligament of the anterior teeth, tongue tip, and mucosa, was acute. There is a greater concentration of sensory receptors in the anterior part of the mouth (Kawamura, 1964), and these signals from the periodontal and mucosal receptors are important in controlling and determining biting force. According to Kawamura, the sensory acuity in the middle part of the mouth, including the molar teeth, was not as definitive. Adler (1947) also assessed load thresholds of human teeth and likewise reported that minimal load thresholds increased from the anterior to the posterior parts of the mouth. Lowenstein and Rathkamp (1955) found that minimal load thresholds increased significantly from the canines to the first molar and that a patient's ability to localize a mechanically stimulated tooth was practically 100% in anterior teeth but less in posterior teeth.

Nishiyama and others (1967) applied 20 gm. loads to 833 natural teeth in thirty-one adults, and discovered that the patient's judgment of the loaded tooth in localizing the stimulated tooth was better among anterior teeth than among posterior teeth.

These studies indicate that the natural anterior teeth exhibit more sensitivity and discrimination than the posterior teeth and, therefore, give more discrete sensory input. However, posterior teeth also should be retained for overdentures when feasible, even though they contribute less to proprioceptive sensibility.

Dimensional perception

Some of the many oral studies of dimensional perception relate to the discrimination of different thicknesses of objects between the occlusal surfaces of the teeth. The term *perception* is used here in these studies of human teeth because comparative evaluation is based on conscious discrimination. In comparing the dimensional perception in patients with natural dentitions to that in patients with artificial dentures, Kawamura and Watanabe (1960) found that patients with natural dentition could discriminate differences at the 2 mm. range better than those with artificial dentures.

Manly and associates selected a parameter for comparing discrete changes in food texture in patients with natural dentitions and artificial dentures. They used graded quantities of calcium carbonate suspended in bland pudding in the following percentages: 0.1, 1.0, 2.0, 2.9, 4.8, 7.4, 9.1, 17, 23, and 29. Almost all patients with natural dentitions could detect 2.9% calcium carbonate or less, whereas the majority of denture patients require more than 9% calcium carbonate for detection. This study indicated that sensitivity of texture judgment of the majority of the denture wearers was considerably less than that of patients with natural dentitions. Manly and associates suggested that the sensory input from the detection of exceedingly small particles might be of vibratory origin. Likewise, Garton (1968) tested load thresholds of patients with natural teeth while they wore earplugs. These patients believed that sensory input of the tooth was more auditory than tactile in origin. These findings emphasized the importance of conservative procedures and the importance of the retention of natural teeth.

Canine response

Several studies related to canine response are accepted as the best studies of this type inasmuch as it is impossible to perform similar human studies. Corbin and Harrison found in their studies of cats' teeth that the canines were the most sensitive of all oral structures. They applied pressure stimulation to the oral region and noted the bursts of potential in the mesencephalic root.

Kruger and Michel (1962) said that the canines had more neurons than any other teeth. They placed microelectrodes in the brains of twenty-three decerebrated cats and applied mechanical stimuli to the teeth by manual pressure. Kawamura and Nishiyama (1966) studied twenty-five decerebrated cats with brain microelectrodes while applying manual stimulation to the incisors, canines, and molars. They made a topographic map of the trigeminal nucleus showing the points at which they noted potentials. The neurons for the canines were the most densely distributed, and sensory information from individual teeth had its own specific reception site in the trigeminal nucleus. In a study Bonaguro and associates (1969) found that patients differentiated with their maxillary canines the smallest relative differences in force applied to the teeth, although the canines had a higher optimal functional range than the maxillary incisors.

Studies of canine response indicate that the canine may be the most important proprioceptive organ. The results of this research emphasize the significance of the sensory ability of the canine teeth and lend support to their retention for overdentures.

Directional sensitivity

Several animal studies of directional sensitivity have been done. This proprioceptive mechanism underscores the true importance of the periodontal ligament. Jerge (1963, 1965) reported that the receptors in the periodontal ligament were directionally sensitive. He said that the receptors are arranged around a tooth in such a way as to respond to pressure regardless of the direction from which it is applied. Kubota and Kawamura (1964) did research in which they applied pressure stimulus to cats' teeth and recorded the activity from the trigeminal sensory nucleus. They found that the specific sites in the bulbar and spinal trigeminal nuclei responded to pressure on the tooth from a specific direction. Kruger and Michel also reported that the teeth had excellent directional sensitivity.

It appears that there are specific sensory nerve endings for various kinds of force, that is, a lingual force or a buccal force. Kawamura (1964) believed that this was a valuable finding. Directional sensitivity is one of the most important elements in the interaction of the masticatory system. It means that the periodontal receptors have a functional individuality and that the relationship of the tooth to its periodontal ligament is highly important from a sensory standpoint. Therefore teeth should be retained for use with an overdenture to preserve the directional sensitivity. This is based on the assumption that some lateral forces are transmitted by the overdenture to the supporting tooth. It has been shown that teeth are more sensitive to lateral forces than to those in the long axis (Adler). This finding reinforces the importance of directional sensitivity.

Muscle changes after natural tooth contacts

Several investigators (Schaerer and associates, 1967; Brenman and co-workers, 1968; Beaudreau and associates, 1969) have found that the periodontal receptors are related to the activity of the masticatory muscles. Beaudreau and co-workers reported finding silent periods produced bilaterally in human temporal and masseter muscles by tapping individual teeth. They found that local anesthesia to the stimulated tooth eliminated the pauses in muscle activity. It was believed that the action of the local anesthesia in the abolition of the muscle inhibition implicated the input from the periodontal receptors as being responsible for the inhibition. Schaerer and associates did electromyographic recordings of masseter and temporal muscles simultaneously with telemetery. They found that immediate stops or interruptions in electromyographic activity resulted on occurrence of tooth contacts.

Other investigators (Hannam and co-workers, 1969) also observed the activity of the human masseter muscle during mechanical stimulation of the teeth while chewing or tapping on the teeth. They reported that a mechanical stimulus to the patient's forehead also produced a similar muscle inhibition. Hannam and associates found that the use of local anesthesia around the stimulated tooth did not abolish the muscle inhibition. They concluded that the periodontal receptors were not involved in the muscle inhibition.

On the other hand, Sessile and Schmitt (1972) did electromyographic studies of the right and left masseter muscles during tooth tapping. The right maxillary central incisor was tapped by mechanical stimulation that was accurately controlled by electronic calibration. They also found that there was an inhibition of muscle activity after tooth stimulation. However, they reported that the use of local anesthesia around the tooth abolished the inhibition that had been elicited by stimulation of this tooth. They did not find any clear evidence of an inhibitory period produced by forehead stimulation. They concluded that the receptors in and around the teeth were responsible for the inhibition of jaw muscle activity by the tapping of teeth.

It has been suggested by Jerge (1965) and Kawamura (1964, 1967) that the periodontal receptors are actively involved in cyclic jaw movements during mastication. Jerge states that the activity of specific muscles or parts of muscles attached to the mandible is directed by specific receptors of specific teeth. Kawamura says that the sensory input from the periodontal structures always inhibits the activity of some of the motor neurons of the muscles that close the jaw. It was mentioned previously that nerve cells from muscle spindles in masticatory muscles and from receptors in the periodontal ligament have both been found in the mesencephalic nucleus (Jerge, 1963).

Proprioception and salivary secretion

Kapur and Collister (1970) studied food texture discrimination and concluded that the periodontal receptors played an indirect role in the masticatory salivary reflex by regulating the range and type of the masticatory stroke. The muscle activity determined by this masticatory stroke controlled the parotid gland secretion during mastication. They stated that absence of the periodontal ligament in denture wearers appeared to result in impairment of the mechanism regulating parotid gland stimulation during mastication. This research showed the importance of the interaction between the periodontal ligament receptors and the other components of the masticatory system.

Perception of nonvital teeth

The majority of natural teeth used to support overdentures are devitalized and treated endodontically. Perceptive studies showed that vital and devitalized teeth had equal sensory input capabilities (Stewart, 1927; Adler).

Perception of teeth with reduced alveolar support

Studies on animals indicated continuous sensory input from small roots. In his animal studies, Hannam (1968a) found that after removal of all but a small portion of the root, extremely light pressure on the remaining portion gave a neural response. Edel and Willis (1973) compared perception of occlusal forces in an axial direction in two groups of patients; one had normal bone support around the teeth, and the other had reduced alveolar support due to periodontitis. They found little difference between the two groups.

Often teeth selected for use with overdentures may have lost bone support. These studies showed that the tooth still had a proprioceptive input capability even though much of the bone support was lost.

Decrease of perception in older individuals

Perceptive ability appears to decrease with age. MacDonald and Aungst (1970) found that the ability to identify forms in the mouth remained stable in young adults and then deteriorated with age. Litvak and associates (1971) also reported that the level of perception decreased as age increased and believed that an overall decrease in sensory capacity occurred in the edentulous patient. Use of the overdenture is an attempt to retain every possible sensory element at the time the patient may experience a generalized decrease in sensory capacity.

OCCLUSAL FORCES IN OVERDENTURES AND CONVENTIONAL DENTURES

Fenton (1973) studied the ability of human subjects to perceive thin objects between the occlusal surfaces of their teeth. He compared occlusal thickness perception in patients with natural dentitions, conventional complete dentures, and overdentures. Varying thickness of mylar triacetate strips were placed between the occlusal surfaces of the teeth in the area of the first bicuspids, and the subjects were asked to respond when they felt something between their teeth. The thickness of the plastic strips ranged from 12.7 to 343 μ. He found that the occlusal thickness limen for subjects with overdentures opposing a complete denture was the highest of all groups tested. He concluded that the overdenture patients in the study had less occlusal thickness perception than patients with conventional complete dentures.

On the other hand, Pacer (1971) found that the overdenture patients could discriminate measured occlusal forces better at the higher levels than patients with conventional dentures. He compared the ability of two groups of patients to discriminate between various calibrated occlusal loads. One group had conventional mandibular dentures and the other had mandibular overdentures supported by at least two reduced teeth. Calibrated, perpendicular forces in the range of 100 to 2000 gm. were applied to the dynamic center of the occlusal tables of each denture.

Conventional denture wearers had lower discriminatory thresholds (just noticeable differences) at the 100, 200, and 500 gm. force levels, whereas the overdenture wearers discriminated occlusal forces better at the 2000 gm. level. Pacer postulated that during light occlusal loads, the overdenture base probably made light contact or none with the retainer teeth because of the resilient effect of the edentulous saddle.

On application of heavier occlusal forces, there was firm contact between the overdenture and the retained teeth. This brought into action the proprioceptive receptors of the periodontal ligament. Probably the greater sensory input from the periodontal receptors was responsible for the better discriminatory ability of the overdenture wearers at the higher occlusal values. Pacer believed that the better response of the overdenture wearer indicated that this type of denture approached more closely the response of patients with natural dentition. Pacer also thought that the poorer discrimination of the conventional denture wearers at the higher level of 2000 gm. was associated with the possibility that the mucosal receptors under the conventional denture were approaching the limit of their discrimination capability.

It could be theorized that herein lies one of the answers of the question, "Why does alveolar bone resorption occur under conventional dentures?" The answer can be postulated that the mucosal receptors under conventional dentures may reach their upper limit of discrimination during mastication and consequently are unable to warn against occlusal overloading. With natural teeth, the proprioceptive input from the periodontal ligament receptors is so discrete that excessive occlusal loads probably signal the muscles to let up on their contractions.

ALVEOLAR BONE PRESERVATION IN OVERDENTURES

Miller (1958), one of the first dentists to use overdentures in recent times, stated that the maxillae and mandible were designed to house the teeth and not to support artificial dentures. He believed that no support for the occlusal forces was as adequate as the roots of the natural teeth. Apparently, the alveolar processes of the maxillae and mandible do not respond positively to occlusal forces by the use of artificial dentures.

A recent study compares alveolar bone loss in patients with mandibular overdentures to that in patients with conventional mandibular dentures. Crum and Rooney (1975), in a 4-year study, found that the retention of mandibular canines for overdentures led to preservation of alveolar bone. Using comparative cephalometric radiographs and study casts, they found an average of 0.6 mm. vertical loss of alveolar bone in the anterior part of the mandible in the overdenture patients. The vertical bone loss in the anterior part of the mandible in patients with conventional dentures was an average of 5 mm., that is, eight times as much bone loss as in patients with overdentures. They also observed that the use of the overdenture preserved the alveolar bone between the canines in both height and width. The overdenture patients also exhibited less alveolar bone loss in the area immediately posterior to the canines.

From this study it was apparent that the use of the overdenture, in contrast to the conventional mandibular denture, preserved alveolar bone. The alveolar bone was preserved even though the retained canines were involved with periodontitis and hypermobility prior to the start of treatment. The overdenture patient gained other advantages as a result of the bone preservation. These advantages were better masticatory function and less loss of overall face height. The study showed that the presence of the roots of the teeth in the alveolar bone was important to the preservation of the alveolar bone.

Numerous studies have been made of alveolar bone loss after extraction of the natural teeth and replacement by complete conventional dentures. Several studies revealed that the alveolar process was resorbed much faster in the anterior part of the mandible than in the anterior part of the maxillae.

Tallgren (1967, 1969) found that the mean resorption of the anterior height of the mandibular process during the first 6 months of denture use was approximately twice the mean maxillary resorption. This resorption of the alveolar process continued, and, at the 7-year stage, the mandible loss was approximately four times that in the maxillae. The total linear vertical resorption of the anterior maxillary and mandibular process during the 7-year period was a mean of 8.3 mm., that is, 6.6 mm. of the mandibular process was resorbed, whereas the maxillae lost 1.7 mm. of alveolar bone.

Tallgren's findings that the anterior height of the mandibular process was resorbed four times faster than the maxillary process with complete dentures clearly indicated the need for any procedure that would slow down this loss. Tallgren (1972) stated that the bone loss patterns seemed to indicate that the mandibular ridge was more likely to respond to various functional forces transmitted through the dentures than the maxillary ridge. She reasoned also that this difference in response occurred because of the smaller area and less advantageous shape of the lower basal seat.

The results of Tallgren's 7-year studies of alveolar bone loss around the mandibular natural teeth in patients with partial dentures and in patients with complete dentures are interesting. The vertical loss of only 0.8 mm. of bone in the natural dentition areas of the partial denture cases was slight when compared to the 6.6 mm. loss of bone in the complete denture cases.

Research on the patterns of alveolar bone loss in patients with overdentures and in those with conventional dentures clearly indicates that use of the overdenture preserves alveolar bone, especially in the area of the retained teeth. In this area resorption occurs at an exceedingly rapid rate after extraction of the teeth. These observations reinforce the need to retain mandibular canines for overdentures.

SUMMARY

The rationale for the retention of teeth for overdentures has been presented in this chapter. The results of numerous studies on the sensory input from the periodontal ligament and on alveolar bone loss have also been presented. There is a need for more research in fields relating to proprioception, alveolar bone loss, and the overdenture.

REFERENCES

Adler, P.: Sensibility of teeth to loads applied in different directions, J. Dent. Res. **26**:279-289, 1947.

Anderson, D. J., Hannam, A. G., and Matthews, B.: Sensory mechanisms in mammalian teeth and their supporting structures, Physiol. Rev. **50**:171-195, 1970.

Beaudreau, D. E., Daugherty, W. F., and Masland, W. S.: Two types of motor pause in masticatory muscles, Am. J. Physiol. **216**:16-21, 1969.

Bonaguro, J. G., Dusza, G. R., and Bowman, D. C.: Ability of human subjects to differentiate forces applied to certain teeth, J. Dent. Res. **48**:236-241, 1969

Brenman, H. S., Black, M. A., Coslet, J. G.: Interrelationship between the electromyographic silent period and dental occlusion, J. Dent. Res. **47**:502, 1968.

Corbin, K. B., and Harrison, F.: Function of the mesencephalic root of fifth cranial nerve, J. Neurophysiol. **3**:423-435, 1940.

Crum, R. J., and Loiselle, R. J.: Oral perception and proprioception: a review of the literature and its significance to prosthodontics, J. Prosthet. Dent. **28**:215-230, 1972.

Crum, R. J., and Rooney, G. E.: Comparative alveolar bone loss in patients with mandibular overdentures, J.A.D.A. (In press.)

Edel, A., and Willis, D. J.: Effects of reduced alveolar support on the sensibility of the incisors of humans to axial pressure, J. Dent. Res. **52**:946, 1973 (abst.).

Fenton, A. H.: Studies of the effects of denture and overdenture therapy on occlusal thickness perception, M.S. Thesis, Rochester, N. Y., 1973, Eastman Dental Center and University of Rochester.

Garton, C. P.: 1968. Quoted in Anderson, D. J., Hannam, A. G., and Matthews, B.: Sensory mechanisms in mammalian teeth and their supporting structures, Physiol. Rev. **50**:171-195, 1970.

Grossman, R. C.: Oral sensory threshold determination methods, J. Dent. Res. (supp.) **43**:833, 1964a.

Grossman, R. C.: Sensory innervation of the oral mucosae: a review, J. South. Calif. Dent. Assoc. **32**:128-133, 1964b.

Grossman, R. C., Hattis, B. F., and Ringel, R. L.: Oral tactile experience, Arch. Oral Biol. **10**:691-705, 1965.

Hannam, A. G.: An electrophysiological study of periodontal mechano-receptors, Ph.D. thesis, Bristol, England, 1968a, University of Bristol. In Anderson, D. J., Hannam, A. G., and Matthews, B.: Sensory mechanisms in mammalian teeth and their supporting structures, Physiol. Rev. **50**:171-195, 1970.

Hannam, A. G.: Spontaneous activity in the dental mechano-receptor units, J. Dent. Res. (supp.) **47**:969, 1968b.

Hannam, A. G., Matthews, B., and Yemm, R.: The response of the masseter muscle following tooth contact in man, J. Physiol. (London) **203**:25-26, 1969.

Jerge, C. R.: Organization and function of the trigeminal mesencephalic Nucleus, J. Neurophysiol. **26**:379-392, 1963.

Jerge, C. R.: Comments on the innervation of the teeth, Dent. Clin. N. Amer., pp. 117-127, March, 1965.

Kapur, K. K., and Collister, T.: A study of food textural discrimination in persons with natural and artificial dentitions. In Bosma, J. F., editor: Second Symposium on Oral Sensation and Perception, Springfield, Ill., 1970, Charles C Thomas, Publisher.

Kawamura, Y.: Neurophysiologic background of occlusion, Periodontics **5**:175-183, 1967.

Kawamura, Y.: Recent concepts of the physiology of mastication. In Advances in oral biology, vol. 1, New York, 1964, Academic Press, Inc.

Kawamura, Y., and Nishiyama, T.: Projection of dental afferent impulses to the trigeminal nuclei of the cat, Jap. J. Physiol. **16**:584-597, 1966.

Kawamura, Y., and Watanabe, M.: Studies on oral sensory thresholds, Med. J. Osaka Univ. **10**:291-301, 1960.

Kruger, L., and Michel, F.: A single neuron analysis of buccal cavity representation in the sensory trigeminal complex of the cat, Arch. Oral Biol. **7**:491-503, 1962.

Kubota and Kawamura, Y.: Quoted in Advances in oral biology, New York, 1964, Academic Press, Inc.

Litvak, H., Silverman, S. I., and Garfinkel, M. H.: Oral stereognosis in dentulous and edentulous subjects, J. Prosthet. Dent. **25**:139-151, 1971.

Loewenstein, W. R., and Rathkamp, R.: A study of the pressoreceptive sensibility of the tooth, J. Dent. Res. **34**:287-294, 1955.

MacDonald, E. T., and Aungst, L. F.: Apparent independence of oral sensory functions and articulatory proficiency. In Bosma, J. F., editor: Second Symposium on Oral Sensation and Perception, Springfield, Ill., 1970, Charles C Thomas, Publisher.

Manly, R. S., Pfaffman, C., Lathrop, D. D., and Keyser, J.: Oral sensory thresholds of persons with natural and artificial dentitions, J. Dent. Res. **31**:305-312, 1952.

Miller, P. A.: Complete dentures supported by natural teeth, J. Prosthet. Dent. **8**:924-928, 1958.

Nishiyama, T., Funakoshi, M., and Kawamura, Y.: A study of sensitivity of the human tooth, J. Dent. Res. (supp.) **46**:136, 1967.

Pacer, F. J.: An evaluation of occlusal force discrimination by denture wearers, M. S. Thesis. Maywood, Ill., 1971, Loyola Univ. School of Dentistry.

Posselt, U.: The physiology of occlusion and rehabilitation, ed. 2, Philadelphia, 1968, F. A. Davis Co.

Ramfjord, S. P., and Ash, M. M.: Occlusion, ed. 2, Philadelphia, 1971, W. B. Saunders Co.

Schaerer, P., Stallard, R. E., and Zander, N. A.: Occlusal interferences and mastication: an electromyographic study, J. Prosthet. Dent. **17**:438-449, 1967.

Sessile, B. J., and Schmitt, A.: Effects of controlled tooth stimulation on jaw muscle activity in man, Arch. Oral Biol. **17**:1597-1607, 1972.

Sicher, H.: The biologic significance of hinge axis determination, J. Prosthet. Dent. **6**:616-620, 1956.

Sicher, H., and Bhaskar, S. N., editors: Orban's oral histology and embryology, ed. 7, St. Louis, 1972, The C. V. Mosby Co.

Stewart, D.: Some aspects of the innervation of the teeth, Proc. Roy. Soc. Med. (Sect. Odontol.) **20**:55-66, 1927.

Tallgren, A.: The effect of denture wearing on facial morphology, Acta Odont. Scand. **25**:563-592, 1967.

Tallgren, A.: Positional changes of complete dentures—a 7 year longitudinal study, Acta Odontol. Scand. **27**:539-561, 1969.

Tallgren, A.: The continuing reduction of the residual alveolar ridges in complete denture wearers: a mixed longitudinal study covering 25 years, J. Prosthet, Dent. **27**:120-132, 1972.

Yemm, R., Hannam, A. G., and Matthews, B.: Changes in the activity of the masseter muscle following tooth contact, J. Dent. Res. **48**:1131, 1969.

2

ADVANTAGES, DISADVANTAGES, INDICATIONS, AND CONTRAINDICATIONS

ALLEN A. BREWER

In the past only three procedures for restoring inadequate, mutilated, or diseased dentitions were considered when teeth were to be retained. They were fixed or removable prosthesis or both and teeth restored with fillings or onlays and crowns. The overdenture with its many advantages and few disadvantages is now considered as a means of treatment.

ADVANTAGES

Equally effective or superior method of treatment. In many situations the overdenture gives better service than alternative methods of treatment. It is particularly useful for patients with congenital defects, such as oligodontia, microdontia, cleft palate, and cleidocranial dysostosis, and for Class III patients, i.e., a prognathic jaw not amenable to surgical or orthodontic treatment. It is possible to restore occlusion and improve esthetics tremendously by proper positioning of teeth and support of soft tissues. Frequently overdentures are superior to fixed prosthesis or conventional removable partial dentures when a patient has few remaining teeth, none of which is adequately supported by bone.

Simplicity of construction. The procedures used in creating overdentures are the same as those for conventional complete dentures. Additionally, the retained teeth or roots or both provide stability to the bases during registration of maxillomandibular records. They also aid in determining the correct vertical dimension of occlusion and in proper tooth placement.

Ease of maintenance. Repairs, alterations, or refitting of the overdenture can be accomplished readily in the same manner as with conventional complete dentures.

Stability. Stability is comparable to that obtained with fixed or removable partial dentures. The retention of four abutments, such as two cuspids and two molars in each arch, contributes greatly to this stability.

Retention. Generally retention is excellent because of the better stability of overdentures. However, relief of the denture in some areas may be necessitated by pronounced tissue or bony protuberances adjacent to the retained teeth (usually cuspids). Although the seal is broken, use of one of the available attachments or of a soft liner such as Molloplast-b* overcomes this problem.

Esthetic excellence. The extensive selection of artificial denture teeth and the many possible arrangements for them aid in creating an esthetic effect. The possibility of restoring bony defects and altering the matrix enables the dentist to produce better results with the overdenture than with more conventional prostheses.

Open palate possible. The maxillary overdenture of many patients can be "roofless" if neces-

---

*K. G. Kostner & Co., 6370 Obersursel/Taunus, Postfach 271, West Germany.

sary, especially when both anterior and posterior teeth are saved.

Reasonable cost. Fees are based on treatment provided rather than on procedures accomplished. The time required for creating an overdenture and thus the cost can be less than for alternative procedures such as fixed partial dentures.

Familiar procedures. The procedures are similar to those used for conventional complete dentures. Adequately oriented dentists and technicians with no special training can accomplish them with ease.

Ease in making measurements. When teeth are retained for immediate insertion of an overdenture, the vertical dimension of occlusion can be maintained with a high degree of accuracy. These teeth also contribute to the stabilization of the recording bases. As with any immediate denture, restoring the existing composition or improving on it is simplified. Even the retention of one or two roots for a remote overdenture aids considerably in proper placement of teeth.

Ideal occlusion. The dentist is better able to provide not only an adequate occlusion, but also one that is acceptable esthetically. It is possible to have a pronounced vertical overlap of the anterior teeth and still avoid displacing the dentures in function. Therefore a special effort is made to save a few maxillary anterior teeth when the patient has either a completely dentulous mandible or one in which the anterior teeth are intact and the posterior teeth are replaced by a distal extension partial denture. The organic type of occlusion that many patients have with natural teeth can be incorporated into the overdenture.

Excellent patient acceptance. Probably the major factor that contributes to patient acceptance is the knowledge that he still has his own teeth. Loss of all teeth at an advanced age seems to be much more traumatic than at a younger age. Frequently young patients request that all of their teeth be removed and that complete dentures be substituted, whereas older patients, and rightly so, have a horror of losing all of their teeth.

Less trauma to supporting tissues. One of the leading advantages of retaining teeth is that a hard tooth surface supports the denture. This situation prevents resorption of the residual ridge that occurs when all teeth are removed and complete dentures are provided. In addition the soft tissues experience less trauma.

Stabilization of existing structures. Although the tissues under a long span without tooth support may resorb, little change occurs at the site of the retained teeth. Therefore the vertical dimension and the lip and face support are maintained, and settling is minimized.

Minimal adjustments. Little adjustment is required because of the stability and support provided to the overdenture by the retained teeth.

Possibility of using attachments or soft liners. When soft tissue or bony protuberances necessitate considerable relief of the denture, it is difficult to maintain a "seal." However, attachments or soft liners can be incorporated into the existing overdenture. These procedures may be accomplished subsequent to initial insertion, since the need for additional retention may not become apparent until the patient has worn the overdenture.

Transitional or training denture. Even though the patient may lose the retained teeth or roots or both in a relatively short time, the overdenture is not only stable and retentive for the period of use, but it is also excellent for transitional or training purposes in preparation for receiving a complete denture.

Conversion to complete denture. Inasmuch as the tissue coverage and border extensions are usually the same for overdentures as for complete dentures, it is easy to compensate for the loss of one or all of the retained teeth. Either the spaces can be filled in or the denture can be relined or rebased.

Reversibility. When making overdentures over a complete natural dentition, it is is seldom necessary to alter the existing teeth. Therefore the procedure is completely reversible; removal of the denture puts the patient's teeth back to their original status.

Ease in cleaning. All surfaces of isolated abutments are readily accessible for cleaning, and the denture, being removable, is easier to clean than is a fixed prosthesis.

DISADVANTAGES

Overdenture treatment is more expensive than conventional denture treatment because of the endodontic therapy usually required and the subsequent restoration of the teeth with alloys or gold copings. Frequently the teeth to be retained also need periodontal therapy.

The overdenture is bulkier than fixed or removable partial dentures.

Many patients do not like anything that is removable and therefore prefer fixed partial dentures. Generally the overdenture patient is not a suitable candidate for fixed partial dentures.

If the patient does not keep the retained roots or teeth and the overdenture clean, caries and periodontal disease may still progress.

INDICATIONS

Consideration should be given to using the overdenture for a patient when the result would be equal or superior to that provided by another method of treatment. Although the presence of few remaining teeth is one of the major indications for the overdenture, as many abutments as possible are retained in the arch.

In our practice, overdentures may be made for patients with only one tooth or root remaining and even for those with a complete complement of teeth. Examples of this type of overdenture are seen in Chapter 8.

Overdentures are indicated especially for patients with a poor prognosis for complete dentures. When the palatal vault is high and the ridges slope, it may be difficult to make a stable retentive maxillary denture. When the mandible has a poorly defined sublingual fold space, the floor of the mouth drapes, and the tongue falls back, positive retention and stability can be hard to attain. For these patients every effort is made to save teeth for an overdenture.

Retention of a few teeth in the maxilla for an overdenture is highly important when a pronounced vertical overlap of the anterior teeth is required to produce a good esthetic result.

When teeth are of questionable value as conventional abutments because of an unfavorable crown-root ratio, they can be treated endodontically, and the clinical crown can be reduced almost to the ridge. This procedure improves the crown-root ratio tremendously, and these teeth serve as overdenture abutments for years.

Use of an endosseous endodontic implant is considered when bone loss around the teeth to be retained is extensive.

In many situations removable partial dentures are better when fabricated over some teeth that have been retained and reduced. They add support and stability to the prosthesis, and they greatly prolong the life of teeth used in this manner.

Teeth with little bony support have been used for fabricating a removable partial denture in some instances. If they become mobile, they can be reduced, and the prosthesis can be altered to cover them. This procedure increases stability and delays residual ridge resorption.

A unilateral overdenture can be used to provide good function and esthetics when a large amount of bone and soft tissue have been lost on one side of the arch.

CONTRAINDICATIONS

The overdenture is contraindicated when another method promises to give superior results unless the patient cannot afford the alternative treatment.

Psychologically some patients cannot accept a denture. They have only three or four teeth left in an arch, but they insist on having "anything but a complete denture."

When a patient cannot maintain abutment teeth and periodontal tissues surrounding them, he will inevitably lose the teeth. Therefore it is impractical to undertake the additional work and expense required to make the overdenture unless the patient is fully aware of his responsibilities.

PART TWO
PRELIMINARY PROCEDURES

3
SPECIAL RELATIONSHIP BETWEEN DENTIST AND PROSTHODONTIC PATIENT

JOHN D. LARKIN

The relationship between the dentist and the patient is never more important than in prosthodontic treatment. Several factors may contribute to the unusual sensitivity of this relationship. For some patients, total tooth loss can have an emotional impact equivalent to that of an amputation or other major surgical procedure. For *most* patients, emotions about aging and body image changes are involved. These and numerous other special factors intensify the necessity that this be a long, continuing relationship. It is axiomatic that denture treatment is completed only when the patient dies.

The relationship is of long duration whether the patient requires extensive fixed restorative treatment, removable partial dentures, complete dentures, overdentures, or some combination of treatments. The patient will never have more teeth or more supportive tissue than are present at the time of the initial visit. Although research in implantology is still progressing, no predictably successful method of providing a substitute for the natural tooth root is available now. The residual alveolar bone and its soft tissue covering are subject to deterioration and loss. The rate of these changes appears to be related to the degree of tissue abuse. Additional support made possible by remaining teeth or roots helps to minimize abusive stresses. The preservation of residual structures necessitates a continuing plan of treatment for all of these patients.

Maintenance of the patient's comfort, appearance, and function requires continuing care. Interference with any of these factors usually makes the patient aware of the need for treatment. Frequently the absence of symptoms is accepted by patients as an indication of the lack of need for professional care. This attitude is dangerous for the patient in view of possible sequelae; treatment needs can become acute and more extensive. Negligence in the presence of malignant lesions can even threaten the life of the patient.

TREATMENT OPTIONS

Treatment of prosthodontic patients can be planned with various objectives, and plans can be modified for an infinite number of reasons related to the patient's welfare, physical condition, and other personal details.

It is a rare situation that does not offer some treatment options. An adequate examination, which includes diagnostic casts and, in many instances, diagnostic bases, radiographs, photographs of similar treatment situations, or even simple pencil sketches can aid in developing and explaining the dentist's recommendations as to the best treatment procedure. Thorough exploration can require three or more appointments, and none can be hurried. After arriving at a decision on the available treatment options and preparing properly for a *treatment conference,* the dentist sees the patient. Use of this term is preferable to *case presentation,* since it avoids the implication of a commercial sales pitch.

SPECIAL FACTORS RELATED TO PROSTHODONTIC PATIENT

On a long-term basis, the prosthodontic patient, more than any other, can demand the maximum effort and capability of the dentist to understand the numerous special problems. Following are a few of the factors requiring special consideration for the prosthodontic patient:

1. Bone and joint pathology, especially in relation to the temporomandibular joint. Being one of the most complicated joints in the body, it can give rise to symptoms ranging from minor to bizarre.

2. Bone maintenance related to nutrition, stress, endocrine dysfunction, and other possible systemic disease.

3. Biologic factors in the aging process in health and disease.

4. Special nutritional problems in aging patients and in some younger ones requiring prosthodontic treatment.

5. The physiology of mastication involving all the related bone and joint structures, musculature, and proprioceptor mechanism.

6. Pathology of the central nervous system or local nerve involvements with motor or sensory dysfunction or both. Early manifestation of neurologic disorders may involve oral, facial, and adjacent areas. Effects can vary from minor problems to those leading to death. Progressive bulbar paralysis, amyotrophic lateral sclerosis, myasthenia gravis, multiple sclerosis, and peripheral facial paralysis are a few of the disorders that may first be observed by the prosthodontist.

7. Variance in oral tissue health or disease, tissue tolerance, and pain threshold may all possibly be influenced by local or systemic factors. In this area alone many problems can create extreme difficulty for the patient and the dentist. In the absence of a positive diagnosis, it may be advisable to recommend consultation. Other prosthodontists, oral pathologists, and some physicians may provide diagnostic aid and valuable opinions about additional treatment. Experience has proved that such efforts help to maintain good patient relationships even if the results are less than satisfactory to the dentist and the patient.

8. Selection of an occlusion concept and responsibility for producing appliances that conform to the concept chosen.

9. Necessity for determining, recording, transferring, and maintaining acceptable jaw relations in the completed restorations.

10. The need for appropriate dental education to enable the patient to make demands and expectations of the prosthesis no greater than structural or functional limitations permit.

Psychologic problems

Patients experiencing psychologic and emotional problems can make the prognosis unfavorable for any type of denture treatment. Proper timing is the essential element. Psychologic problems can be related to oral problems and can influence acceptance or rejection of the denture.

The emotional impact of tooth loss can be extremely traumatic to the patient involved. The effect on body image plus the deep emotions associated with the oral area tend to exaggerate the problem. These factors can increase enormously the time demands and the stress for the dentist (Moulton, 1946; Collett, 1955).

A patient under considerable stress in everyday life situations may believe that direct expression of aggression or hostility is not acceptable. However, if he or she is receiving prosthodontic treatment at this time, the restoration and the dentist may seem to be causes for justifiable complaint, thereby precluding satisfactory results.

Clear distinctions are essential before pronouncing judgment in apparently similar situations. Patients have been referred for psychiatric therapy when adequate denture treatment was their only need. Consultations with other specialists, as suggested previously, minimizes the risk of making such errors.

A psychologic problem can arise as the result of an excellent dentist-patient relationship. Some patients apparently become socially dependent on the dentist and his office personnel. They tend to return for minor reasons and overdo their expressions of gratitude for the results and the considerate treatment. It is possible that these patients are willing to pay for treatment time primarily to receive a measure of attention from someone because others do not extend such kindness. The dentist may wish to exercise controls to ensure that such treatment is provided only to the appropriate extent.

Some patients accept the dentist but are unable psychologically to surrender authority to the full extent of accepting all of his recommendations. Therefore they may insist on retaining or duplicating undesirable features of existing restorations. Confrontation and insistence on winning a point at the wrong time can result in the dentist losing the opportunity to help the misguided patient. At least in some instances the dentist's temporary acquiescence gains acceptance by the patient now and full cooperation later.

The situations discussed are not the only ones that can arise, but they serve to illustrate potential special problem areas in denture treatment.

HUMAN RELATIONS VS. PRACTICE MANAGEMENT

Discussions on patient relationships often are modified to relate to patient *management* or even to practice management. However, such labels may imply an undesirable attitude, and no one desires to acknowledge that he/she has deep interest in a study that implies the desire to manipulate people in a commercial manner for personal aggrandizement. Most dentists consider themselves stigmatized by such an accusation.

These comments on practice management are not intended to be an attack on legitimate ethical applications of the term. Most dentists need advice and consistent counseling by capable, trained, and qualified experts. One course sponsored by a university is described as follows: "Office management, accounting, tax and investments and financial management, insurance, estate planning and practice organization format." Extremely valuable information is presented on the physical layout of offices and equipment and on the effective use of auxiliaries.

The large number of books, journal articles, lectures, and courses on related subjects indicate the demand for assistance with what may preferably be referred to as "people relations."

The Golden Rule, which is understood and respected in most parts of the world, is the underlying principle and basic guide in all relations between people.

PATIENT RELATIONSHIPS
Establishing the relationship

The dentist establishes the approach to the patient relationship and care during the initial appointments, which correspond to the examination, diagnosis, and treatment planning stages. All the requirements are summed up in the word *rapport*. In too many instances this becomes only a word and is not descriptive of a relationship between two concerned individuals acting jointly to best meet the treatment needs. The denture patient especially requires this favorable relationship, which is sometimes elusive, difficult, or seemingly impossible. We must remind ourselves that we are involving at least two human personalities with all their frailties, prejudices, and complications, including inherent and acquired susceptibilities of misunderstanding and being misunderstood. Additionally, prior unhappy dental experiences may cause a patient to approach the first appointment with apprehension.

Patients begin to form their impressions when they first hear about the dentist, whether it is in casual conversation at a bridge game or by the direct referral of a friend or a professional colleague. At this point it is the responsibility of the dentist and the other personnel in his office to maintain and further each patient's confidence. It is possible for this confidence to be so thoroughly established by the referral source that it may require only that we avoid destroying it.

When patients telephone or come to the office to make the initial appointment, it is imperative that their convenience and comfort be given every possible consideration. It is agreed generally that the "voice with a smile" type of greeting can set the mood for future contacts. Patients should be received with warmth and friendliness and be made aware that they are recognized as individuals and human beings, not merely denture "cases." The manner in which they are dismissed after each appointment is equally important; they should be made to feel that everyone involved is sincerely interested in their well-being. No patient should be dismissed without a specific plan for future contact.

The need for preparatory treatment of prosthodontic patients has been recognized for a long time, and acceptable procedures for the conditioning of tissues, muscles, and joints have been recommended. In addition, denture construction should not be undertaken until the patient has been prepared emotionally and psychologically to participate in the endeavor.

Varied procedures in initial appointments

Dentists use what they consider the appropriate approach to each patient. Generally, they ask specific questions during the initial appointment. The detail with which they record the patient's medical and dental history varies considerably. Health, age, complaints about present dentures, reasons for seeking additional service, and occupational and social needs related to the use of dentures are all related specifically to the demands placed on a dentist undertaking treatment in any given instance. Other questions can be directed toward determining the relative importance to the patient of esthetics, comfort, and function in speech as well as mastication. The patient may have nutritional deficiencies and be ready to accept advice or referral for supportive therapy in this area. Vitamins, food supplements, and exercise can be discussed. A simple question as to the date of the last medical checkup may reveal the information necessary to obtain effective cooperation from the patient's physician.

One or more visits should be exploratory; however, pain or other conditions may require immediate treatment. During these visits the dentist can learn something about the patient's personality, attitudes, general demeanor, and physical and dental history, as well as chief complaints and expectations. The dentist also has the opportunity to manifest favorable elements of his personality and treatment philosophy.

Patients have stated explicitly that although they assumed the dentists were not aware of it, their first few visits were aimed principally at evaluating or analyzing them. During these visits, examination and evaluation become a mutual experience.

Maintaining a desirable patient relationship

To maintain the relationship with the patient on a professional level, it is imperative that emphasis be placed on treating the patient in contrast to selling him some type of oral device. Also, despite accelerating third-party influences, dentists must avoid a vendor-consumer situation. They must by specific effort establish and maintain a valid, realistic, and recognizable doctor-patient feeling and atmosphere. This, of necessity, brings the discussion back to the key word *rapport,* which is defined as a relation of harmony, conformity, accord or affinity. The means of achieving this will be as varied in number as there are dentists and patients.

The dentist is assumed to be a well-trained and capable person of high moral standards and good will. The dentist's qualifications have been called "competency with a conscience" (Fleming, 1956). It is the dentist's responsibility to communicate to the patient a feeling of competence and conscience. The key word is *communicate;* an old maxim about speech states the objectives as "to be heard, understood, and believed." Another requirement is the all-important element of sincerity; the dentist must have a sincere desire to meet the needs of the patient by the most effective possible means in every situation. Sincerity is as difficult to conceal as insincerity; people readily sense the difference. It is evidenced in a willingness to listen sufficiently and attentively to whatever the patient desires to relate. The dentist can ask questions to indicate interest, as well as offer some words of encouragement and state a desire to be of assistance.

Maintenance needs of the overdenture

At this point it is appropriate to explain in detail some of the developments that can be anticipated, the patient's responsibility as to home care, supplemental treatments required, and methods of maintaining the restoration as a result of tissue changes. It should be recognized and made clear to the patient that all restorations are subject to mechanical wear in addition to the influence of tissue changes. Some breakage can be anticipated especially in instances in which limited vertical dimension or unusual tissue contours may require minimal bulk of the restorations. Special emphasis is placed on home care and supportive professional care for maximum control of potential areas of caries or periodontal involvement.

Consideration is given to corrective treatment, which is required in the event of loss of one or more supportive teeth. The possibility of loosening of special attachments, bars, or copings is explained when applicable. In addition, possible methods of treatment for overcoming problems that may arise are discussed. If all potentials are explained and if the patient is aware of possible problems before they occur, this procedure can aid the dentist if some of these events happen. Any explanation after their occurrence may be viewed by the patient as merely an alibi.

The light touch

The enormous value of "the light touch" in improving the dentist-patient relationship is not to be overlooked. Many years ago, Kells (1925) wrote about the desirability of a dentist's touch being worthy of the description, "touche de velour." Gentle treatment of a patient's oral tissues is certain to be appreciated. Most patients appreciate and respond well to the verbal "touch of velvet," that is, words of kindness and thoughtfulness. Often it is necessary to search for something about which to compliment a patient, but a "Thank you for . . ." is worth the effort. If the dentist fails to control his temper on occasion, an "I'm sorry I . . ." can make a friend, even though it may be embarrassing. The numerous lists of preferred words and phrases deserve study and appropriate application.

The verbal light touch does not require any breakdown of professional stature. It has been said that laughter is one of the principal characteristics that distinguishes human beings from lower animals. The professional person is supposed to be human and humane to a greater degree than other people. There is a time and a place for everything; laughter can be inappropriate under a variety of circumstances. However, there is nothing wrong with the effort to create an atmosphere of hospitality, warmth, friendliness, and light-heartedness. By no means should a dentist attempt to assume an artificial personality pose or behave in any manner out of character, for it is likely to appear false. Most of the time it is possible to manage a smile and even a friendly word when greeting or dismissing a patient. Properly trained and motivated, all personnel in the office can reinforce this effort. After the pleasant greeting, an offer to assist patients in removing hats, coats, or packages is appreciated. When the schedule permits or when an appointment is lengthy, the offer of a cold drink, hot coffee, or even a restroom break is especially welcome. If telling a joke does not conflict with the dentist's personality, most patients appreciate the relief from the tension of the charged atmosphere that often accompanies the usual concentration required during many dental procedures.

As stated previously, most dentists are essentially good people, qualified, concerned, and eager to serve the patient's needs to the limit of their capability. However, most can improve their techniques or effectiveness in making patients aware of their interest and qualifications. It requires many talents to make what Pankey* calls a dental missionary, that is, a missionary for the benefits of good dentistry in general and for the motivating dentist in particular. The benefits to the patient and to the dentist are mutual.

FEES
Factors in fee determination

Although it might be preferable to omit any reference to fees and their collection, this subject can be crucial in a practice and in the dentist-patient relationship. Cost is generally a significant consideration during the discussion of plans with patients in almost all situations. The old saw, "good judgment comes from bad experience" leads to the following statement: A fee should not be offered until both the dentist and the patient know and understand the extent and character of the treatment. Many factors influence the choice of treatment and the nature of the demands placed on the dentist.

Consideration of time, cost, and degree of potential stress on the dentist, as well as degree of skill, care, and judgment required, usually arouses an entirely new area of thinking in patients accustomed to viewing a denture as an entity with a known fixed cost, and, ergo, a fixed fee. A brief period of thought, accompanied by a limited amount of information, should be sufficient for anyone to realize that there is no way to make a fixed fee fair to the patient and the dentist. It may appear to work well in some practices, but it necessitates the equalizing of procedures and limitations of treatment. The results in terms of quality

---

*Pankey, L. D.: Personal communication, Nov. 20, 1973.

of patient care vary with the limitations imposed. It is reasonable to assume that the effectiveness of treatment is directly proportionate to the level of the fixed fee.

Often in the postinsertion phase of treatment, stress on the dentist-patient relationship reaches its maximum. During the initial restoration effort, appliances can be completed and put in place before the dentist recognizes the need for modifications. Therefore the diagnosis can continue into what ordinarily is considered the postinsertion treatment phase. If limitations in treatment and results produce unlimited annoyance, nuisance, and unhappiness for the patient, the dentist, or both, a favorable relationship often collapses. Censor grievance committees can attest to the need for improved dentist-patient understanding and planning to minimize such occurrences. Although it is not generally true, payment of the fee alone can become the dominant factor in these conflicts. The uninformed patient can become the most uncooperative. Admittedly, education of the patient takes time, and some patients apparently cannot accept or understand the efforts of the dentist to inform them about factors that influence the condition and behavior of their structure as well as the potential variances in the results of treatment. The variables previously described indicate why it is impossible to render adequate treatment to patients on a routine fixed plan or at a fixed fee.

Plans for payment of fees

The specific arragement for payment of fees can have an immense influence on the dentist-patient relationship as well as on the attitude of the patient toward the treatment and the people involved.

Many dentists have been advised that "a denture never fits until it is paid for." It is appropriate to add that if a denture fits, it is not so merely because it is paid for. Patients who pay for and receive dentures that prove inadequate comprise dentistry's principal detractors. Most practitioners have encountered patients who have one denture or several made in rapid succession with unhappy results. Some patients who have several recently placed unsatisfactory dentures can become satisfactory, cooperative, and appreciative if they receive proper preparation and adequate treatment. Too often these unfortunates are categorized as crackpots, neurotics, or undesirables. Patients can be too ill to receive treatment, but an inconsiderate, hasty decision can be unfair and inaccurate.

The traditional requirement for cash payment on denture service has added to the woes of some patients. They report that postinsertion care or adjustments were provided grudgingly, hurriedly, for too short a time, or not at all in previous instances. Advance planning and specific detailed agreement on treatment exclusions can minimize disagreements. If the unhappy experience is repeated, one can understand readily why the patient becomes skeptical and apprehensive and tends to inquire about guaranteed results.

An approach that shows the dentist's concern with achieving helpful results rather than with collecting a fee aids in building up confidence. Appropriate preparatory treament can convince the dentist and the patient that the results will be successful. This should be accomplished before definitive treatment is undertaken.

Strict, short-term payment schedules can aggravate patients and stimulate their apprehension and skepticism. They may believe that these dentists lack confidence in their ability or intention to pay for the services and conclude that their honesty is questioned. They may even believe that the dentists lack confidence in their own ability to produce satisfactory results.

Experience has demonstrated that in a practice devoted exclusively to removable prosthodontics, a seemingly loose and liberal approach to financial planning with patients has merit. Apparently when emphasis can be placed on exploring treatment benefits, rapport is developed more readily. Most patients become faithful friends of the dentist. A large number of patients who were treated in previous years return for additional treatment. Financial losses are surprisingly low and have usually provided a means of achieving a more selective practice.

The foregoing can be construed as an indication that no problems arise or that an authoritarian attitude is never used. There are exceptions to any plan for patient relationship handling, and occasionally there is need for establishing a firm policy.

As a result of insufficient information, some patients may not have total confidence in the dentist. Occasionally, patients request "testimonials" directly or indirectly because they need reassurance from successfully treated patients. Although such requests are refused, this need indicates the patients' lack of confidence. The dentist explains that the code of ethics prohibits release of such information and recommends another competent dentist. The patient is also advised to consult other professional personnel in whom he/she has confidence before seeing the other dentist. Frequently this approach has made the patient aware that the dentist is not offering encouragement to continue treatment, but is encouraging him/her to go elsewhere. This procedure tends to have a reverse effect.

Occasionally a portion of the fee has been paid and the dental work is in progress before signs of hostility or uncooperative behavior appear. In some instances an offer to refund the fee and the suggestion that another dentist might be selected for the patient can be a gesture of good will. It can also change a patient's attitude from one of hostility to that of cooperative behavior.

Situations can develop in which anger is manifested by the dentist, the patient, or both. This destroys rapport and must not be allowed to occur. Definite decisions must on occasion be firmly stated. Any necessary explanations should be made but courtesy and consideration are still required.

Most important of all, a demonstrated attitude of mutual trust, with the patient's welfare being the primary concern, provides a solid foundation for the dentist's objective, that is, a satisfactory dentist-patient relationship conducive to optimal results in the immediate future and in the years to come.

REFERENCES

Collett, H. A.: Psychodynamic study of abnormal reaction to dentures, J. Am. Dent. Assoc. **51**:451-546, 1955.

Fleming, W. C.: Human relations: one more river to cross, J. Am. Coll. Dent. **23**:312-316, 1956.

Kells, C. E : The dentist's own book, St. Louis, 1925, The C. V. Mosby Co.

Moulton, R.: Psychological problems associated with complete denture service, J. Am. Dent. Assoc. **33**:476-485, 1946.

4
EXAMINATION, DIAGNOSIS, TREATMENT PLANNING, AND PROGNOSIS

ROBERT M. MORROW
ALLEN A. BREWER

Thorough examination, accurate diagnosis, and rational treatment planning are prerequisites for success with overdenture treatment.

HISTORY AND RECORDS
Medical history

A medical history should be obtained from each patient being considered for overdentures because of the importance of his general health. Use of a health questionnaire expedites the recording of medical and psychiatric data pertinent to the treatment. Bolender and associates (1969) found the Cornell Medical Index Health Questionnaire (Cornell University Medical College, New York) reliable in identifying patients who might have difficulty with new dentures, and they reported a positive correlation between emotional and denture problems. The grouping of questions about the various systems also minimizes the possibility of a dentist overlooking pertinent symptoms. Debilitating medical or psychiatric disorders, which rule out essential clinical procedures or seriously compromise the patient's ability to maintain an adequate level of oral hygiene, are contraindications for overdentures.

Dental history

A record of the patient's past dental history often contains meaningful information about previous experiences that may consciously or subconsciously influence his attitudes, motivation, and expectations. The success or failure of earlier prostheses is especially significant, and instances of unsatisfactory results deserve careful exploration. Why did the patient lose teeth, and what difficulties did he have with replacements? Occasionally a patient may expect too much from proposed prostheses, and the dentist must realign the patient's thinking or expectations within the treatment capabilities to avoid disappointment. A record of home care efforts, including the methods, materials, and frequency, as well as the previous instructions to the patient should be obtained and evaluated in relation to the current oral hygiene status. Patients with acceptable oral hygiene have a much better overdenture prognosis than those with a history of many oral hygiene counseling sessions and poor oral hygiene.

Pretreatment records

Accurate diagnostic casts mounted in a suitable articulator supply information pertinent to the patient and the selection of abutments (Fig. 4-1). The occlusion should be analyzed to determine the presence of deflective occlusal contacts. Information disclosed by the diagnostic casts includes tooth positions, jaw relationships, tuberosity impingement, tori, available denture space,

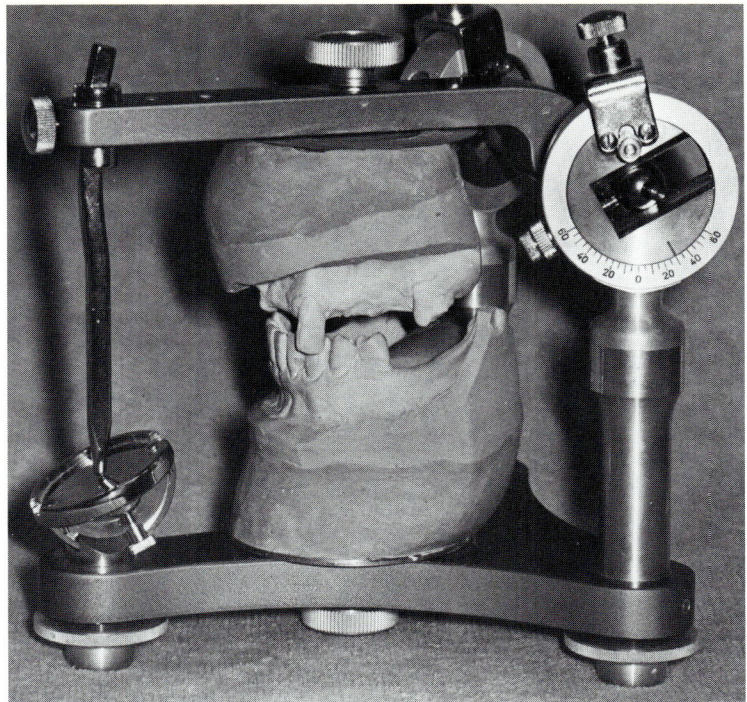

Fig. 4-1. Diagnostic casts mounted in articulator.

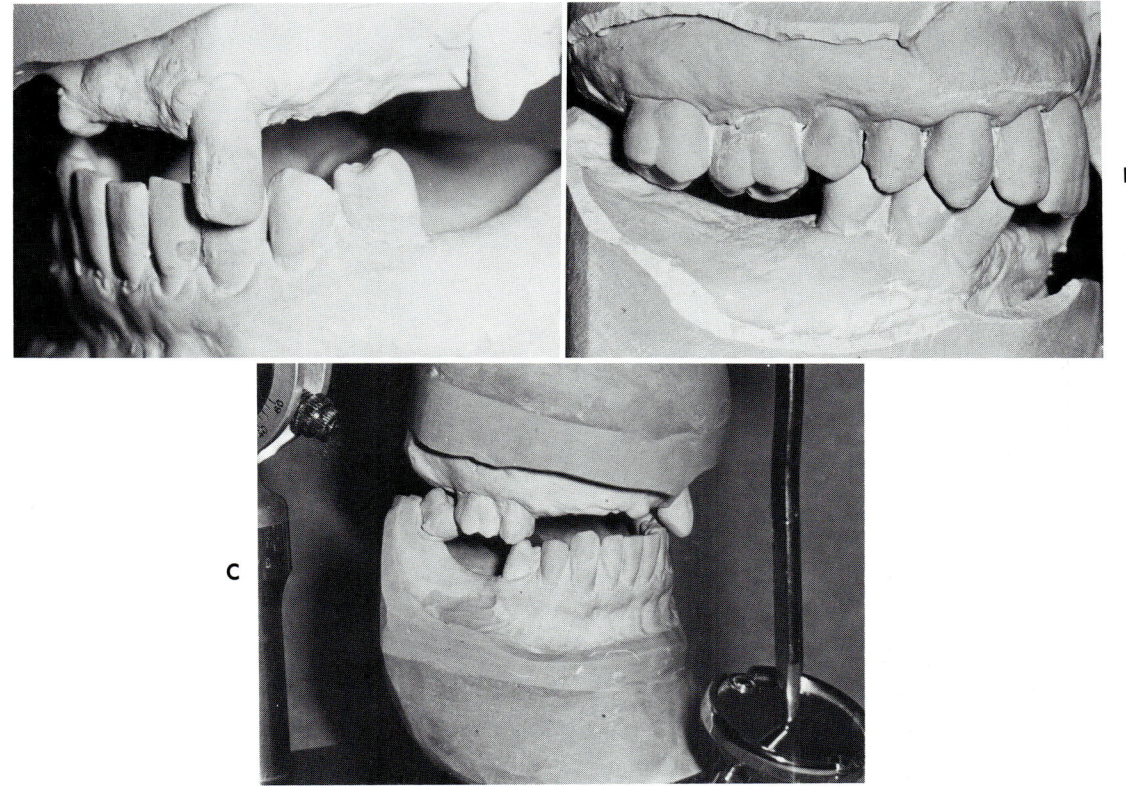

Fig. 4-2. **A,** Diagnostic casts indicating presence of adequate denture space. Maxillary cuspid will serve as overdenture abutment. **B,** Extrusion of maxillary molars encroaching on available denture space and producing unfavorable occlusal "plane." **C,** Tissue undercut results from labial position of maxillary left cuspid.

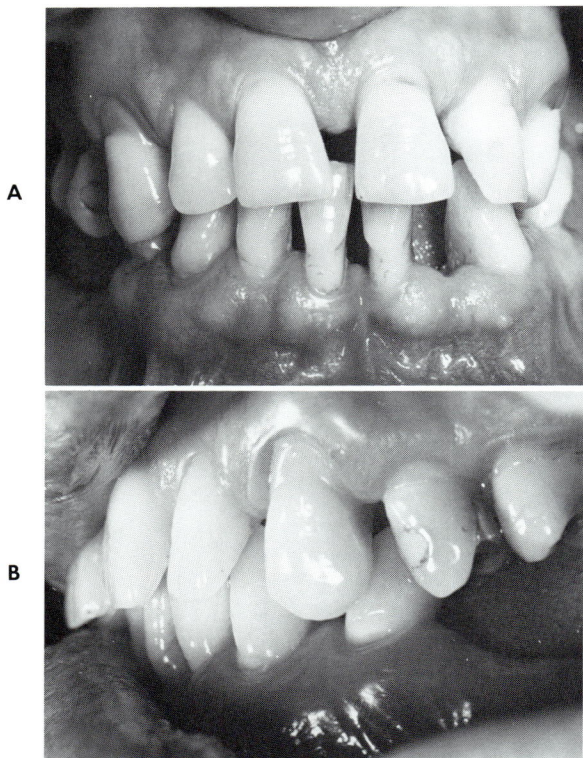

Fig. 4-3. **A,** Excellent photographic pretreatment records of position, size, and shape of teeth supplement but do not replace diagnostic casts. **B,** Lateral view of maxillary cuspid proposed for overdenture abutment. Note severe vertical overlap, which can cause space problems for overdenture base.

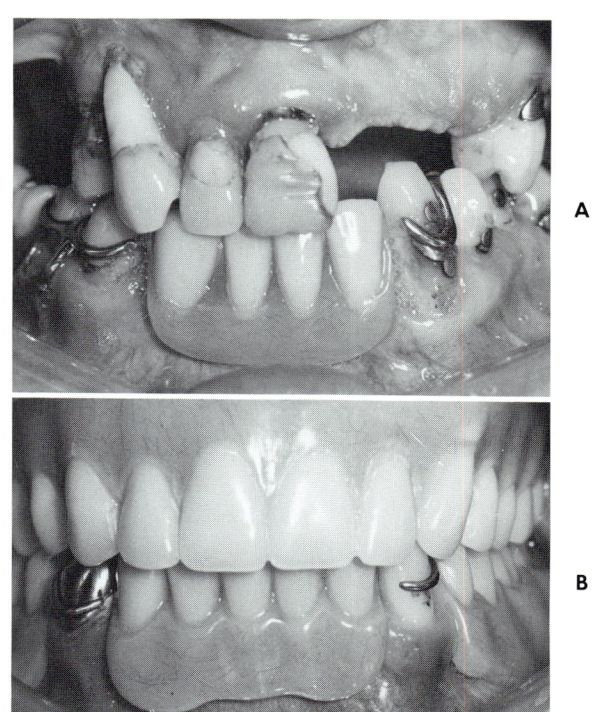

Fig. 4-4. **A,** Patient with prosthesis and evidence of poor oral hygiene, numerous defective restorations, and uncontrolled periodontal disease, all of which are negative factors for proposed overdenture. **B,** Patient wth denture and removable partial denture worn satisfactorily for several years and with good prognosis for overdenture because of excellent oral hygiene and denture cleanliness.

tissue undercuts, and size as well as arrangement of teeth (Fig. 4-2). These casts should be retained as a permanent record and should not be used in making prostheses. Color transparencies or photographs of the teeth and adjacent structures, including frontal, side, and occlusal views, can supplement the diagnostic casts as a part of the pretreatment record (Fig. 4-3). Profile registrations (Turner, 1969), moulages, and cephalometric radiographs may be required for unusual treatment situations.

EXAMINATION
Visual and digital examination

Thorough visual and digital examinations of the oral cavity, tongue, and teeth should be made. The lips, buccal mucosa, gingiva, floor of the mouth, hard and soft palates, and fauces should be examined carefully for possible pathologic changes that might be much more important to the patient's health than other findings. It is of particular importance to evaluate the response of supporting tissues to existing prostheses, such as inflammation and hyperplastic tissue associated with denture abuse (Fig. 4-4). Digital examination of the soft and hard tissues might indicate exostoses, sharp mylohyoid ridges, and displaceable tuberosity tissues otherwise missed during visual examination alone. Other information about the denture-supporting tissues could be obtained by digital examination; there might be freely displaceable tissues on residual ridges and tissue undercut areas in need of surgical correction before overdenture treatment (Fig. 4-5, *A* and *B*).

EXAMINATION, DIAGNOSIS, TREATMENT PLANNING, AND PROGNOSIS   27

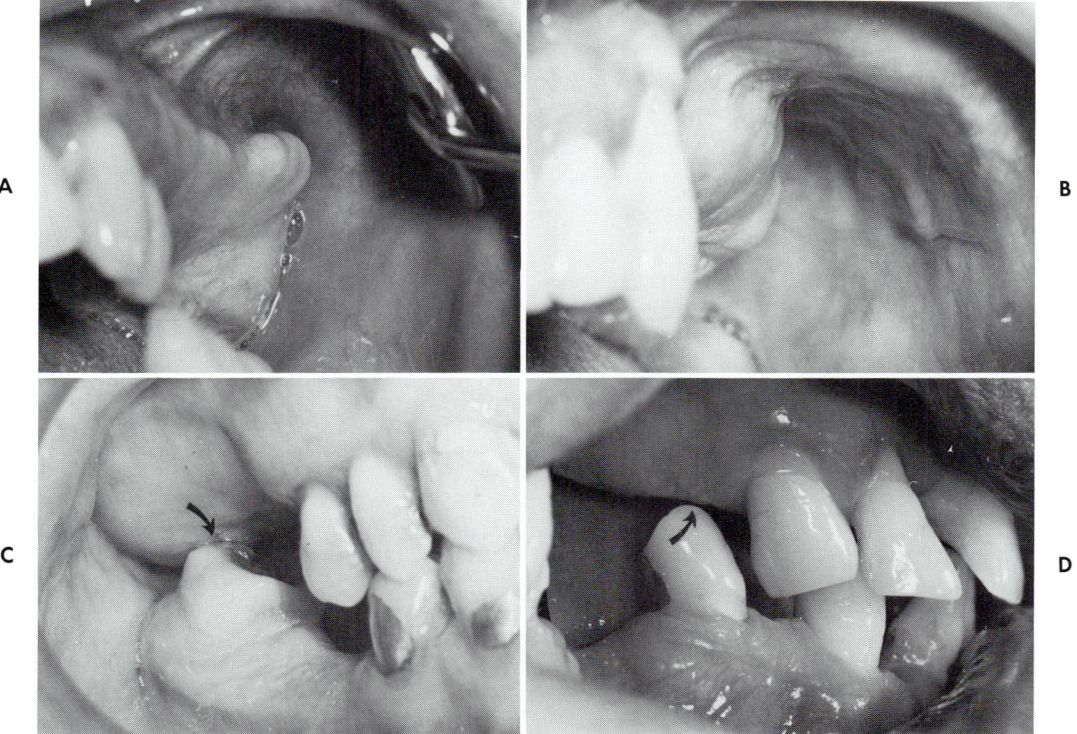

Fig. 4-5. **A,** Severe bony exostoses revealed by examination and needing recontouring. **B,** Same patient after surgical procedure that contributed significantly to success of overdenture. **C,** Recontouring of malposed mandibular molar or reduction of maxillary tuberosity or both are required to provide space for overdenture base. **D,** Minimal space is available for overdenture base.

Dental examination

Carious lesions and defective restorations should be charted and vitality tests made when indicated. Missing teeth and the condition of replacements should be noted. The occlusion should be evaluated in relation to the findings from the diagnostic casts (Fig. 4-5, *C*). It is important to determine the presence of adequate denture space (Fig. 4-5, *D*). Indications of clenching or bruxing and of abnormal tongue or lip habits should be observed. The oral hygiene status and, if pertinent, the patient's denture-cleaning methods should be studied by using disclosing tablets or solutions. Poor oral hygiene and unhygienic removable prostheses with attendant inflammation of the denture-supporting tissues indicate a poor prognosis for an overdenture unless corrective procedures are effective.

Periodontal examination

Although the majority of patients who are candidates for overdentures have signs and symptoms of chronic periodontal disease, some have deformities that are congenital or that result from traumatic incidents. Generalized bone loss, increased periodontal pocket depths, and hypermobility are characteristic of periodontal disease. Crevicular and pocket depths as well as furcations should be probed and the findings recorded. The magnitude and direction of mobility patterns should be recorded and correlated with the functional demands of individual teeth. Some increase in mobility is not in itself contraindicative of selection for overdenture abutments, but teeth with horizontal and vertical displacement are poor choices. Teeth retainable after periodontal therapy and those with a hopeless prognosis should be identified and charted. It is essential to evaluate the patient's oral hygiene efforts in relation to the periodontal status and to assess both motivation and interest in preserving the remaining teeth. Establishing and maintaining an adequate oral hygiene regimen are singularly important in achieving a reasonable service life for an overdenture.

Radiographic examination

Findings from a complete periapical radiographic survey are usually the basis for abutment selection. If only a few natural teeth remain, individual periapical films supplemented by a panoramic radiograph are adequate. It is of prime importance to ascertain what bone support is available for the prospective abutment. Attention should be paid to retained roots, impacted teeth, crown-root ratios, carious lesions, apical pathology, radiolucent and radiopaque lesions of the jaws, the status of previous endodontic treatments, potential for endodontic treatment, and the status of the periodontium. Appropriate decisions about treatment should be made on the basis of this information.

CONSULTATIONS

After examining a prospective overdenture patient, frequently it is prudent to obtain consultations from a periodontist and an endodontist prior to the selection and treatment of abutment teeth. Consultation with an oral surgeon may be indicated if a large number of hopeless teeth are to be removed or if surgical procedures to correct residual ridge deformities are required. When indicated, consultations should be obtained from appropriate medical specialists prior to the initiation of overdenture treatment.

DIAGNOSIS

The data from diagnostic casts, radiographs, histories, laboratory reports, examinations, and consultations are the basis for the diagnosis. The majority of prospective overdenture patients have chronic, generalized periodontal disease. Other patients may have congenital deformities such as a cleft palate, orthodontic problems, or loss of teeth from a traumatic incident. The number of patients with multiple hopeless teeth because of rampant caries seems to be decreasing and may reflect the growing emphasis on treatment oriented toward prevention.

TREATMENT PLANNING

The patient who has only a few retainable natural teeth may present difficult treatment questions for the dentist. Should fixed partial dentures be used? Should removable partial dentures be considered? Should both fixed and removable partial dentures be used? Should complete dentures be recommended? Should an overdenture be used? If so, what type should be used, and how should it be implemented? All these questions should be considered, and the treatment options should be discussed candidly with the patient. Johnston and associates (1965) offer the following advice: "A bridge is indicated whenever there are properly distributed and healthy teeth to serve as the abutments, provided that these teeth have suitable crown-root ratios and that after radiographic, diagnostic cast, and oral examinations seem capable of sustaining the additional load."[*] When indicated, fixed partial dentures are the treatment of choice; however, the prospective overdenture patient usually does not have properly distributed, healthy teeth with suitable crown-root ratios. The few retainable teeth generally are scattered throughout the arch, and invariably they are involved periodontally with unfavorable crown-root ratios. Should removable partial dentures be used? Often they are used when a fixed partial denture is contraindicated. McCracken (1961) gives several specific indications for use of a removable partial denture, including "distal extension situations, after recent extractions, long spans, where there is a need for bilateral bracing, esthetics in anterior region and the excessive loss of residual bone."

We consider the use of overdentures if four or fewer retainable teeth are present in an arch, and we consider removable partial dentures or other fixed or removable combinations if more than four retainable teeth are present. However, the number four is not immutable, and a rational treatment approach requires flexibility as to the number and position of abutments for overdentures.

---

[*]From Johnston, J. F., Phillips, R. W., and Dykema, R. W.: Modern practice in crown and bridge prosthodontics, Philadelphia, 1965, W. B. Saunders Co.

For some patients with orthodontic problems or congenital deformities, such as cleft palate, an overdenture can be constructed over a complete or nearly complete dentition. Overdentures can also be used over a number of maxillary abutment teeth as a compensating prosthetic treatment for some Class III malocclusions.

There are few situations in which a complete denture is preferable to an overdenture. For the uncooperative, disinterested patient, the prognosis for overdentures is guarded; when no retainable teeth are present, a complete denture may be indicated. However, the majority of patients benefit from the preservation of teeth to serve as abutments for an overdenture. Younger patients particularly deserve every treatment consideration to prevent the removal of natural teeth and the associated bone changes. For the patient with few retainable teeth, an overdenture usually is indicated (Fig. 4-6). It should be considered also when an inadequate number of retainable teeth are present to support a conventional type of restoration or to meet specific treatment requisites, such as the aforementioned congenital deformities. Other types of patients suitable for overdentures are those destined to lose teeth in one arch while the other arch remains dentulous and those with malrelated ridges, unfavorable tongue positions or muscle attachments, or any situation in which stability or retention would be a serious problem with complete dentures.

Patient conference

All findings should be discussed at a patient conference, during which treatment options and recommendations are presented. The type of overdenture that best satisfies the patient's needs should be selected, and all treatment procedures should be explained in clearly understandable terms. The need for service and maintenance after placement of the overdenture should be emphasized.

Type of overdenture

The type of overdenture depends primarily on the status of the patient's dentition at the start of treatment.

Immediate overdenture. An immediate overdenture is constructed for insertion immediately after the removal of some natural teeth. Immediate overdentures are used when the patient has

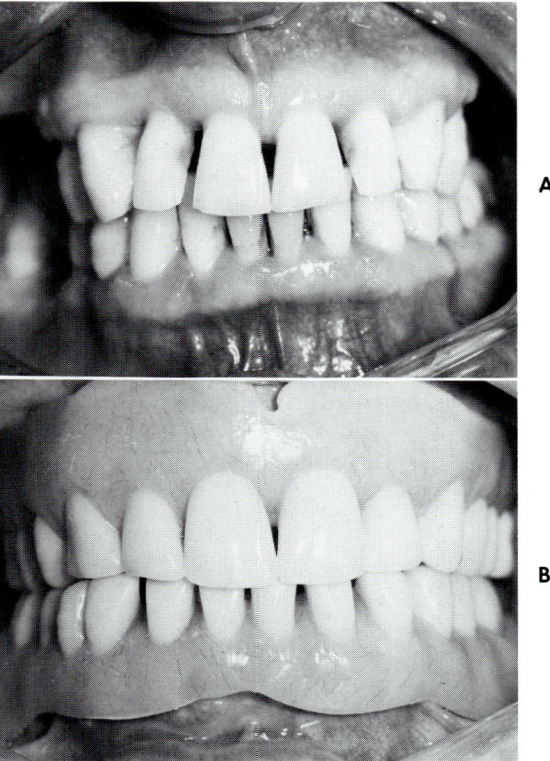

Fig. 4-7. **A,** Many hopeless, periodontally involved teeth, resulting in patient receiving immediate overdenture. **B,** Immediate overdenture in place, with cuspids and second premolars used as abutments.

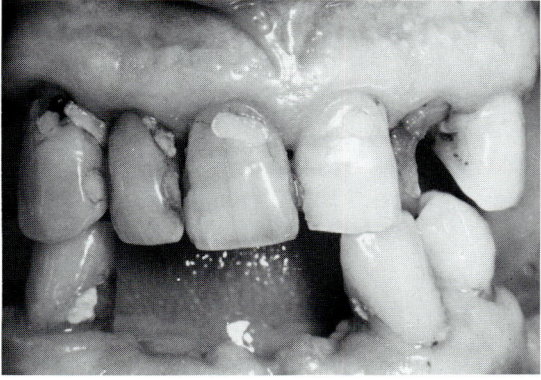

Fig. 4-6. Only a few remaining teeth are retainable, making overdenture the treatment of choice.

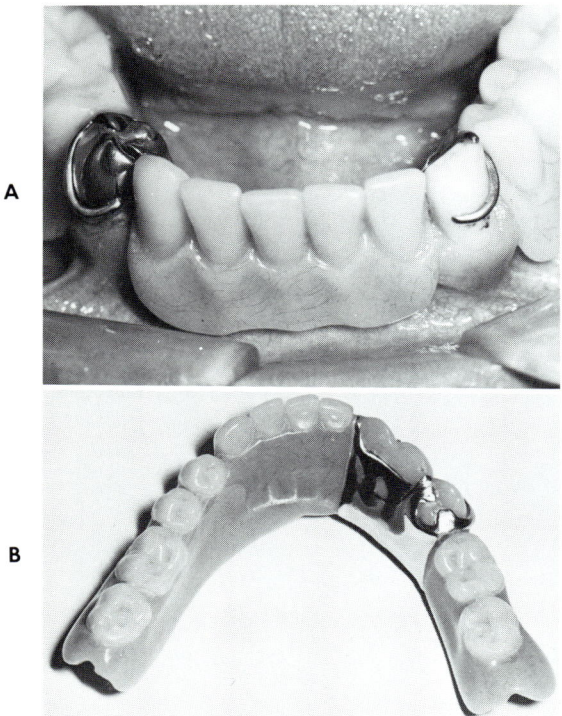

Fig. 4-8. A, Conversion of removable partial denture to transitional overdenture is often beneficial to patient for whom overdenture is planned. **B,** Existing mandibular removable partial denture has been modified to serve as transitional overdenture.

many hopeless teeth (Fig. 4-7). Abutment teeth are selected and treated, and the overdenture is inserted as an immediate replacement. The immediate overdenture, modified as required, can be worn for several years under favorable circumstances. The majority of our patients receive immediate overdentures initially. Immediate overdentures are discussed in Chapter 10.

Transitional overdenture. A transitional overdenture is obtained by converting an existing removable partial denture to overdenture status. A patient who has removable partial dentures can be phased into an overdenture if the partial denture is modified into a transitional overdenture (Fig. 4-8). Transitional overdentures are discussed in Chapter 9.

Remote overdenture. A remote overdenture is an overdenture other than transitional or immediate. It is usually constructed for insertion at some time "remote" from the removal of hopeless natural teeth. For the patient with only a few remaining teeth, all of which are to be abutments, a more definitive or remote overdenture can be considered (Fig. 4-9). The abutment teeth can be treated endodontically, prepared, and given protective copings before the remote overdenture is constructed. Remote overdentures are discussed in Chapter 11.

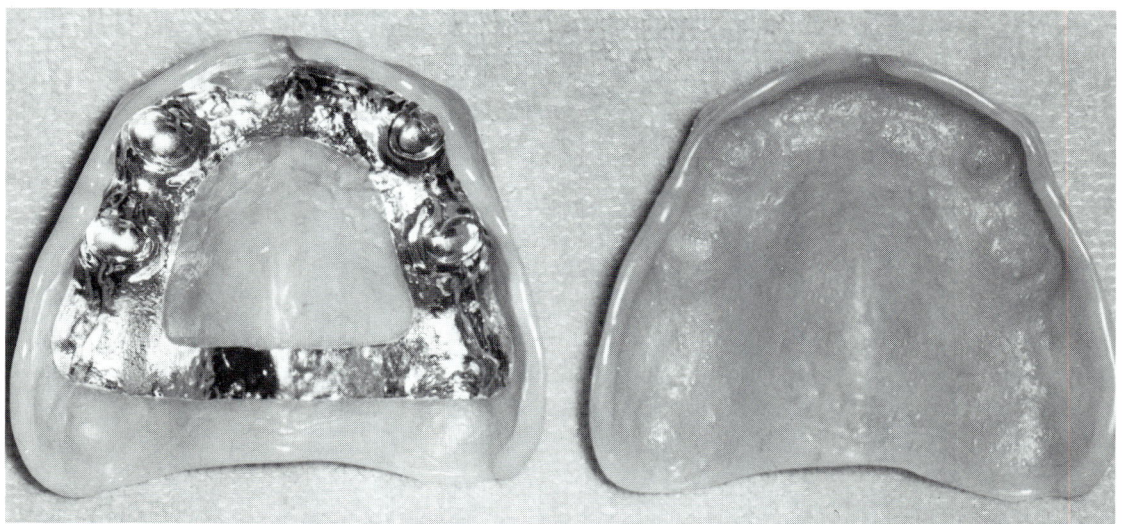

Fig. 4-9. Remote overdenture can be constructed of resin or reinforced with metal base.

Abutment selection

The loss of natural teeth by a patient usually follows a characteristic pattern. Maxillary teeth are lost before the mandibular teeth. An all too typical restorative sequence for a hypothetical patient consists of (1) loss of the maxillary posterior teeth and replacement with a maxillary removable partial denture, (2) loss of the remaining maxillary anterior teeth and restoration with a conventional maxillary denture, (3) loss of the mandibular posterior teeth and replacement with a mandibular removable partial denture, and (4) loss of the remaining mandibular anterior teeth and restoration with complete dentures.

The chronology of tooth loss and the method of replacement vary considerably, but the overall pattern is characteristic. If the patient is seen early in the chronology of tooth loss, abutments will be selected for a maxillary overdenture opposed by a natural mandibular dentition. At later stages abutments will be selected for a mandibular overdenture opposed by an already edentulous maxillary arch. However, the basic objective is still to prevent the loss of natural teeth and the consequent need for complete dentures.

During the examination, all potential abutment teeth should be evaluated carefully from the viewpoints of (1) periodontal status, (2) caries activity, (3) potential for endodontic treatment, and (4) positional considerations.

Periodontal status. Since overdentures rely on abutment teeth for support and stability, it is axiomatic that these teeth must be in an acceptable state of periodontal health prior to completion of the overdenture. The achievement and maintenance of abutment periodontal health is affected by the overdenture. The most important factors are (1) conical shape of the abutment, (2) masticatory stimulation, and (3) oral hygiene of isolated teeth. Loss of the normal protective contours of the natural tooth from the conical shaping may contribute to an unfavorable gingival response. After the overdenture is inserted, the frictional forces of mastication and of the tongue are not applied to the gingival tissues. The reduction in functional stimulation can cause a decrease in keratinization and thereby can make these tissues more susceptible to injury. Clinical experience has shown that patients find it difficult to maintain acceptable oral hygiene around isolated teeth. Routine use of the toothbrush alone is inadequate for achieving the desired level of oral hygiene.

It is best to select abutments that are in an acceptable state of periodontal health initially, but often it is necessary to use teeth that are less than ideal. Prospective abutments should have minimal mobility, have adequate bone support, and be amenable to any indicated periodontal treatment (Fig. 4-10). Although mobility patterns are important in selecting abutments, the improvement of clinical crown-root ratios (with the aid of successful endodontic treatment) can reduce apparent clinical mobility significantly.

Caries activity. Ideally, teeth with minimal or no caries involvement should be selected for abutments. Although carious teeth can be used after successful restorative procedures, it must be em-

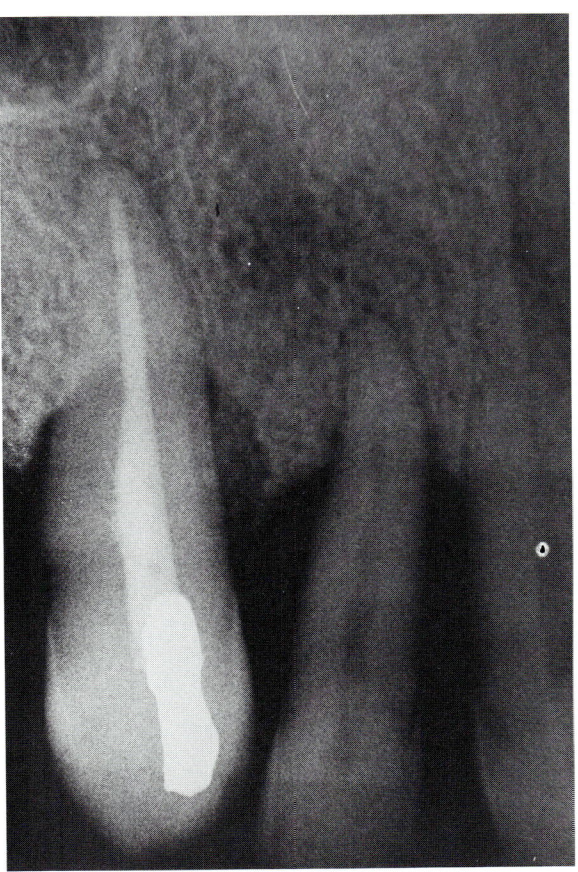

Fig. 4-10. Prospective abutment, which should be amenable to endodontic treatment and have adequate bone support (generally 6 mm.).

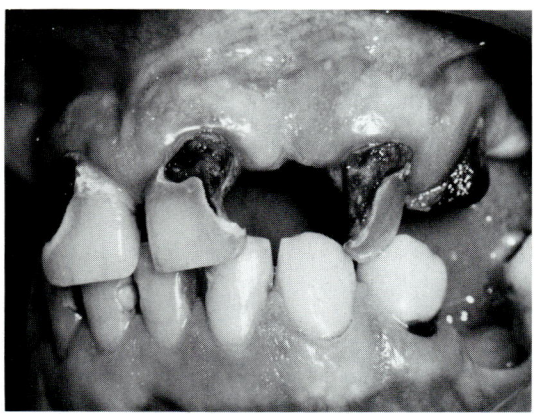

Fig. 4-11. Rampant caries is a negative factor for success of overdentures.

phasized that caries activity in a prospective overdenture patient is undesirable for reasons other than the technical problems of restoration (Fig. 4-11). An active caries process can lead to a recurrence of caries in unprotected abutment teeth or gingival to coping margins, and this can lead to failure of the overdenture.

Potential for endodontic treatment. Endodontic treatment is recommended for overdenture abutments, and its advantages outweigh its disadvantages (Fig. 4-12). Successful endodontic treatment contributes to the esthetic result by allowing sufficient reduction of the abutment tooth and replacement with one of similar size and shape. Crown-root ratios are improved by reducing the crown after endodontic treatment. This treatment permits the use of tilted or malposed teeth and hemisectioned or root-amputated molar teeth as abutments for overdentures. Clinical observation indicates that postinsertion losses of abutment teeth related to endodontic treatment are rare.

Positional considerations. Overdentures should be considered for a patient with four or fewer retainable teeth. This is particularly true when these teeth have less than ideal periodontal support. Depending on the distribution, four abutments in one arch can represent an ideal stress distribution, such as two cuspids and two second premolar abutments (Fig. 4-13, *A*). This distribution provides maximal stability and support for the overdenture, which is truly tooth-supported. Our clinical experience indicates that this number and dis-

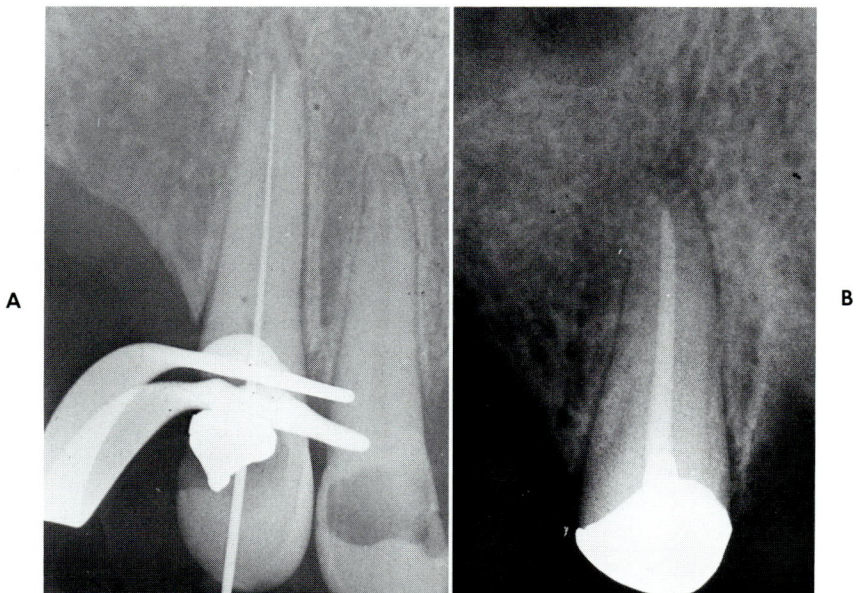

Fig. 4-12. A, Endodontic treatment contributes to success of overdentures. **B,** Clinical crown-root ratios are significantly improved and provision of good esthetics for completed overdenture is facilitated.

tribution of abutments is not the most common pattern (Fig. 4-14). The position of three abutment teeth in the arch may give unbalanced support if two abutments are on one side of the arch and one is on the other side (Fig. 4-13, *B*). This distribution pattern, although unbalanced, does not seem to cause the patient any untoward difficulty. A better distribution pattern for three abutments consists of two cuspids and a central incisor, which provide a tripod of support in the anterior

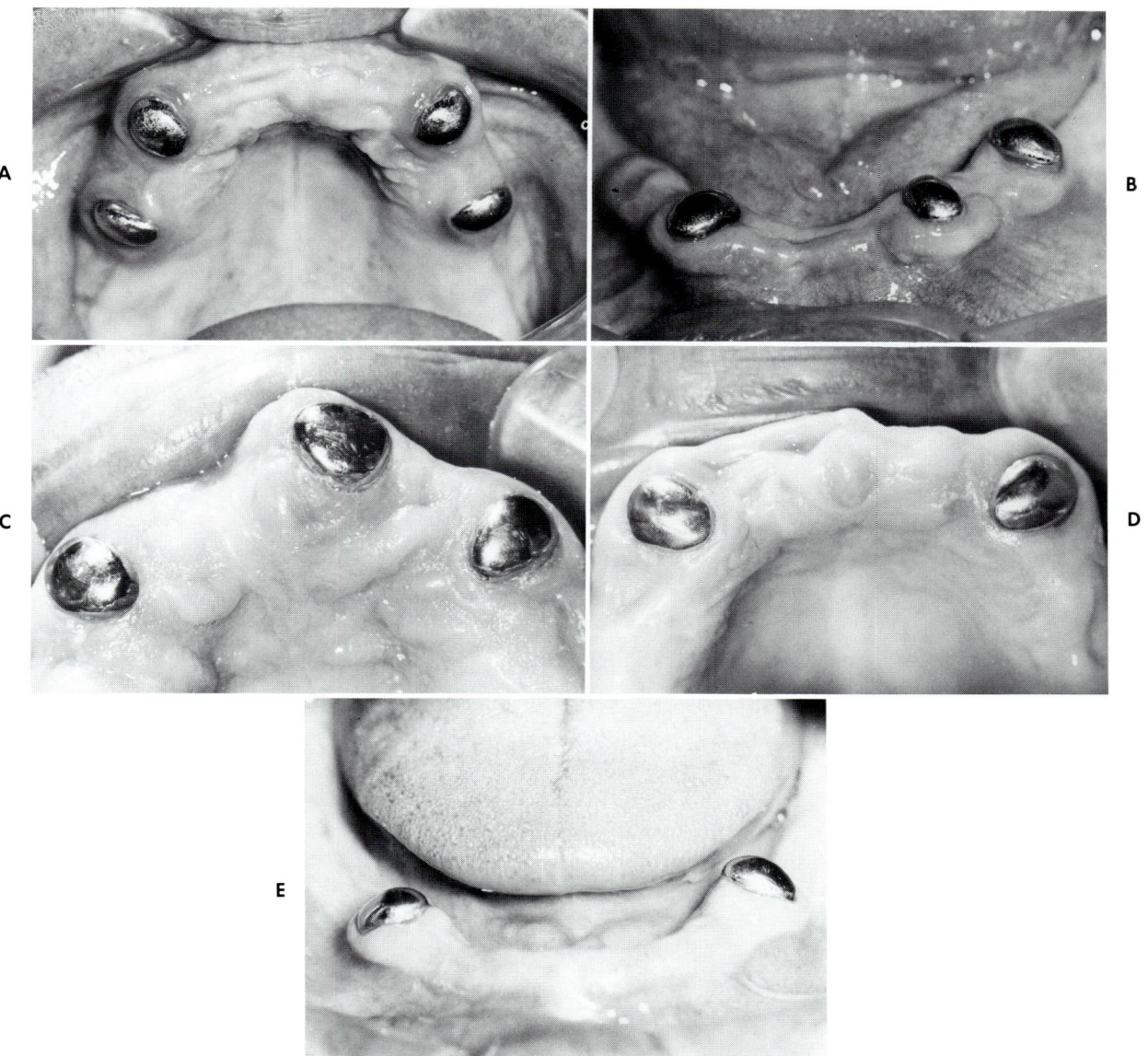

Fig. 4-13. **A,** Four abutments in an arch is the ideal distribution. Cuspids and second premolars were used here. **B,** Three abutments, a cuspid on the right and a cuspid and second premolar on the left, made an unbalanced distribution with which patient had no difficulty. **C,** Better distribution pattern for three abutments, two cuspids and one maxillary central incisor, provides a tripod of support in anterior arch that is particularly effective when it is opposed by a natural dentition. **D,** Common distribution for overdenture abutments is two cuspids in maxillary or mandibular arch. **E,** Less common distribution pattern is two premolars.

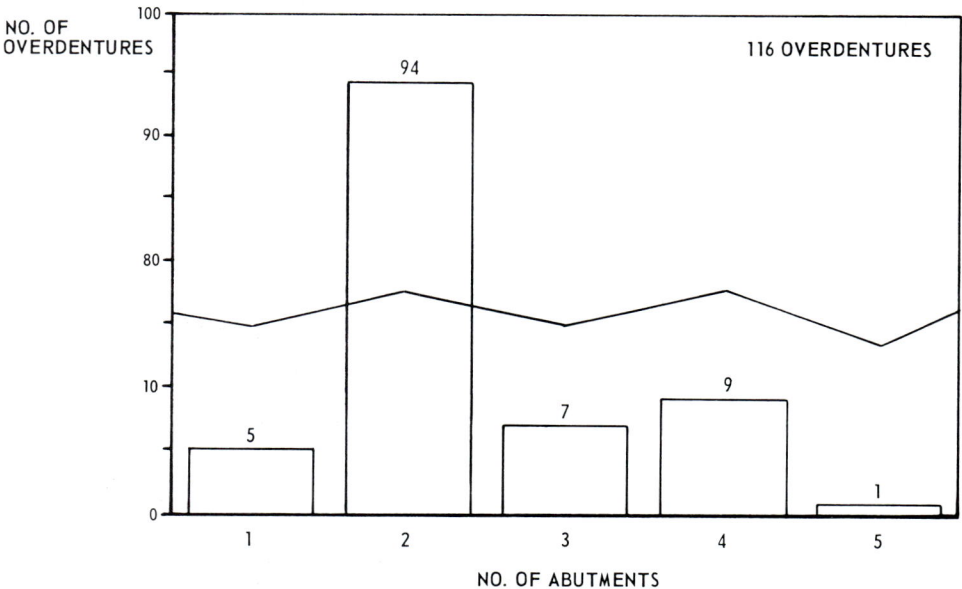

Fig. 4-14. Overdentures by number of supporting abutments. Two abutments are used most frequently.

jaw (Fig. 4-13, *C*). This distribution is particularly effective for a maxillary overdenture opposed by mandibular natural teeth.

In the most frequent distribution pattern two abutment teeth are present; usually they are cuspids, but they can be premolars (Fig. 4-13, *D* and *E*). Cuspids are selected more often than any other teeth, since they generally are amenable to endodontic treatment, have an adequate periodontal attachment area, and are in strategic positions in the arch. Table 4-1 shows the distribution of teeth used as abutments for more than a hundred overdentures. If only two abutment teeth are available, they should be situated bilaterally for optimum support. A cuspid and a premolar on the same side used for unilateral support are less desirable. Two cuspids, a cuspid and a premolar, or two premolars are preferred to molars for two abutments, since the anterior position of the cuspids minimizes the soft tissue loading in the anterior arch. Usually the results are better if the abutments are not approximating (Fig. 4-15). A cuspid and an approximating first premolar do not give much more support than one abutment. Sometimes approximating abutments are more difficult for the patient to clean, and their presence may make tooth positioning on the overdenture more difficult. Even overdentures supported by only one abutment function satisfactorily; in this instance it is best to use a cuspid, although others may be used (Fig. 4-16). When the opposing arch is restored with a conventional complete denture, the service life seems to be lengthened.

It is essential to consider occlusion in selecting abutments for overdentures. One should avoid a great disparity in the strength of opposing arches when constructing a prosthetic restoration. If an

Table 4-1. Teeth used as abutments for overdentures*

Maxillary	
Cuspids	114
Incisors	18
Premolars	19
Molars	0
Mandibular	
Cuspids	67
Incisors	1
Premolars	23
Molars	3
Total	245

*Cuspids are used most often for maxillary and mandibular overdentures.

EXAMINATION, DIAGNOSIS, TREATMENT PLANNING, AND PROGNOSIS 35

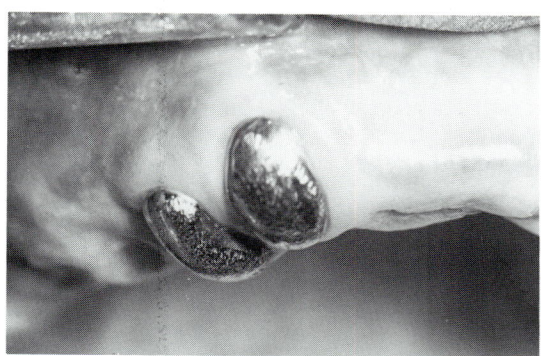

Fig. 4-15. Better results are usually obtained when approximating abutments are not used.

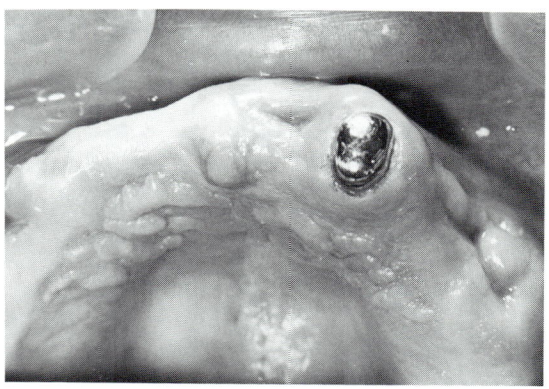

Fig. 4-16. Lateral incisor, the only available tooth, was used as the one abutment to support and stabilize an overdenture, which was satisfactory although not ideal.

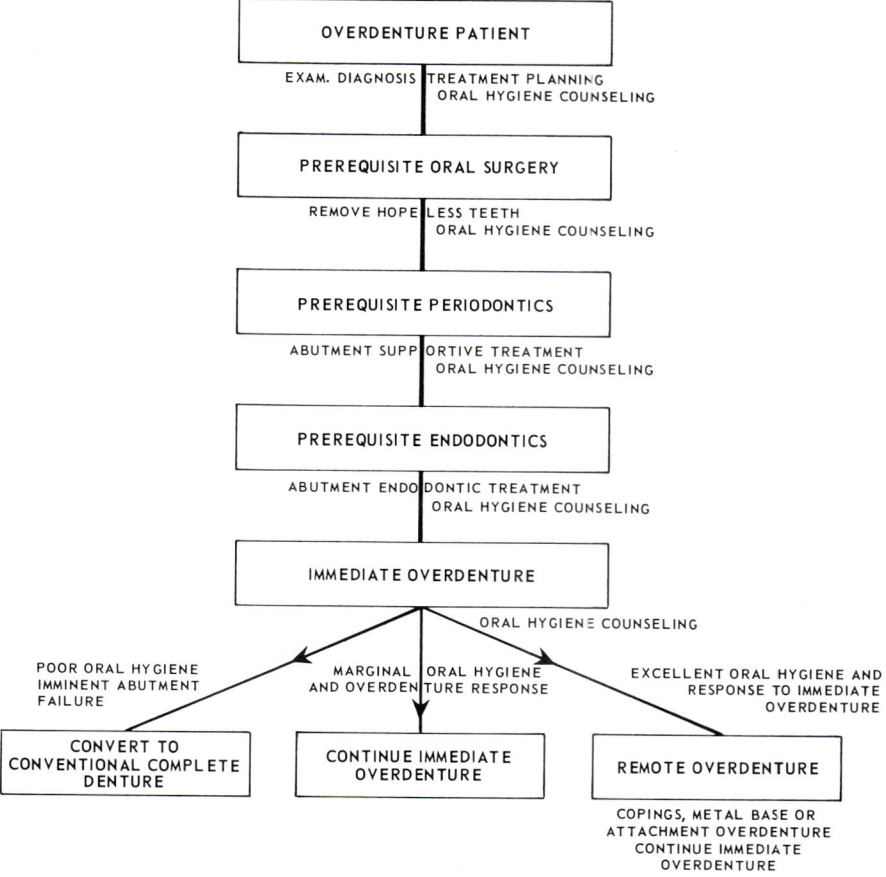

Fig. 4-17. Treatment sequence for overdenture patient. Although patients differ in their needs for treatment and the sequence of treatment, this chart is typical of many and indicates potential results.

overdenture is opposed by a complete denture or a removable partial denture with a large number of artificial teeth, the functional forces on the overdenture usually will be less than if the overdenture is opposed by an intact natural dentition with, perhaps, a heavy masticatory musculature. Therefore abutments for overdentures opposed by a natural dentition should be selected to reflect the increased need for support and stability. Development of a logical treatment sequence follows the selection of the abutment teeth.

Prerequisite treatment

The sequence of treatment procedures varies according to the needs of the patient and the type of overdenture (Fig. 4-17). An immediate overdenture is the usual introductory prosthesis. Posterior hopeless teeth are removed first to allow for longer healing and better access for periodontic and endodontic procedures on the retained teeth. The periodontal therapy indicated should be completed for all abutment teeth, and then the endodontic treatment would be done. Impressions of the arches are made with alginate irreversible hydrocolloid, and an immediate overdenture is constructed. Directly prior to insertion of the immediate overdenture, the abutment teeth are reduced, and the remaining hopeless teeth are removed. Adjunctive periodontal surgical procedures can often be completed in conjunction with tooth removal. Then the immediate overdenture is inserted; 6 to 8 weeks later it usually requires relining. In other instances, endodontic therapy can be accomplished, and a complete immediate overdenture can be placed. In this case posterior teeth also are removed at the time of insertion, and the periodontal treatment is completed later. The number and distribution of teeth to be removed as well as the physical condition of the patient influence the type of immediate overdenture to be used. A patient can wear the immediate overdenture for several months to several years; however, after a year of satisfactory experience, a more definitive overdenture usually is made. In this manner, the immediate overdenture becomes a valid prognostic aid for a more definitive prosthesis.

PROGNOSIS

A thorough examination and an accurate diagnosis are the foundation for determining the prognosis for an overdenture. The information collected aids in selection of patients and abutment teeth. Perhaps the most important factor for a favorable prognosis is an adequate oral hygiene level maintained by an interested and motivated patient. The skillful execution of clinical and laboratory procedures, although important, cannot compensate for poor home care.

The prognosis for overdentures is also related to postinsertion service and maintenance, and the need for both must be understood thoroughly by the patient. In instances when the oral hygiene efforts of the patient are inadequate or the required service and maintenance are not given, the prognosis for an overdenture is guarded. Effective oral hygiene procedures and regular follow-up care make the prognosis favorable and invariably lead to a longer service life for the overdenture.

REFERENCES

Bolender, C. L., Swoope, C. C., and Smith, D. E.: The Cornell Medical Index as a prognostic aid for complete denture patients, J. Prosthet. Dent. **22**:20-29, 1969.

Johnston, J. F., Phillips, R. W., and Dykema, R. W.: Modern practice in crown and bridge prosthodontics, ed. 2, Philadelphia, 1965, W. B. Saunders Co.

McCracken, W. L.: Differential diagnosis, fixed or removable partial dentures, J. Am. Dent. Assoc. **63**:767-775, 1961.

Turner, L. C.: The profile tracer: method for obtaining accurate pre-extraction records, J. Prosthet. Dent. **21**: 364-370, 1969.

5

PERIODONTICS AND THE OVERDENTURE PATIENT

LEONARD G. JEWSON

Periodontology can be defined as the science and study of the periodontium and periodontal disease. This specialty of dentistry encompasses the treatment of defects of the supporting structures of the teeth, including the attachment apparatus, that is, cementum, alveolar bone, and periodontal ligament.

In every dental practice (including a periodontal practice), there is a point at which it is impractical to salvage the entire natural dentition. Advancing periodontal destruction may necessitate the removal of several or many teeth. At this stage in the treatment of a periodontal patient, the dentist must decide whether (1) to condemn him to a complete denture and thereby commit him to becoming a more difficult patient or (2) to attempt to save strategic teeth on which to construct an overdenture. If one or more natural teeth are saved, the periodontist still plays a vital role in treating the patient and fulfills the primary objective by maintaining at least part of the natural dentition in a state of health.

In an everyday dental practice the dentist encounters several types of patients. One type may have an almost hopeless dental condition and may make the all too frequent comment, "Doctor, I would prefer to have all my teeth removed and have dentures constructed so that I will not have any more dental problems." Unfortunately, the majority of these patients are not fully aware of the many ramifications of this course of treatment when they make this decision. Another type of patient may have equally serious dental conditions but may say, "Doctor, I will do anything to save my teeth; please help me." Although both are candidates for complete dentures, the dentist must decide how to provide the best dental service to each patient.

From previous experience, the dentist knows that once teeth have been removed, ultimate loss of the alveolar ridge height is inevitable (Sicher and DuBrul, 1975; Brash and Jamieson, 1947), and in time the denture wearer will have more dental problems, but of a different nature. Even in this day of blade, subperiosteal, endosteal, and carbon implants, no established technique can duplicate the function and efficiency of the natural dentition. An element of risk is involved in any implant technique, and some have a higher rate of failure than others. Retention of natural teeth leaves a ligamentous attachment of the abutment tooth to the bone and avoids rejection of the

---

I wish to express my appreciation to Mr. Jack Gillenwater (Medical Photography Section, USAF Medical Center, Wright-Patterson Air Force Base, Dayton, Ohio) for his technical assistance.

foreign body and possible sequestration, which are occasionally observed with some implants.

Patients committed to a complete denture may become poor denture patients tomorrow, even though they are good denture patients today. Many dentists have observed that youthful patients in their twenties or early thirties are frequently ideal complete denture patients. Their tissues and muscle tone adapt easily, and they usually adjust readily to wearing a prosthesis. However, these patients are now committed to wearing artificial teeth for the rest of their lives, generally 40 to 60 years. After many years have elapsed, these people often become poor denture patients who need constant adjustments and are no longer contented with the dentures. They may then spend a large part of their lives going edentulous or, at best, wearing dentures merely for esthetics. On the other hand, if a patient is 60 years of age or older when the remaining natural teeth are lost, an adequate denture can be constructed, and the denture-wearing period is much shorter.

PERIODONTAL BASIS FOR THE OVERDENTURE

The basic concept of the overdenture is valid because it is based on the sound physiologic contention that the presence of healthy teeth in the mouth is essential for maintaining the alveolar ridge. Instead of the functional forces of the denture base being applied directly and solely to the soft tissue and underlying bone, the functional forces of the overdenture are shared by the remaining roots of the abutment teeth. These occlusal forces (when applied within physiologic limits) appear to stimulate the underlying supporting bone and therefore maintain the ridge height (Bunting, 1954) (Fig. 5-1). This same concept applies to the various abutments used in all tooth-borne prostheses.

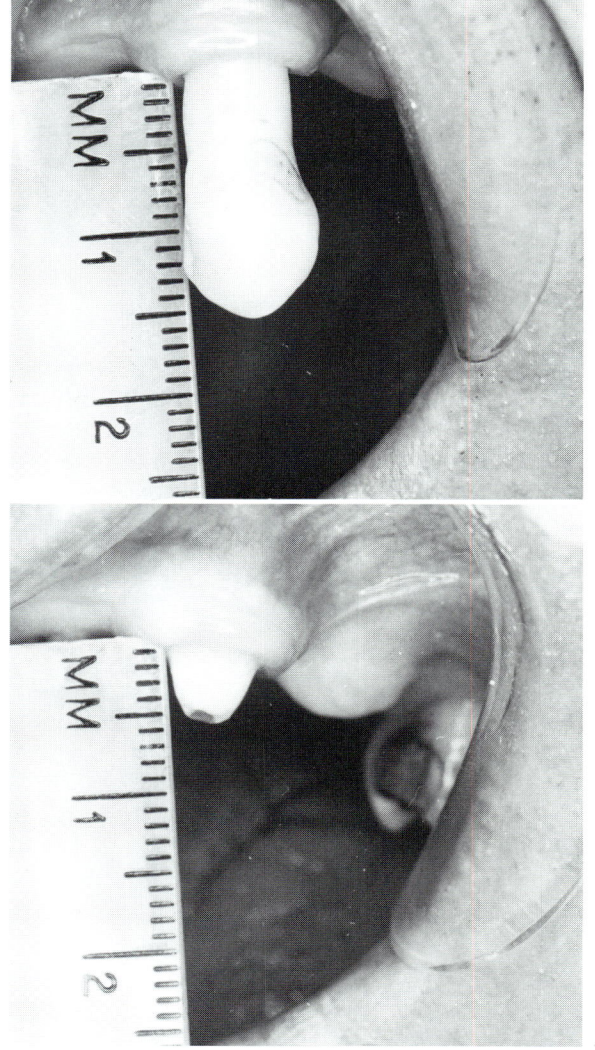

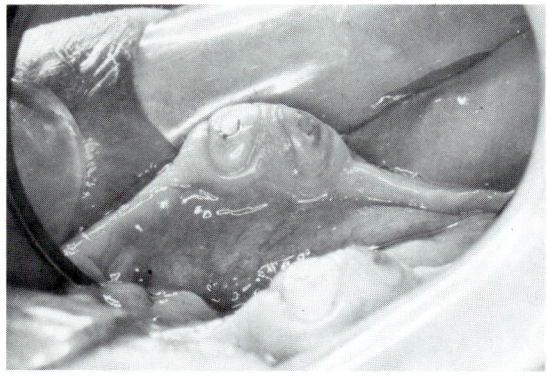

Fig. 5-1. Alveolar ridge height being maintained by retention of two adjacent overdenture abutments.

Fig. 5-2. A, Maxillary left cuspid before being prepared as an overdenture abutment. Clinical crown measures approximately 16 mm. **B,** Maxillary left cuspid after being prepared as an overdenture abutment. Clinical crown now measures approximately 6 mm. The crown-root ratio has been improved dramatically. (Courtesy Dr. Donald C. Kramer, Fairborn, Ohio.)

Earlier overdenture concepts relied on vital teeth for abutments. The teeth were prepared, and gold copings were constructed over the remaining tooth structure (Miller, 1958). Later modifications brought into use teeth that had been devitalized by root canal therapy, so that the clinical crown could be reduced sufficiently to improve the crown-root ratio (Fig. 5-2) and to facilitate the esthetics of the overdenture (Morrow and co-workers, 1969). The various methods of tooth preparation are discussed in other sections of the text.

ANATOMIC BASIS FOR THE OVERDENTURE

From a physiologic point of view, the overdenture is a rational approach to denture construction and maintenance of the alveolar ridge. There are two areas in the jaw proper, the basal bone and the alveolar bone. An apical portion, often referred to as basal bone (the body), is the portion of the maxillae or mandible that remains relatively stable regardless of whether teeth are present in the arch. Unless it is destroyed by some pathologic entity, the basal bone appears to be unaffected by the presence or absence of the teeth. The alveolar bone, the portion of bone coronal to the basal area of bone, is comprised of the alveolus and the surrounding supporting bone (Sicher and DuBrul; Brash and Jamieson). When a tooth is lost or removed, the alveolus is resorbed through disuse atrophy (Sicher and DuBrul). The primary purpose of this bony area is to hold or support teeth. Resorption may continue until eventually most or all of the alveolar supporting bone is resorbed down to the basal area (Prichard, 1972) (Fig. 5-3). On account of this supporting function, the crestal height of the alveolar bone is maintained in the absence of periodontal disease. The actual force of occlusion is applied to the alveolar bone by the fibers attached to the cementum of the root surface and the cortical bone lining the alveolus or socket. These principal fibers are functional elements of the periodontal ligament and, when anchored into the cementum and alveolar bone, are called Sharpey's fibers. They are collagenous, nonelastic filaments that are arranged in such a manner as to resist functional stress (Sicher and DuBrul). Occlusal function stimulates the maintenance of the crestal bone

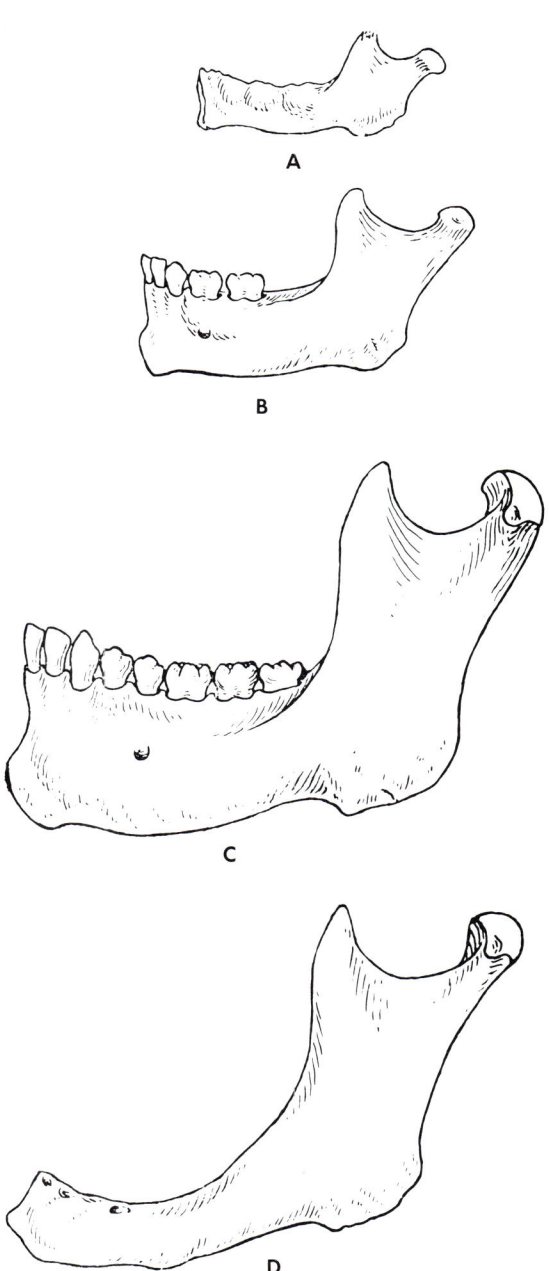

Fig. 5-3. Mandible in four stages of development. **A,** Mandible at birth. **B,** Mandible at 6 years of age. **C,** Mandible in adult life. **D,** Edentulous mandible. This figure shows loss of alveolar bone after removal of dentition. (Redrawn from Goss, C. M., editor: In Gray, H.: Anatomy of the human body, ed. 27, Philadelphia, Lea & Febiger; from Boucher, C. O., editor: Swenson's complete dentures, ed. 6, St. Louis, 1970, The C. V. Mosby Co.)

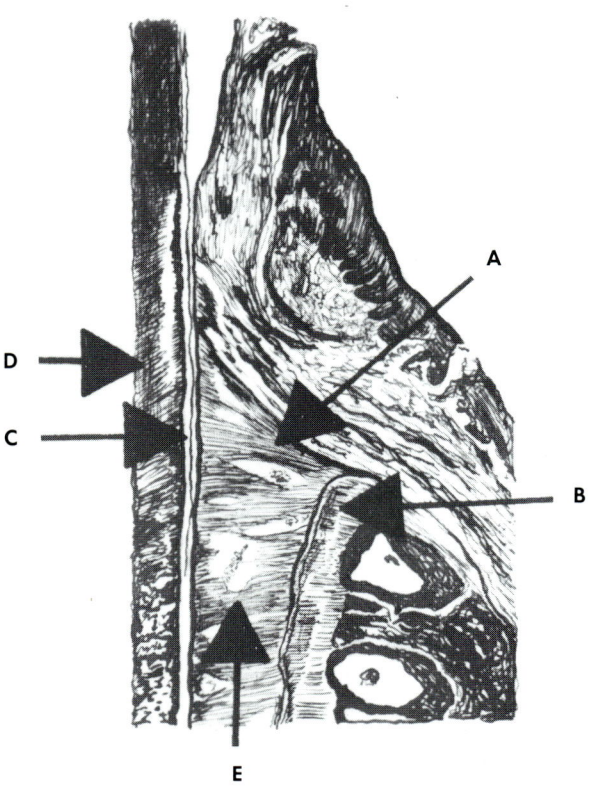

Fig. 5-4. Periodontium. **A,** Alveolar crest fibers. **B,** Alveolar crest. **C,** Cementum. **D,** Dentin. **E,** Periodontal ligament space. (Diagramed by Medical Illustration Section, USAF Medical Center, Wright-Patterson Air Force Base, Dayton, Ohio.)

(Bunting).* This stimulation is transferred through all groups of periodontal fibers, especially the crestal fiber group, which is apical to the cementoenamel junction, and traverses from the cementum to the crest of the alveolus (Fig. 5-4). The transeptal fibers connect two adjacent teeth and extend from the cementum of one tooth, which they traverse coronal to the interproximal alveolar crest, and attach to the cementum of the other tooth (Glickman, 1964).

PERIODONTAL PATHOLOGY

If the crestal or transeptal fibers are destroyed, a periodontal pocket is formed with the apical proliferation of the epithelial attachment. Deepening of the pocket depends on the migration of the epithelial attachment apically along the cementum, accompanied by separation of the gingiva as a result of inflammation (Goldman and Cohen, 1973). When a pocket forms with its base apical to the crestal bone, the crestal bone no longer functions and is therefore resorbed. It is axiomatic that function determines bone morphology. An example of physiologic reaction to loss of function is observed in a patient with poliomyelitis that has affected the legs. When steel braces are used to support the legs, the diameter of the legs soon decreases. Although this disease affects the muscle, not the bone, the bone decreases in size from the lack of functional pull by the muscles; the braces provide the support previously given by the long bones. Therefore, when in function (within the range of physiologic limits), the teeth stimulate the alveolar crest to remain at a desirable level in relation to the root surface (Bunting). This same stimulation is maintained when the tooth is devitalized, reduced in height, and used as an abutment for an overdenture. The crestal fibers are stimulated by the apical forces applied to the root through the overdenture base. Without the retained root, the portion of the alveolus that supports the root undoubtedly would undergo resorption. The presence of even one root seems to reduce or delay resorption of the adjacent alveolar bone.

PATIENT EVALUATION
Medical history

It is imperative that every dental patient complete a health questionnaire. It can vary in length and complexity with the type of treatment performed. Oral surgical and periodontal procedures often involve extensive preoperative and postoperative medications (with possible allergic manifestations) and surgical intervention, which depend on the patient's overall health for the necessary healing factors. A more extensive health background is required to ascertain the patient's response to the various procedures to eliminate unnecessary risks in the course of treatment. A typical health questionnaire that should be adequate for the majority of dental office procedures is published in Accepted Dental Therapeutics. Any systemic condition that can alter the pa-

---

*Hurt, W. C. (Chairman, Department of Periodontics, Baylor College of Dentistry, Dallas): Personal communication, 1973.

tient's treatment requires evaluation and medical consultation prior to the initiation of therapy.

Oral examination

The dentist who treats the patient assumes responsibility not only for correcting his dental deficiencies but also for evaluating his complete health as viewed orally. A thorough intraoral and extraoral examination is essential prior to any definitive therapy. This examination pertains to the head, face, neck, and all intraoral areas, including the mouth proper and oropharynx. Often the dentist is the first person to observe abnormalities unknown even to the patient.

Radiographic examination

Prior to establishing a definitive treatment plan, a full series of intraoral radiographs is obtained (Fig. 5-5). It is suggested that periapical radiographs of all remaining teeth be included in the examination and that the long-cone technique be used. This technique eliminates much of the distortion observed in radiographs taken by the angle bisection method. Accuracy without distortion, particularly vertical distortion, is extremely important when attempting to determine the crown-root ratio of teeth. In addition to the periapical radiographs, it is preferable to make a panoramic survey (Fig. 5-6) for a full overview of the entire mouth, including the maxillary sinuses and the temporomandibular joints. Many pathologic entities such as impactions, cysts, fractures, and foreign body masses can be overlooked on periapical radiographs. The dentist must recognize that a diagnosis cannot be made from a cursory glance at the patient's radiographs, which are merely two-dimensional pictures of three-dimensional objects. A periodontal probe must be used

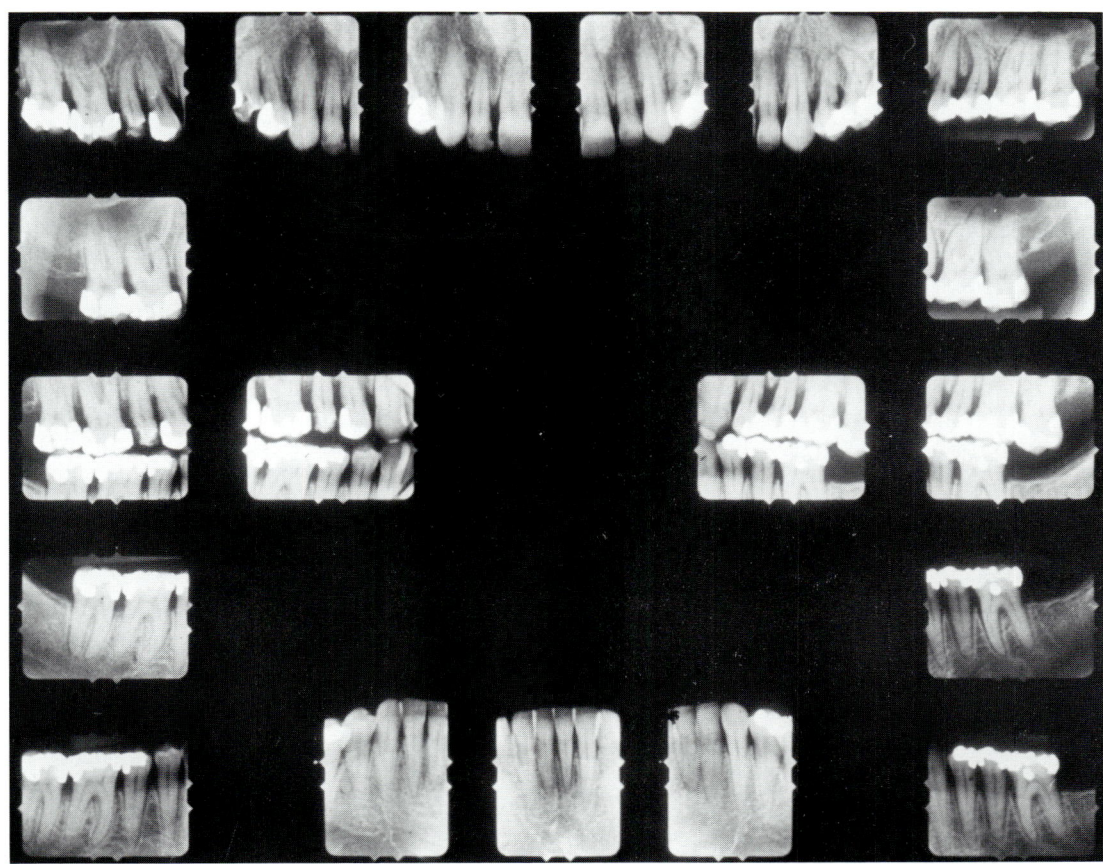

Fig. 5-5. Full-mouth radiographic series (nineteen radiographs) using split-maxillary central incisor view and four periapical bite-wing exposures.

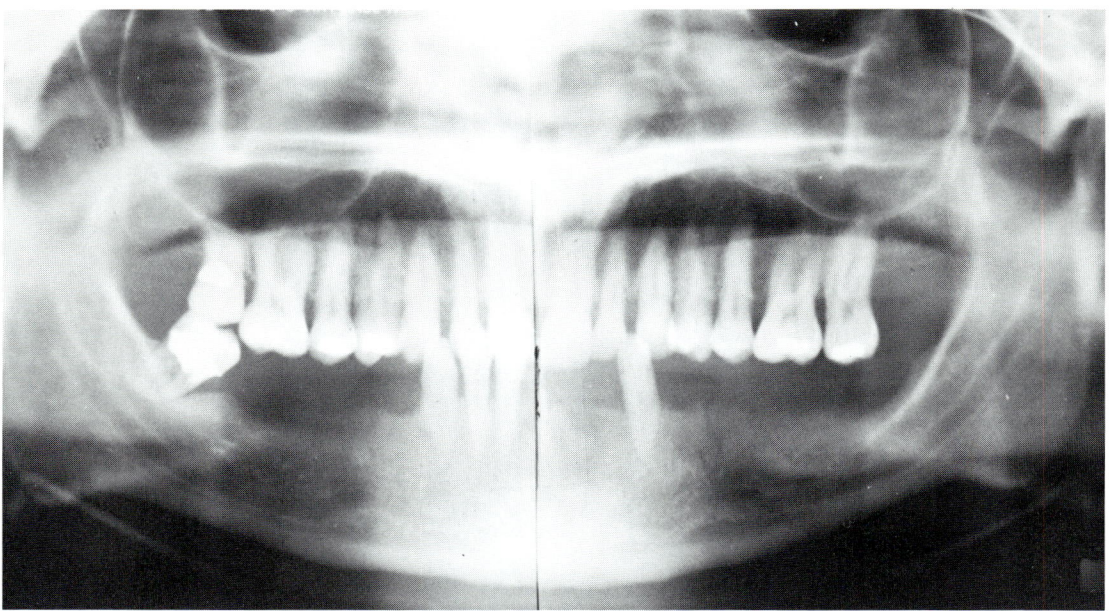

Fig. 5-6. Panoramic radiograph, providing an overall view of oral and surrounding structures.

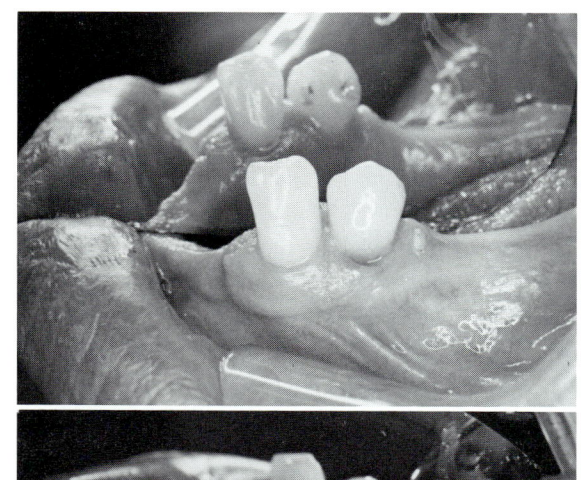

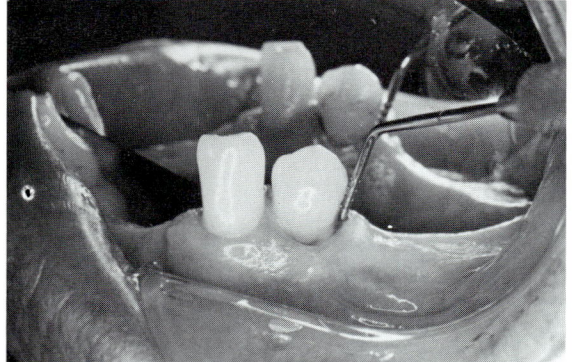

to evaluate the amount of supporting attachment that remains. Often buccal and lingual defects are overlooked on radiographs because the tooth structure and calcified structures, such as the mylohyoid ridge, the external oblique ridge, and the malar process are superimposed over the defects. If the dentist had only one aid in making the proper diagnosis, the periodontal probe would be much more reliable than the radiograph; the appearance of the tissues, the presence or absence of an exudate, and tooth mobility as well as pocket depth must be considered in making the proper diagnosis and prognosis (Fig. 5-7).

Probing

Many periodontal probes are on the market; some have flat sides, whereas others have different styles of round probing surfaces. Some probes

Fig. 5-7. A, Cuspid and first bicuspid teeth to be considered for overdenture abutments; without a thorough radiographic and clinical examination, these teeth appear to be unaffected by periodontal disease. B, Cuspid and first bicuspid teeth, A, with periodontal probe in place, revealing a moderate to severe pocket on distal aspect of first bicuspid tooth.

have a calibrated probe on one end and an explorer on the other end. However, I prefer the double-ended Williams probe by Hu-Friedy (Fig. 5-8). This probe allows easy access to all areas of the mouth and to the sulcus because of the small diameter and tapered shape of the probe and the offset angle of the probing surface to the handle of the instrument. When probing for periodontal defects, at least eight readings are taken around each tooth: three on the facial aspect, three on the lingual aspects, and one on both the mesial and distal aspects of the tooth. This procedure can be accomplished with minimal discomfort to the patient if the probe is inserted into the gingival crevice (or pocket) and all readings are taken without withdrawing the probe from the confines of the crevice except to move it to the buccal or lingual surfaces. When a molar or a maxillary first bicuspid tooth is considered for an overdenture abutment, a curved probe or a curved periodontal curette is used to determine the possible presence of a furcation involvement (Figs. 5-9 and 5-10).

DIAGNOSIS

After a thorough perusal of the patient's medical and dental histories and a complete clinical evaluation from the radiographs, pocket readings, and mobility patterns, the dentist makes the final diagnosis that will enable him to formulate his final treatment plan. Factors such as the patient's attitude, ability to maintain his oral health after treatment, and desire to retain his natural teeth, coupled with the dentist's ability, influence selection of the final treatment plan. Usually the diagnosis of periodontal disease is not difficult. The radiographic appearance of bone loss, presence of pocket depth, poor tissue tone and appearance, abnormal mobility patterns, and presence of an exudate are signs of periodontal disease. These findings, in conjunction with the dentist's knowledge and experience, permit him to arrive at a diagnosis. Treatment of the findings appears to be more difficult, for success of the overdenture depends on the retainability of the abutments.

Ideally, all periodontal pathology is eliminated prior to construction of the overdenture. Occasionally, periodontal therapy can be accomplished in conjunction with construction of the overdenture. However, it is recommended that transitional overdentures be used, since they can be functional and provide the patient with an acceptable pros-

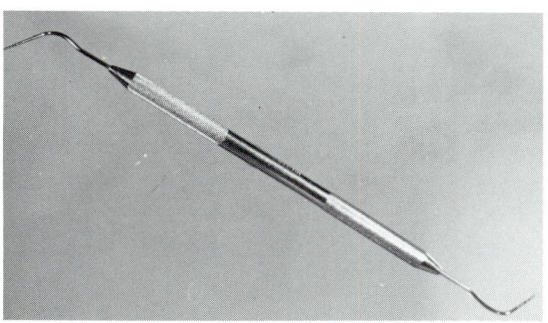

Fig. 5-8. Double-ended Williams periodontal probe (Hu-Friedy Mfg. Co., Inc., Chicago).

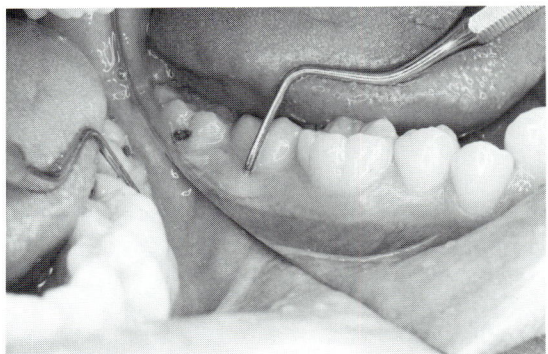

Fig. 5-9. Mandibular second molar showing a curved periodontal curette inserted into facial gingival sulcus, revealing a furcation involvement.

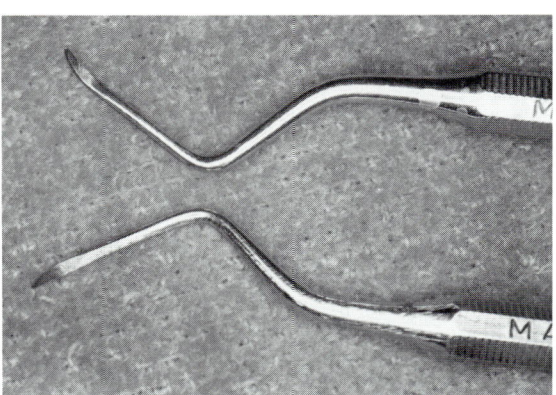

Fig. 5-10. Curved periodontal curettes (Columbia 4R and 4L), which may be used to probe furcation involvements on molar teeth.

thesis until the periodontal status of the abutments is determined. The transitional overdentures can also be used as a periodontal dressing when lined with tissue conditioners such as Hydrocast (Frisch and associates, 1968). The final overdenture is not fabricated until the periodontal therapy is completed; a failure in abutment retention at this stage of treatment would be disheartening.

PROGNOSIS

The overdenture patient is like any other periodontal patient. The success of the treatment depends strictly on the patient's ability to maintain the teeth (abutments) in a state of health. If bacterial plaque is permitted to accumulate on the abutments, an inflammatory condition will arise again, eventual loss of the abutments is inevitable, and the overdenture construction becomes an expensive, time-consuming failure. Patients must be instructed in the various methods of oral hygiene and must be seen on a regular periodontal maintenance schedule to permit periodic examination of the abutments for periodontal destruction and elimination of the destructive condition, if present, before a hopeless state is reached and a conventional complete denture must be fabricated.

TREATMENT PLANNING

Once the decision on construction of an overdenture has been made, a definitive treatment plan is formulated. This plan is established in such a manner that each step will be accomplished in a logical sequence that expedites the therapy and requires of the patient the minimal amount of time, expense, and discomfort.

Tooth selection

Cuspid teeth are used for overdenture abutments more frequently than any other teeth, probably because they have a larger surface area for attaching the periodontal fibers and are among the last teeth removed from a mouth with periodontal disease (Fig. 5-11). The shape and position of the cuspid teeth make them less likely to become victims of tooth decay than posterior teeth, which have a large interproximal contact area. Cuspids are in the corner of the arch, where the posterior segments join the anterior component and act as the keystone of the arch; hence they are in a strategic position for use as abut-

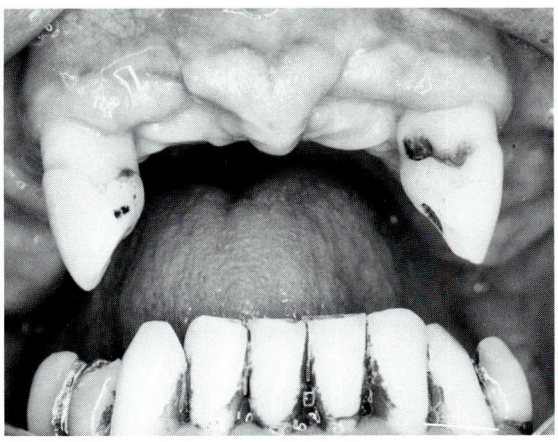

Fig. 5-11. After periodontal therapy, maxillary cuspid teeth will be used as overdenture abutments. Maxillary overdenture will occlude against patient's remaining natural dentition, a condition that would ordinarily cause rapid resorption of the maxillary anterior ridge if overdenture abutments were not retained.

ments. Anterior teeth (incisors), having small conical roots with minimal attachment area, often are lost earlier in the progression of disease and seldom are available to serve as abutments for the overdenture. Molar teeth, being multirooted, have a large surface root area for attachment, but they often show severe bone loss involving the furcation areas that renders them unsuitable for overdenture abutments unless they are sectioned. Single roots of molar teeth can be treated as single-rooted teeth, and they make excellent abutments in selected instances.

Recently, prosthodontists have used more bicuspid teeth for abutments because they are in the middle of the ridge and provide support for both the anterior and posterior segments of the denture base. The second bicuspids usually are single rooted, and, therefore, have no furcation involvements, as is occasionally true of the maxillary first bicuspids. The second bicuspids usually are centered approximately equidistant between the buccal and lingual cortical plates of the arch, whereas the first bicuspids and the cuspid teeth often are in a slightly labial position with a minimal amount of bone over the facial aspect. From strictly a periodontal point of view, the cuspid teeth usually are not as satisfactory for periodontal treatment

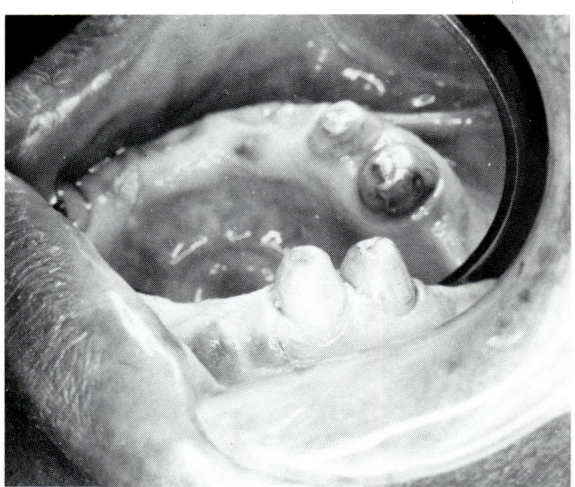

Fig. 5-12. Adjacent overdenture abutments.

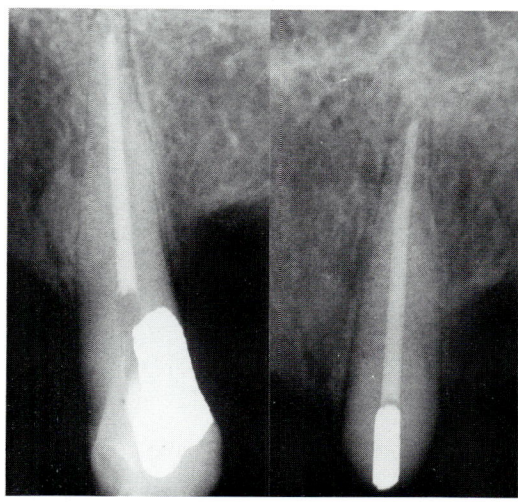

Fig. 5-13. Radiographs of maxillary left cuspid before and after being prepared for an overdenture abutment, showing improved crown-root ratio after abutment preparation. (Courtesy Dr. Donald C. Kramer, Fairborn, Ohio.)

as the second bicuspid teeth, since the labial position of the cuspids often results in a fusion of their facial cortical plate of bone with the alveolar bone. Therefore the cuspids may have a facial dehiscence or fenestration that cannot be repaired adequately by periodontal therapy; the weakened attachment area that remains is subject to further breakdown (Clarke and Bueltmann, 1971). A good combination for overdenture abutments (when they are available with good periodontal support), appears to consist of cuspids and second bicuspids, making four abutments that give uniform support to the denture base. Since these teeth are not adjacent to each other, the edentulous area between them permits better maintenance of the encircling periodontal attachment. When two adjacent teeth are used, the small interproximal area can make cleansing difficult, and, if proper relief of the denture base is not provided, the pressure of the base material can cause atrophy of the marginal tissues (Fig. 5-12).

The shape and form of the periodontal osseous defects in advancing periodontal disease depend on the position of the tooth in the arch and the surrounding osseous topography. Infrabony defects (pockets with their base apical to the alveolar crest) usually are not found in the anterior portion of the mouth because the cortical plate and alveolar housing (the supporting bone in this area) often are fused together without any spongy bone between them. In this instance, as the periodontal disease progresses, both layers of bone are lost. However, in the posterior segments, the distance between the buccal and lingual cortical plates and the cortical layer lining the alveolus is greater, and the amount of interproximal bone due to the shape of the crowns of the posterior teeth is increased; therefore when periodontal destruction occurs, osseous defects or craters are produced (Prichard, 1965). When selecting abutments for overdentures, the position of the tooth in the arch and its position between the buccal and lingual cortical plates should be evaluated carefully. The clinical crown to clinical root ratio, which is also important, must show that the bone remaining is sufficient to support the tooth and the additional stress of the overlying denture base. The crown-root ratio is improved considerably by reducing the clinical crown height when preparing the tooth for its role as an abutment (Fig. 5-13). The anatomic crown of the tooth is the portion of the crown coronal to the cementoenamel junction, and the anatomic root is the area apical to the junction. The clinical crown is the portion of the crown (and possibly some root area) that is coronal to the attachment apparatus. When periodontal disease produces bone loss and recession, the clinical crown may be of much greater length than the anatomic crown

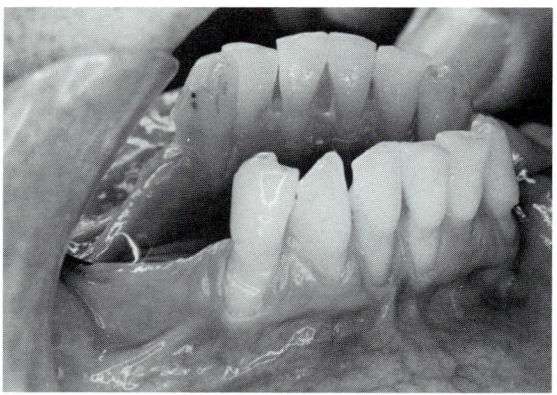

Fig. 5-14. Gingival recession with concomitant bone loss on facial aspect of mandibular anterior teeth, thereby increasing length of clinical crown and worsening crown-root ratio.

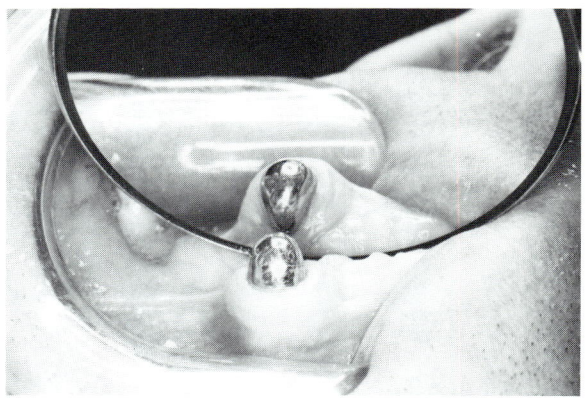

Fig. 5-15. Completed overdenture abutment after periodontal therapy, obturation of root canal, and final cementation of cast gold coping. Short clinical crown and dome shape of abutment establish that occlusal forces of denture base will be in an axial direction with minimal lateral displacement. (Courtesy Dr. Donald C. Kramer, Fairborn, Ohio.)

(Fig. 5-14). Therefore, in abutment selection, adequate supporting bone should be present, even though the crown-root ratio will be improved later. Although no specific numerical values can be assigned to the desired amount of supporting bone necessary for the overdenture abutment, an approximation can be made by careful evaluation of tooth mobility and pocket depth as well as by radiographic evaluation. Severely mobile teeth or teeth with severe osseous defects are poor candidates for abutments. Once the tooth has been prepared for an abutment, the decrease in crown height will make it much more stable, for the fulcrum point of the tooth within the alveolus is moved apically and the corresponding lever arm length is shortened; less torque is applied to the shortened crown and less lateral force is applied to the contents of the periodontal space (Fig. 5-15).

In discussing the crown-root ratio and the attachment apparatus and surface area, the root shape also must be considered. Conical roots of mandibular central incisors have an extremely limited area of attachment compared to multirooted molars. The number of individual periodontal ligament fibers that can be attached to the cementum of the root surface is directly proportionate to the surface area of a specific root. Therefore a mandibular incisor with a short cone-shaped root would have a much smaller overall surface area available for attachment than a tooth with a broad flat root or a multirooted tooth. However, mandibular incisors can be used successfully as overdenture abutments, particularly when they are opposed by a maxillary complete denture. The angulation of the tooth to be used for an abutment is also considered. To distribute most effectively the functional forces applied to the remaining root, ideally the root should be in an axial position perpendicular to the direction of the occlusal forces. This position seems to facilitate distribution of forces in such a manner as to be absorbed by the oblique fibers, which constitute the majority of the fibers in the ligament space. The oblique group of fibers withstand vertical occlusal forces and prevent intrusion of the tooth within the alveolus. If the tooth root is angled or is not perpendicular to the alveolar ridge, the distribution of forces is not directed along the long axis of the root, and possible damage to the supporting structures could result. Molar teeth are used infrequently as abutments for overdentures because of the presence of possible furcation involvement. Most likely molar teeth will show bone loss in the presence of generalized periodontal destruction, and invasion of one or more furcations can be expected in most instances. This involvement is difficult to treat periodontally, and, even when treated, it often has a questionable prognosis. Hemisection and root amputation can be used to salvage an otherwise hopeless molar tooth for use as an overdenture abutment; however, its usefulness must be questioned extensively because of the root canal therapy, the periodontal treatment, and the prosthodontic treatment required.

Extraction of hopeless teeth

In most instances, when posterior support is not a factor or when esthetics are not paramount, it is usually advisable to extract as many hopeless teeth as possible at the earliest possible time. Since the patient may forget the original treatment plan or change his mind after the dentist has started, complications can arise if the patient suddenly decides to retain teeth already declared hopeless. Also, early extraction of hopeless teeth permits edentulous areas to heal and ridge tissues to mature to accommodate the denture base while periodontal therapy around the abutment teeth is being completed. In addition, removal of hopeless teeth, especially those adjacent to the selected abutments, makes it possible to obtain additional support from the extraction site after healing. Another advantage of early extraction of these teeth is that performing the necessary periodontal corrections around isolated abutments often is easier, and the patient can become acclimated to wearing an overdenture (transitional overdenture) prior to preparation of the final abutments. One disadvantage of the early extraction of hopeless teeth is that when corrective periodontal therapy is performed on isolated teeth, it is often difficult to retain any type of dressing around a single tooth, especially if crown reduction techniques have been used in the preparation.

Transitional or intermediate overdentures

Various types of transitional dentures can be used in the treatment plan for the overdenture patient. Some prostheses merely have holes in the full denture to permit the unprepared abutments to extend through it, whereas other types use clasps or cut-out sections of the denture base. A transitional prosthesis performs the following functions:

1. Esthetics. It may permit the patient to have a pleasing appearance during the various stages of therapy before insertion of the final overdenture.

2. Vertical dimension. It helps to maintain the patient's vertical relationship and prevent overclosure, which can occur when all centric occlusal stops are removed.

3. Traumatogenic occlusion. It prevents excessive occlusal forces from being applied to abutments, either by functional movements or possible habit patterns that often develop when a patient attempts to occlude the remaining natural teeth.

4. Protection. It can be used as a covering for surgical sites or as an intraoral bandage to aid in periodontal therapy.

Endodontics

In most instances the time at which the endodontic therapy on the abutment teeth is performed makes little difference. Usually root canal treatment can be accomplished in conjunction with most periodontal procedures, thereby shortening the total treatment time. However, some periodontists believe that if intrabony osseous defects are being managed, the canals should be debrided, but the final canal filling should not be placed until several weeks after intrabony surgery. An intrabony defect is an osseous crater with three bony walls, the fourth wall being the tooth root; generally, if these defects are curetted thoroughly and if the causative factors are eliminated, the defect responds successfully. However, obturation of the root canals in intrabony therapy appears to be detrimental to the success of the therapy (Prichard).

Periodontal therapy

Periodontists can provide support for the dentist constructing the overdenture in many ways, and frequently dentists can perform these services themselves if they have had the necessary background and experience. First, periodontal pockets can be eliminated, for if they remain, the prognosis for an abutment is guarded. Reduction or elimination of pockets is essential for establishing a healthy environment for the abutment tooth. The periodontist also can perform surgical procedures that increase the zone of attached gingiva, increase the depth of the vestibule and, in general, eliminate the inflammation that may surround the teeth to be used as abutments. Areas of attached gingiva (Fig. 5-16) can be increased by using free soft tissue autografts in which keratinized tissue from one area of the mouth is transposed to an area of minimal attached gingival tissue (Sullivan and Atkins, 1968). Generally the masticatory mucosa of the hard palate is the donor site for autografts, but other areas, such as edentulous ridges, have been used successfully (Fig. 5-17). Other methods of therapy can be used to increase the zone of attached gingiva, such as the pedicle graft in which the keratinized mucosal tissue can be rotated from an edentulous ridge area and repositioned over an area of minimal attachment or a denuded root surface (Corn, 1964). Often still other methods are used, such as the double papillae flap (Cohen and Ross, 1968) or the horizontal repositioned flap (Grupe, 1960), both of which aid in covering denuded roots and provide for an increased zone of attached gingiva that is so essential in teeth used for overdenture abutments. Soft tissue defects that do not involve the underlying supporting bone can be eliminated by a gingivectomy (resection) technique in which the superfluous tissue is removed; this procedure is used when the underlying attachment apparatus is intact, no osseous defect is present, and an adequate zone of attached gingiva is found (Fig. 5-18). When the presence of periodontal pockets and osseous defects is observed, flap surgery must be initiated to correct the underlying defect (Fig. 5-19). Many methods of osseous defect therapy are available, such as osteoplasty, osteotomy, different types of osseous graft procedures, and new attachment procedures. The reader is advised to consult a good periodontal text such as Prichard or Goldman and Cohen if he is not familiar with these methods.

The role of the general practitioner during this stage of the construction of the overdenture is debatable. Many necessary periodontal procedures can be accomplished readily by the general dentist; however, each practitioner must judge his own ability and experience in treating both the periodontal condition of his patient and any complications that may arise from the treatment. The most important element in periodontal therapy is

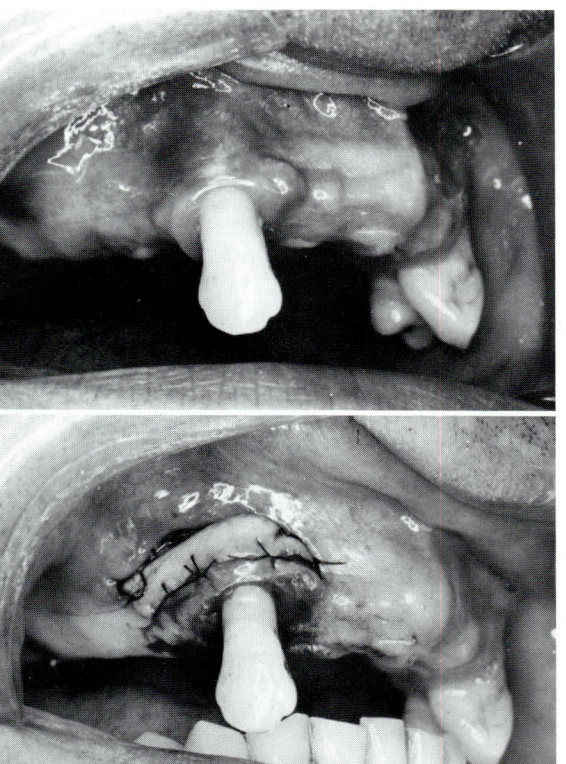

Fig. 5-17. **A,** Maxillary right cuspid tooth, which is to be used as an overdenture abutment. There is an inadequate zone of attached gingiva on facial aspect. **B,** Maxillary right cuspid, **A,** after gingivectomy and gingivoplasty procedures and placement of a free soft tissue autograft to increase zone of attached gingiva. (Courtesy Dr. Glenn Jividen, Dayton, Ohio.)

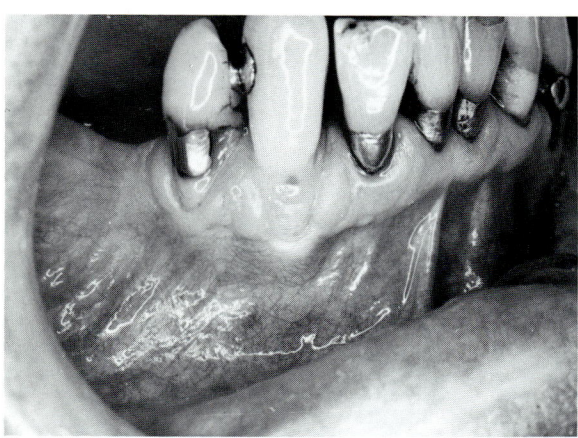

Fig. 5-16. Inadequate zone of attached gingiva on facial aspect of mandibular right cuspid and first bicuspid teeth that will require mucogingival surgery before these teeth can be used successfully as overdenture abutments.

PERIODONTICS AND THE OVERDENTURE PATIENT 49

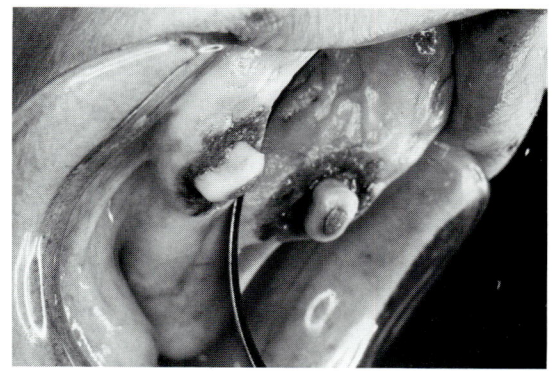

Fig. 5-18. Pocket elimination by simple gingivectomy procedure; no underlying osseous defects were present. (Courtesy Dr. Glenn Jividen, Dayton, Ohio.)

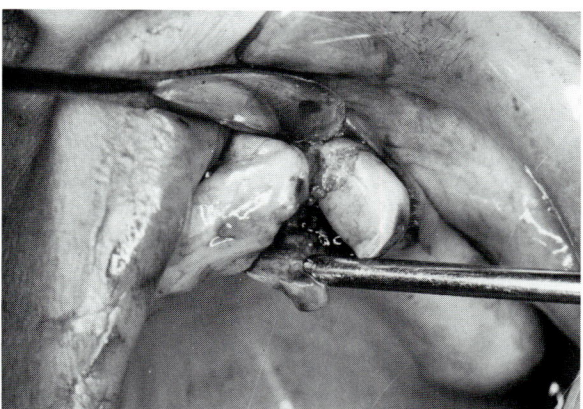

Fig. 5-19. Flap surgery on an overdenture abutment to eliminate osseous defects. (Courtesy Dr. Glenn Jividen, Dayton, Ohio.)

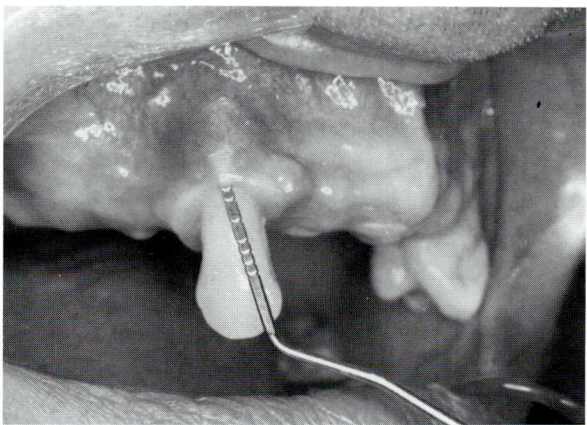

Fig. 5-20. Maxillary right cuspid tooth to be used as an overdenture abutment. Periodontal probe inserted into the pocket extends apically past mucogingival junction, indicating necessity for mucogingival surgery in this area.

the diagnosis. The abnormal sulcus depth may be caused by a hyperplasia of the gingival tissues or by the actual destruction of the periodontal attachment apparatus. The pocket depth can be eliminated by a simple resection of the tissues, or a flap procedure can be used if all of the attached gingival tissues should be retained. Problems involving pocket depths that pass apically to the mucogingival junction present still other complications that make the treatment plan slightly more complex (Fig. 5-20). The various forms of therapy needed to eliminate pockets and establish a healthy oral environment depend on the type of tissue, pocket depth, relation of the base of the pocket to the mucogingival junction, and the extent of involvement of the supporting bone.

Construction of the final prosthesis— the overdenture

When all periodontal therapy has been completed, the root canals have been obturated, and the patient has been instructed in the oral hygiene methods necessary to maintain the abutment teeth in a state of health, the patient is ready for construction of the final overdenture.

MAINTENANCE

Various oral hygiene methods have been recommended for the overdenture patient, but the more effective ones appear to be the simplest and involve the fewest hygiene aids. The frequency and the method are not as important as the cleansing efficiency. A soft multitufted toothbrush placed on approximately a 45-degree angle into the sulcus and used with a vibrating action appears to clean the abutments and allow the tips of the bristles to enter into the crevice to aid in its cleansing (Fig. 5-21). Some patients have used roller bandage or gauze (Fig. 5-22, A) effectively, whereas other patients have become adept at using a soft 4-ply nylon knitting yarn (Fig. 5-22, B) or a toothpick mounted on a handle to perform the necessary hygiene (Fig. 5-23). Patients differ, and each one must be evaluated as to whether he/she is a candidate for an overdenture, each tooth must be evaluated as to whether it can be used for an abutment, and each oral hygiene method must be evaluated for the specific patient.

The overdenture patient must be seen on a periodic maintenance schedule, at which time oral

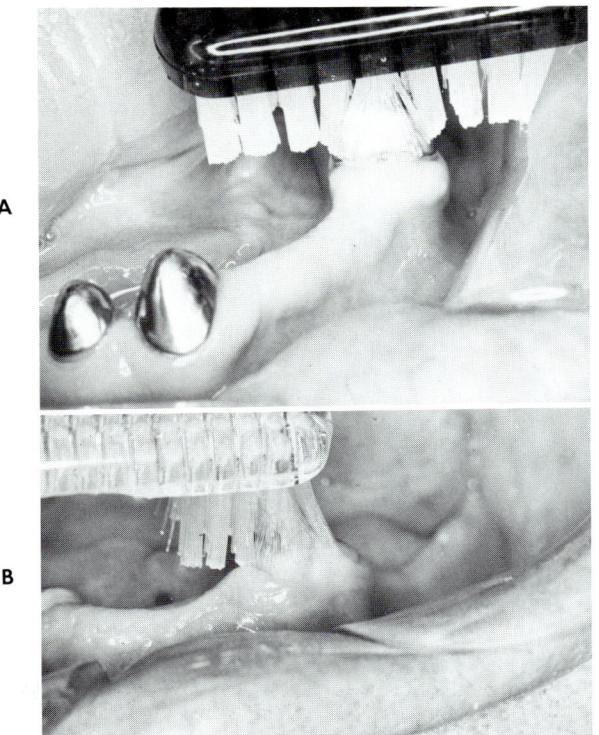

Fig. 5-21. A, Soft multitufted nylon toothbrush with bristles inserted into gingival sulcus to obtain necessary hygiene of overdenture abutment. **B,** Modified soft multitufted nylon toothbrush being used for cleansing of overdenture abutment. (Courtesy Dr. William A. Welker, Dayton, Ohio.)

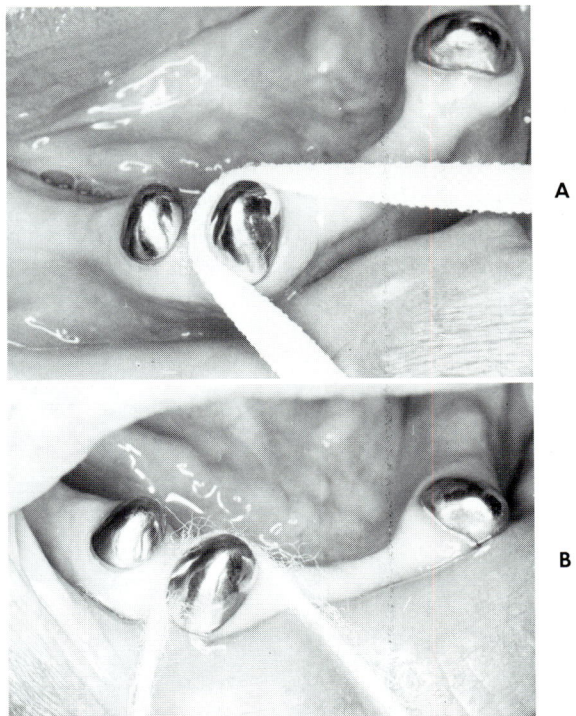

Fig. 5-22. A, One-inch gauze roller bandage being used to clean overdenture abutment in a shoeshine fashion. **B,** Knitting yarn (four-ply, 4 oz. nylon) being used to clean overdenture abutment. (Courtesy Dr. William A. Welker, Dayton, Ohio.)

hygiene is evaluated and reviewed. At this same recall visit the abutment teeth are examined for an indication of recurring periodontal disease, and the denture base is examined carefully to ensure proper adaptation to the abutments and soft tissues to prevent excessive stress on the abutments.

COMPLICATIONS

It is extremely frustrating for both the patient and the dentist constructing the overdenture when complications that can endanger the success of the procedures arise after completion of the prosthesis. The success of the overdenture depends on the success with which the patient retains the abutment teeth. Therefore periodontal complications must be considered and their treatment must be accomplished, or the overdenture will fail.

Irritation of the denture base. It is important to see that the denture base is relieved adequately

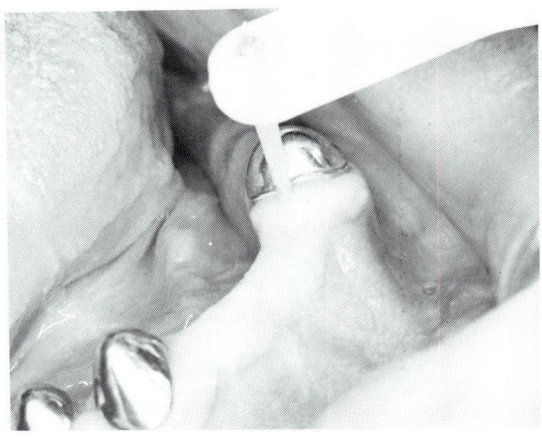

Fig. 5-23. Moist, softened, round toothpick in a convenient handle (Perio-Aid, Marquis Dental Mfg. Co., Denver) being used to cleanse cervical portion of the abutment. (Courtesy Dr. William A. Welker, Dayton, Ohio.)

to avoid impinging on the gingival cuff that surrounds the abutment; pressure atrophy of this collar of tissue can result in subsequent loss of the attached gingival tissue. After loss of this keratinized band, inflammation can rapidly move apically with resultant loss of attachment and, possibly, eventual loss of the abutment.

Poor oral hygiene. If bacterial plaque accumulates on or around the neck of the abutment, a destructive inflammatory condition ensues. The bacterial plaque, with its release of toxic products, can destroy the fibrous attachment and create a destructive periodontal condition with eventual loss of the abutment.

Periodontal abscess. Another complication for the overdenture patient is the periodontal abscess. This condition must be treated as soon as possible, for it is an acute process that can cause irreversible damage to the supporting tissues in an exceedingly short time. An abscess can be recognized by not only the discomfort often produced, but also by the appearance of tissues. The abscess site appears edematous and blue to bluish red in color; it is not uncommon to find a purulent exudate coming from the sulcus. Periodontal abscesses often occur as a result of the embedding of a foreign body within the gingival tissues or after scaling and planing procedures in which a fragment of calculus or tooth structure becomes lodged within the pocket wall. Most periodontal abscesses can be treated adequately by thorough curettage through the sulcus. However, if the periodontal pocket or defect involving the underlying bony structures or the pocket is tortuous in nature, a flap procedure is necessary.

SUMMARY AND CONCLUSIONS

Just as a chain is only as strong as its weakest link, the success of the overdenture depends on every step of the treatment plan from beginning to end. However, the overdenture concept is based on retention of the tooth structure on which to build the denture. The retention of this tooth structure depends on the periodontal status of the tooth, and the periodontal condition of the abutments can determine the strength of the chain (the completed treatment).

REFERENCES

Accepted dental therapeutics, ed. 35, Chicago, 1973, American Dental Association.

Brash, J. C., and Jamieson, E. B., editors: Cunningham's textbook of anatomy, ed. 8, London, 1947, Oxford University Press.

Bunting, R. W.: Oral hygiene, ed. 2, Philadelphia, 1954, Lea & Febiger.

Clarke, M. S., and Bueltmann, K. W.: Anatomical considerations in periodontal surgery, J. Periodont. 42:613, 1971.

Cohen, D. W., and Ross, S. E.: The double papillae repositioned flap in periodontal therapy, J. Periodont. 39:65-70, 1968.

Corn, H.: Edentulous area pedicle grafts in mucogingival surgery, Periodontics 2:229-242, 1964.

Frisch, J., Levin, M. P., and Bhaskar, S. N.: The use of tissue conditioners in periodontics, J. Periodont. 39:359-361, 1968.

Glickman, I.: Clinical periodontology, ed. 3, Philadelphia, 1964, W. B. Saunders Co.

Goldman, H. M., and Cohen, D. W.: Periodontal therapy, ed. 5, St. Louis, 1973, The C. V. Mosby Co.

Grupe, H. E.: Horizontal sliding flap operation, Dent. Clin. North Am., pp. 43-46, March, 1960.

Miller, P. O.: Complete dentures supported by natural teeth, J. Prosthet. Dent. 8:924-928, 1958.

Morrow, R. M., Feldmann, E. E., Rudd, K. D., and Trovillion, H. M.: Tooth-supported complete dentures: an approach to preventive prosthodontics, J. Prosthet. Dent. 21:513-522, 1969.

Prichard, J. F.: Advanced periodontal disease—surgical and prosthetic management, Philadelphia, 1965, W. B. Saunders Co.

Prichard, J. F.: Advanced periodontal disease—surgical and prosthetic management, ed. 2, Philadelphia, 1972, W. B. Saunders Co.

Sicher, H., and DuBrul, E. L.: Oral anatomy, ed. 6, St. Louis, 1975, The C. V. Mosby Co.

Sullivan, H. C., and Atkins, J. H.: Free autogenous gingival grafts. I. Principles of successful grafting, Periodontics 6:121-129, 1968.

6

ENDODONTIC CONSIDERATIONS AND TREATMENT OF OVERDENTURE ABUTMENTS

JOHN W. MYERS
WILLIAM F. BOURNE

The overdenture, well established as a preventive prosthodontic technique, merits consideration for patients who are about to lose their natural teeth or who have extensive prostheses. This prosthesis can be used even though too few teeth will be retained to support a conventional restoration. In the ideal situation, the retained teeth are distributed similarly on both sides. Being readily amenable to both endodontic and periodontic therapy, cuspids and single-rooted premolars usually serve as abutments for overdentures. Before preparation as abutments, the teeth usually first receive the necessary periodontal treatment and then the endodontic treatment. The latter therapy facilitates the development of more favorable clinical crown-root ratios, makes possible a better esthetic result and, in many instances, permits use of tilted or malposed abutment teeth (Morrow and associates, 1969).

ENDODONTIC EVALUATION OF ABUTMENTS

Endodontic evaluation of potential abutments includes not only a clinical but also a radiographic examination. Root canal patency, tooth mobility, and general health of the patient are of prime importance during this evaluation.

Clinical evaluation

Clinical evaluation of potential abutments should include a determination of access to the root canal. Crowns, large restorations, tilted or rotated teeth, and restricted occlusal openings influence the path of entry into the root canal. If restorations permit, pulpal vitality can be evaluated with an electric pulp tester and the application of a hot or cold stimulus. During the examination, root canal procedures are explained to the patient to decrease apprehension and promote better rapport between the dentist and the patient.

Radiographic evaluation

Single-rooted teeth usually serve as abutments; however, multirooted teeth are often used. The anatomy of the root canal system varies, and radiographs generally detect these variations. Maxillary and mandibular cuspids and second premolars comprise the largest percentage of abutments. Maxillary cuspids have only one root and one root canal. However, approximately 5% of mandibular

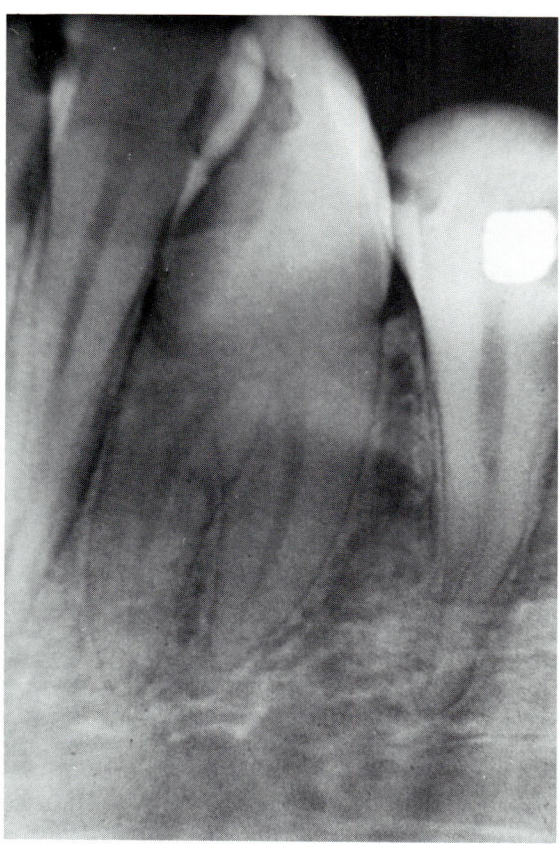

Fig. 6-1. Mandibular cuspid with two separate roots.

cuspids have two separate roots (Carlson, 1968) (Fig. 6-1). Mandibular cuspids also can have two canals in a single root that may or may not join before reaching the apex.

Maxillary second premolars have two separate roots in 15% of the cases (Weine, 1972) (Fig. 6-2). Many second bicuspids have two canals in a single root that may or may not join before reaching the apical foramen. When two root canals are present, the coronal portion of the canals resembles closely a figure eight or a ribbon in cross section. If only one canal is present, it is generally in the center of the access preparation. The root canal system of the maxillary first premolar varies from one to three roots. Carns and Skidmore (1973) have reported that in their cases 37% of maxillary first bicuspids have one root, 57% have two roots, and 6% have three roots (Fig. 6-3).

Split canals. Many single-rooted teeth have split or bifurcated canals; for perhaps two thirds of the root length the tooth has a single canal, which branches into two canals for the apical third. The more apically the canal bifurcates, the more difficult it is to treat endodontically. Approximately 22.7% of the mandibular first premolars have two canals. The mandibular second bicuspid usually has one root and one root canal, but Zillich and Dowson (1973) have reported two canals in 11.7% of their cases (Fig. 6-4).

Molars. Maxillary and mandibular molars are used occasionally for overdenture abutments, gen-

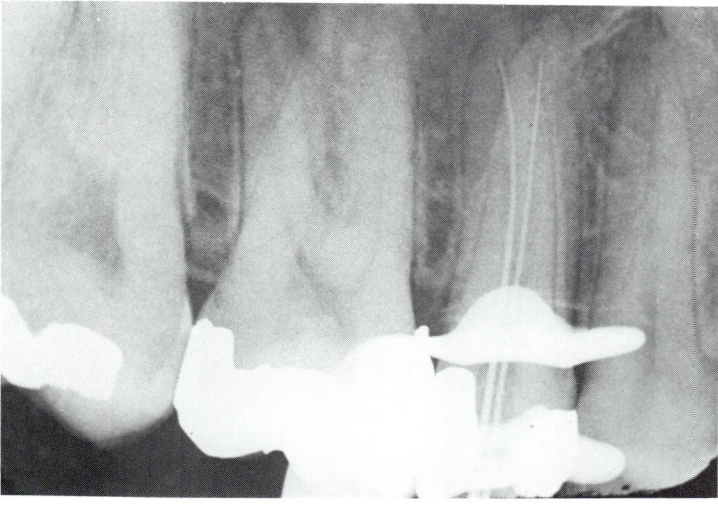

Fig. 6-2. Files placed in each root canal of a maxillary second bicuspid.

54 PRELIMINARY PROCEDURES

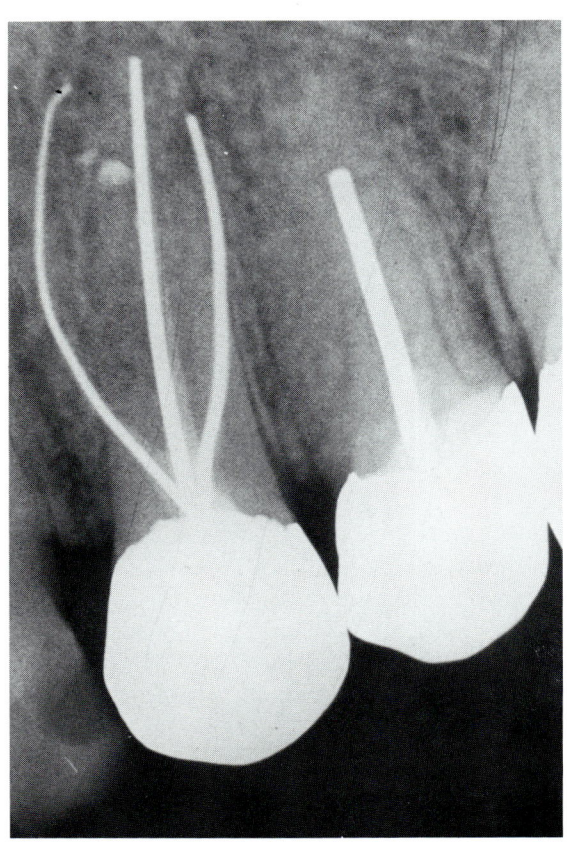

Fig. 6-3. Maxillary first premolar with three roots.

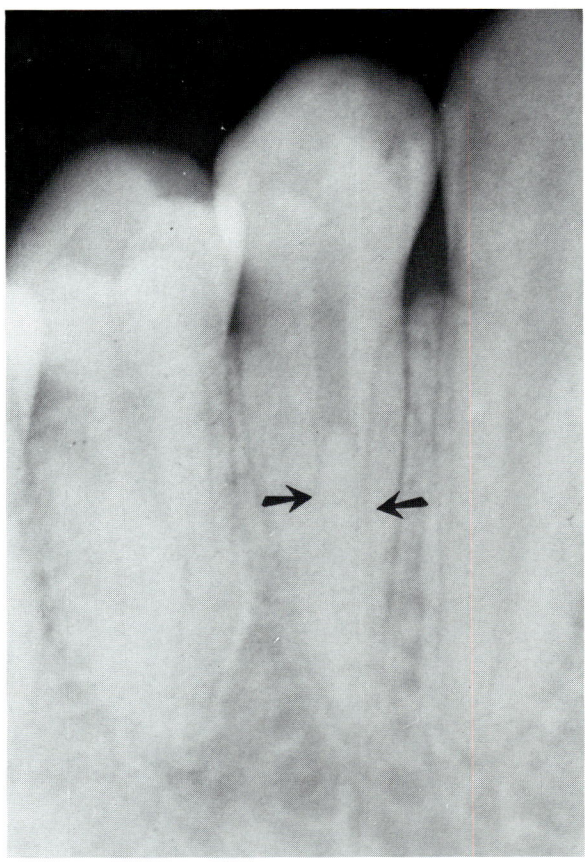

Fig. 6-4. Mandibular bicuspids demonstrating split or bifid root canals.

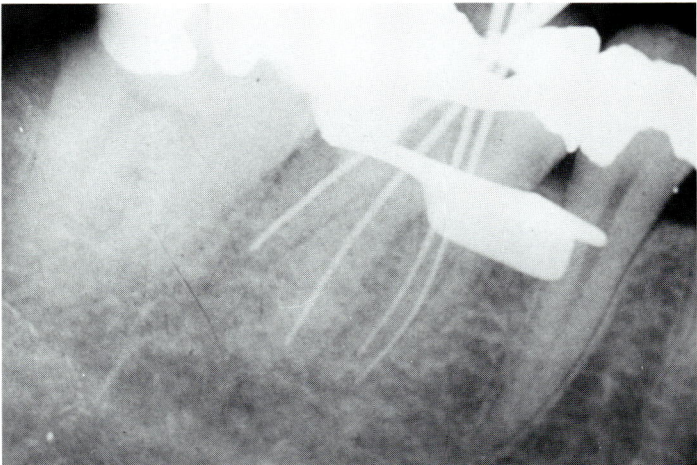

Fig. 6-5. Mandibular first molars can have two separate distal roots.

erally after root amputation or hemisection. Molars also have root canal variations; maxillary first molars can have two separate canals in the mesiobuccal root with two distinct apical foramina as reported by Seidberg and associates (1973) in 25% of their cases. The mesiobuccal root had two canals that joined before the root apex in 37% of their cases. Mandibular first and second molars have two canals in the distal root in 8% of the cases (Green, 1973). In rare instances lower first molars have two distinct distal roots (Fig. 6-5). These variations in the root canal system do not make root canal treatment impractical as long as neither extreme curvatures nor calcifications hinder access to the apex.

Endodontic periodontic considerations

The majority of the teeth used for overdenture abutments have vital pulps and no periapical involvement but some periodontal involvement. The ultimate success of endodontically treated teeth that have periodontal involvement depends on plaque control, pocket depth, the even distribution of the forces of mastication, and the amount of root surface attached through the periodontal ligament. Endodontic treatment is contraindicated when teeth can be depressed in the socket.

Medical history

A complete medical history is taken before any dental treatment. Although no systemic diseases contraindicate endodontic therapy, some precautions are essential.

Rheumatic fever. Patients with a history of rheumatic fever require prophylactic antibiotic coverage before endodontic therapy to prevent subacute bacterial endocarditis in the event of bacteremia during instrumentation. The possibility of bacteremia occurring when instrumentation is confined within the root canal and in an aseptic field is extremely small. However, pulp extirpation and filing beyond the apical foramen can produce a bacteremia (Bender and co-workers, 1963).

The American Heart Association (1965) suggests that 600,000 units of procaine penicillin be given on the day of the procedure and that 600,000 units of crystalline penicillin be given 1 or 2 hours before the procedure. For 2 days after treatment, 600,000 units of procaine penicillin are given intramuscularly daily. If oral penicillin is prescribed, the patient takes 250 mg. of penicillin V four times a day starting on the day of treatment. An extra dose is taken an hour before the endodontic procedure, and four doses are taken daily for 2 days after treatment. If the patient is allergic to penicillin, erythromycin can be substituted, using the same dosage and schedule as for oral penicillin.

Hypertension. Some physicians contraindicate treating hypertensive patients with anesthetic agents containing epinephrine. A vasoconstrictor is essential for the depth of anesthesia necessary for pulp extirpation. Most agree that pain experienced by the patient produces more endogenous epinephrine than would be present in the anesthetic solution. Local anesthetic containing 1:100,000 epinephrine is viewed as safe. However, the anesthetic should be injected slowly and with numerous aspirations to avoid injecting into a blood vessel.

Diabetes. Since diabetics are inclined to have infections and to heal slowly, antibiotics are prescribed if an infection is present. Usually 500 mg. of oral penicillin or erythromycin are given initially and then 250 mg. four times a day for 4 to 6 days. Local anesthetic agents containing epinephrine tend to elevate the blood sugar level by stimulating the sympathetic nervous system (Burket, 1965). If a vasoconstrictor is desired for a diabetic patient, levonordefrin (Cobefrin) can be used, since it does not produce sympathetic stimulation.

Diphenylhydantoin sodium. When a patient is on diphenylhydantoin sodium therapy, overdentures may be contraindicated. Although endodontic treatment can be given, the possibility of hyperplasia of the gingival tissue beneath the denture makes the prognosis equivocal.

ENDODONTIC THERAPY
One-visit endodontic procedures

Usually teeth selected for overdenture abutments are vital but have some degree of periodontal disease. The vitality of these potential abutments makes it possible to treat many of them endodontically at one sitting. Extensive studies have shown that if the pulp is severed in the area of the apical foramen, blood is discharged into the root canal, and the reparative process is aided by this blood coagulum. Additionally, root canal therapy can be completed up to the point of suspected pulp severance during one appointment (Ostby and Hjortdal, 1971). If periapical infection can be expected, immediate filling is contraindicated, and conventional therapy should be instituted.

Anesthesia. Profound local anesthesia, which is necessary for pulp extirpation, usually can be obtained by conduction or infiltration. At times, it is difficult to produce mandibular pulpal anesthesia, and it may be necessary to use two carpules of anesthetic agent and a long buccal injection. However, it is best to delay the long buccal injection until the patient shows signs of mandibular anesthesia because the long buccal injection may mask some lip signs of anesthesia. On occasion, intrapulpal injections are essential.

Access. After anesthesia, the tooth is isolated with a rubber dam, and the area disinfected. Strict asepsis throughout the procedure is imperative. Access to the root canal is gained by using a sterile No. 2 or 4 round bur in a high-speed handpiece. Further refinement is obtained with a tapered fissure bur or a long-shank round bur at reduced speeds. If the abutment is tilted or rotated, the access preparation is started without the rubber dam in place. This procedure allows a better view of the gingiva and bony structure covering the roots and aids in locating the root canal.

Working length. With the aid of parallel radiographs and from a knowledge of the average length of teeth, a tentative working length can be determined. This tentative length is used in placing a standard endodontic file, generally a No. 15, in the root canal, and a radiograph is taken (Fig.

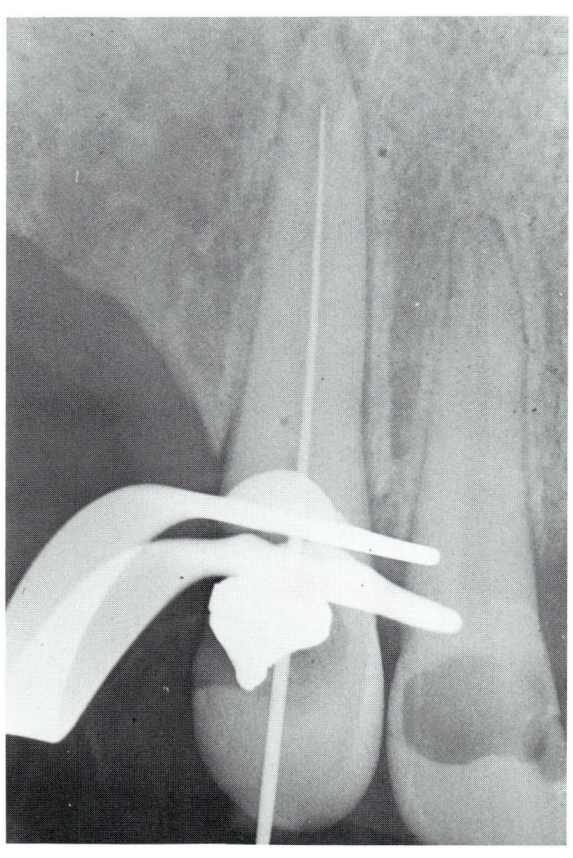

Fig. 6-6. Radiograph of a file at tentative working length.

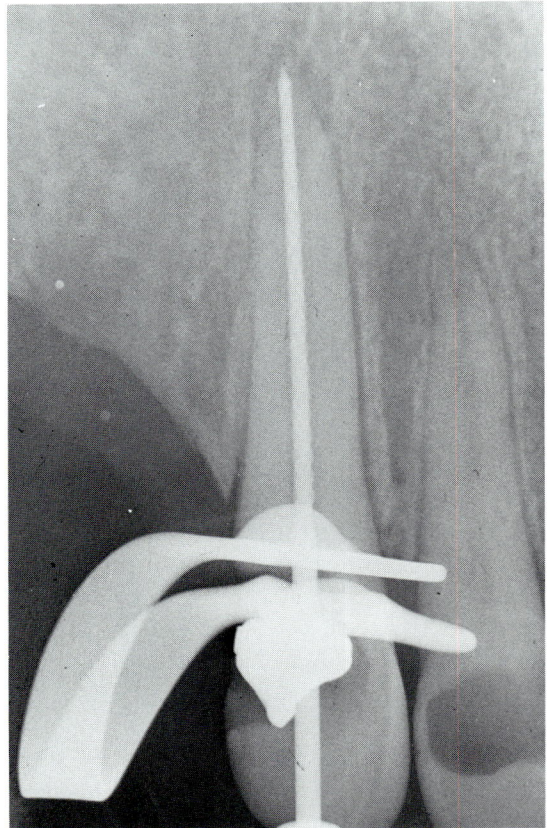

Fig. 6-7. Radiograph of last file that was used to create apical seat.

6-6). The working length should be 1 mm. short of the radiographic apex. If the tentative working length appears to be more than 2 mm. short of the radiographic apex, the length should be adjusted, and a new radiograph should be taken. Several studies indicate that the results are best if the pulp extirpation level is from 1 to 2 mm. short of the root apex (Engstrom and Lundberg, 1965; Stromberg, 1971). To obtain a working length and instrument cuspids, 31 mm. files may be required because the average cuspid is longer than the regular 25 mm. instruments.

Instrumentation. The pulp can be removed with barbed broaches when the root canal is large enough to accommodate a broach without binding. The root canal is instrumented to the working length by using sterile premeasured files in an orderly progression of size. A vertical filing motion is maintained throughout the lateral surfaces of the canal. During filing the root canal is irrigated frequently with 5.25% sodium hypochlorite (Clorox). The biomechanical enlargement of the root canal proceeds until all visible fragments of pulp tissue are removed and the desired apical seat is created. After the apical seat or "stop" has been formed, an evenly tapered canal is created with instruments successively sized 1 mm. short of the previous instrument. For example, if the apical seat was formed with a No. 40 file, a No. 45 file would be 1 mm. short, and a No. 50 file would be 2 mm. short (Wakai and Naito, 1973). Hemorrhage usually stops when all pulpal tissue is removed. A radiograph is taken with the last file used in preparing the apical seat in place to verify the prepared length (Fig. 6-7). The root canal can be dried with sterile paper points. If the root canal is not to be completed in one sitting, then a mild intracanal medicament on a pledget of cotton is placed in the pulp chamber, and the access is closed with a temporary cement. The patient is seen in 5 to 7 days for obturation or remediation.

Obturation. Gutta percha is the filling material of choice for obturating the root canal system. A standard gutta percha cone similar in size to the last file used in preparing the apical seat is selected. The master cone should fit to within 1 mm. of the apical seat, but it is unnecessary to confirm this step by radiograph. A root canal cement is used with the master cone to seal the canal. The next-to-last file used in preparing the apical seat is rotated counterclockwise to streak the walls of the canal with cement. Then the tip of the master cone is coated with the cement and carried to place.

A Kerr No. 3 or a Premier No. 25 or 40 spreader can be used for lateral condensation; a Premier No. 25 is especially useful in finer canals. For posterior teeth the Premier No. 25s or 40s, or the Star D11T is effective (Fig. 6-8). However, any root canal spreader selected should fit loosely in the canal and have a premeasured stop 2 mm. short of the working length. The remaining radicular space can be obturated by using fine accessory cones, a spreader of choice, and lateral condensation. At this time a radiograph is taken to ascertain the completeness of the root canal obturation (Fig. 6-9). Excess gutta percha is removed from the co-

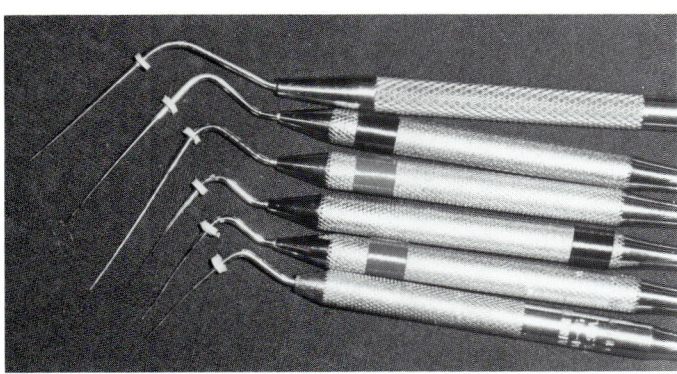

Fig. 6-8. Spreaders used for lateral condensation; bottom to top, star D11T, Premier No. 25s, No. 40s, Premier No. 25, No. 40, and Kerr No. 3.

58 PRELIMINARY PROCEDURES

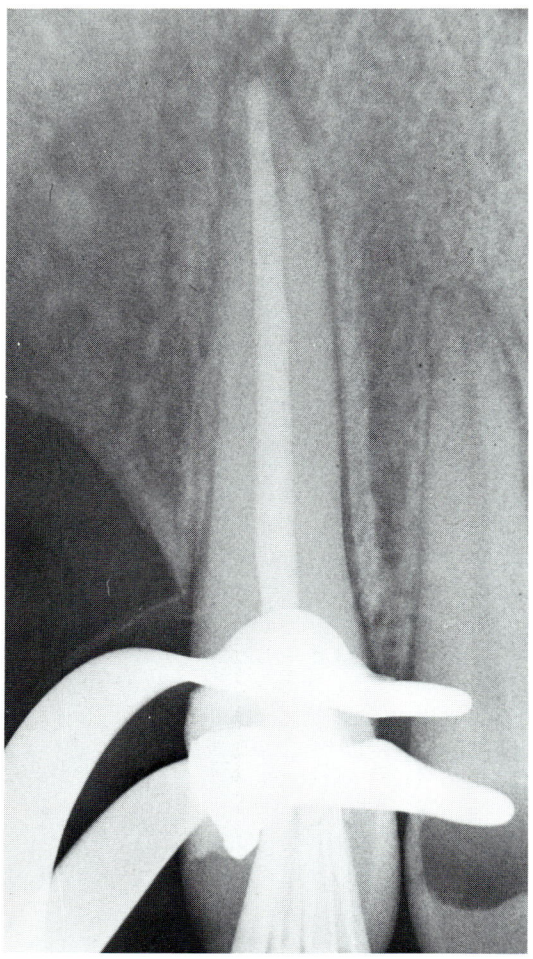

Fig. 6-9. Radiograph is used to inspect completeness of root canal obturation.

ronal portion of the root canal with a heated instrument. The access can be closed with a temporary cement or an amalgam restoration. Often amalgam is the material of choice for closing the access because the coping may not be constructed for several months after the abutments are prepared. A radiograph is taken of the completed root canal, and the patient is instructed to return for a follow-up radiograph in 6 months. The tooth is taken out of occlusion before the patient is dismissed.

Endodontic treatment variations

More than one potential abutment can be treated at a sitting if time and unilateral anesthesia permit. Second bicuspids and cuspids in the same quadrant are the pairs of teeth treated most frequently during the same visit. Maxillary and mandibular cuspids on the same side can also be treated during the same appointment.

On occasion, a mandibular first or second molar that is involved periodontally may have one root with bone support that is acceptable if the crown-root ratio is improved. When the tooth is vital, the acceptable root can be treated endodontically, and the other root can be hemisected at the same sitting (Fig. 6-10).

Incidence of pain after one-appointment endodontics

The incidence of pain after one-appointment endodontic treatment seems to be minimal. Evaluation of 247 teeth in one study indicated that 90% of the patients had little or no spontaneous pain 24 hours after treatment (Fox and associates, 1970). More recently, 65 patients with a total of more than 170 abutments reported minimal or no discomfort after one-visit endodontic therapy in preparation for overdentures. It should be reemphasized that instrumentation and obturation short of the apex not only facilitate repair but also reduce the likelihood of postoperative pain. After one-sitting endodontics, patients are told to expect minor discomfort for 24 to 36 hours, and a mild analgesic is prescribed.

ENDODONTIC IMPLANTS

Endodontic implants can be used to stabilize teeth with extremely short roots or excessive bone loss. They provide the necessary support to a weakened tooth that may serve as an overdenture abutment. Extending the implant from 5 to 10 mm. beyond the apex and reducing the length of the clinical crown can alter the crown-root ratio.

Endodontic implants should not be confused with prosthodontic implants; the latter have a direct communication with the oral cavity through the gingiva. Therefore inflammation can occur around the exposed portions of alloplastic implants. An endodontic implant is a complete implant, for it is entirely within the bone and root canal; it has no direct communication with the oral cavity.

Contraindications

Endodontic implants cannot be used on all teeth. Some contraindications for this procedure follow.

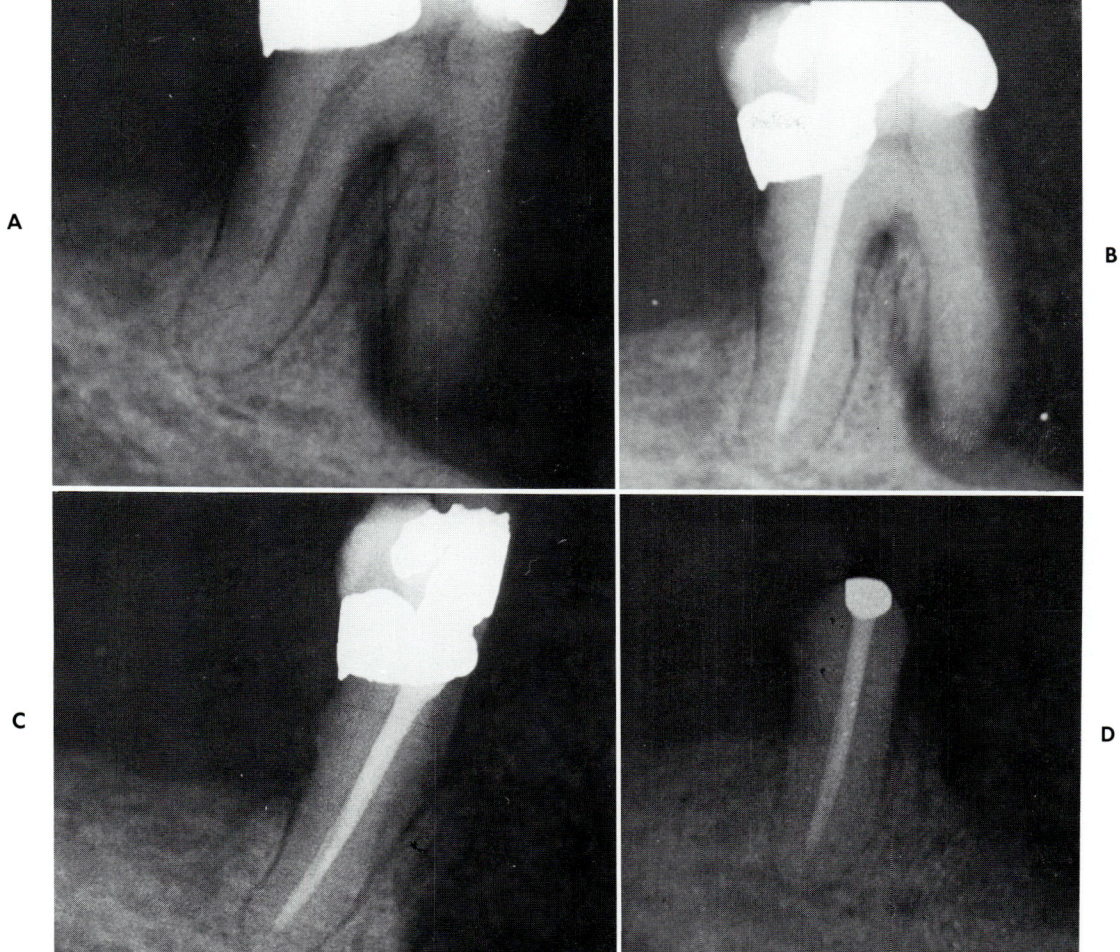

Fig. 6-10. **A,** Preoperative radiograph of mandibular second molar. **B,** Obturation of distal root. **C,** Hemisection of mesial root. **D,** Distal root after preparation as overdenture abutment. Note improved crown-root ratio.

1. When a periodontal pocket extends to the apex of the involved tooth
2. When less than 2 mm. of bone support remains around the root
3. When anatomic structures, such as the maxillary sinus, nares, mandibular canal, and mental foramen cannot be avoided by the implant
4. When the tooth is inclined in such a manner that the implant would penetrate the cortical plate of bone and extend into the soft tissues

Special instruments

In addition to standardized sizes of Vitallium implants, special instruments are essential for endodontic implant procedures; they are 40 mm. intraosseous bone drills (engine reamers) and 40 mm. hand reamers. Threaded Vitallium implants are reported to be more resistant to removal than smooth implants (Judy and co-workers, 1972). In addition, a recent study indicated that Vitallium endodontic implants are not completely resistant to corrosion (Seltzer and associates, 1973).

Technique

The implant procedure can be completed during one visit when the potential abutment is vital. The rubber dam is placed in the usual manner after anesthesia. Strict asepsis should be observed during treatment. Removal of the incisal third to half of the clinical crown allows access to the pulp cham-

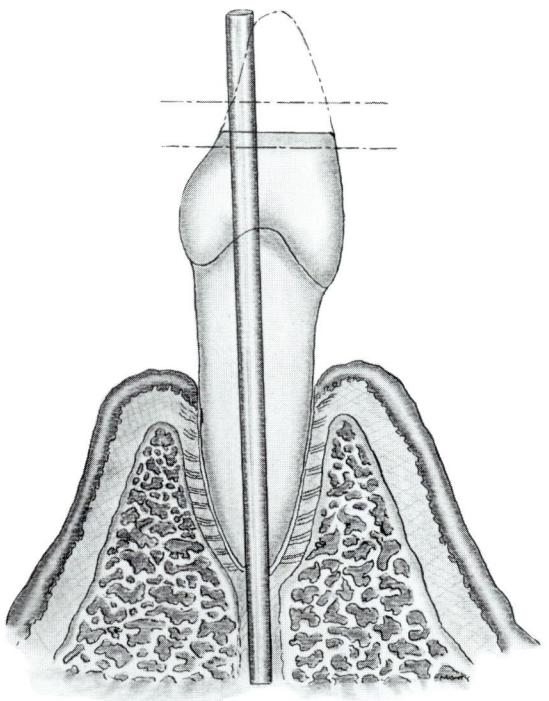

Fig. 6-11. Diagram shows removal of occlusal portion of crown and straight line access for implant.

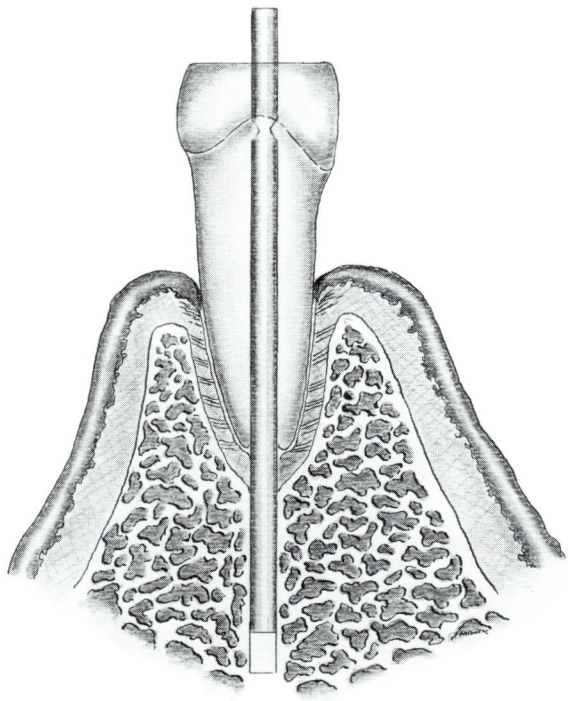

Fig. 6-12. Diagram demonstrates seating implant 1 mm. short of bone and notching of occlusal section of implant.

ber and root canal. Part of the crown is removed to give direct access to the apex and eliminate postoperative occlusal pressures on the tooth; the part of the crown remaining provides adequate retention of the coping (Fig. 6-11).

Preparation. The root canal is prepared at least 2 to 3 mm. beyond the apex with hand reamers to the minimum size of a No. 60 reamer. Then the bone is penetrated with a No. 45 hand reamer, but if the bone is dense, an engine reamer smaller in size than the prepared root canal is used to start the penetration. The osseous preparation is finished with reamers, and care is taken to avoid perforating the cortical plate of bone. The bone is prepared to the minimum size of a No. 60 or 70 reamer approximately 5 to 10 mm. beyond the apex of the tooth. The final instrumentation should produce a continuously tapered preparation from the root canal into the bone. Generally hemorrhage is controlled by using an irrigating solution of sterile saline or lidocaine (Xylocaine) with 1:50,000 epinephrine throughout the biomechanical preparation.

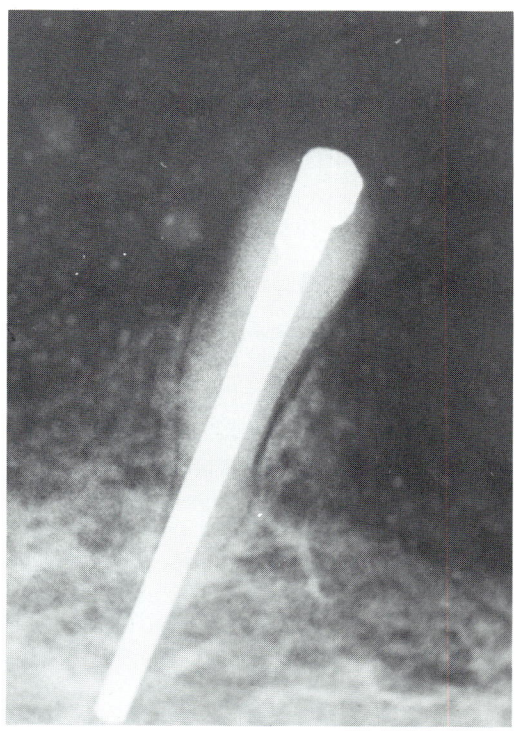

Fig. 6-13. Mandibular bicuspid with endodontic implant used as overdenture abutment.

Fitting the implant. A heavy hemostat is used to fit an implant of the same size and length as the prepared canal and bone. The implant is removed, cut 1 mm. from the tip, and then reseated so that it fits snugly at the apex of the tooth and so that the tip of the implant does not rest on bone. The implant is notched with a bur or disk 2 to 3 mm. from the occlusal or incisal portion of the cut-off crown (Fig. 6-12).

Cementing the implant. The walls of the root canal are coated with sealer, and a layer of root canal sealer is applied to the intracanal part of the implant. Then the implant is cemented into place with firm pressure to assure a good apical seal. The protruding portion of the implant is broken off, and the occlusal opening is filled with zinc phosphate cement (Fig. 6-13).

REFERENCES

Bender, I. B., Seltzer, S., Tashman, S., and Meloff, G.: Dental procedures in patients with rheumatic heart disease, Oral Surg. **16**:466-473, 1963.

Burket, L. W.: Oral medicine, ed. 5, Philadelphia, 1965, J. B. Lippincott Co.

Carlson, O.: Nogle makroskopiske iagttagelser af rodkanalforholdene I humane permanente hjornetaender, Tandlaegebl. **72**:787-817, 1968.

Carns, J. S., and Skidmore, A.: Configurations and deviations of root canals of maxillary first premolars, Oral Surg. **36**:880-886, 1973.

Engstrom, B., and Lundberg, M.: The correlation between positive culture and the prognosis of root canal therapy after pulpectomy, Odont. Revy. **16**:193-203, 1965.

Fox, J., Atkinson, J., Dinin, A., Greenfield, R., Hechtman, E., Reeman, C., Salking, M., and Todaro, C.: Incidence of pain following one-visit endodontic treatment, Oral Surg. **30**:123-130, 1970.

Frank, A. L.: Improvement of the crown root ratio of endodontic endosseous implants, J. Am. Dent. Assoc. **74**:451-462, 1967.

Green, D.: Double canals in single roots, Oral Surg. **35**:689-696, 1973.

Judy, K., Eilberg, R., Lew, I., and Greene, D.: Cement leakage and retention of threaded and non-threaded endodontic implants, Oral Implantol. **3**:28-43, 1972.

Morrow, R. M., Powell, J. M., Jameson, W. S., Jewson, L. G., and Rudd, K. D.: Tooth-supported complete dentures: description and clinical evaluation of a simplified technique, J. Prosthet. Dent. **22**:414-424, 1969.

Morse, D. R.: Endodontic implants: a review and a new approach, N. Y. State Dent. J. **35**:5-12, 1969.

Ostby, N., and Hjortdal, O.: Tissue formation in the root canal following pulp removal, Scand. J. Dent. Res. **79**:333-349, 1971.

Prevention of bacterial endocarditis, 1965, American Heart Association.

Seidberg, B., Altman, M., Guttuso, J., and Suson, M.: Frequency of two mesiobuccal canals in maxillary permanent first molars, J. Am. Dent. Assoc. **87**:852-856, 1973.

Seltzer, S., Green, D., de la Guardia, R., Maggio, J., and Barnett, A.: Vitallium endodontic implants: a scanning electron microscope, electron microprobe, and histologic study, Oral Surg. **35**:828-860, 1973.

Stromberg, T.: Partial pulpectomy at two levels, Odont. Revy. **22**:297-307, 1971.

Wakai, W., and Naito, R.: Filling root canals with gutta percha, Hawaii Dent. J. **6**:8-12, 1973.

Weine, F. S.: Endodontic therapy, St. Louis, 1972, The C. V. Mosby Co.

Zillich, R., and Dowson, J.: Root canal morphology of mandibular first and second premolars, Oral Surg. **36**:738-744, 1973.

7

SURGICAL CONSIDERATIONS IN OVERDENTURE THERAPY

JOHN J. TARSITANO

A LITTLE HISTORY

For many reasons, few of which are valid, patients are separated from their teeth. This event has occurred so often in the population and so early in the lives of patients that an entirely new surgical discipline has come into existence—preprosthetic surgery.

The function of the alveolar process is to support teeth, and it performs this task exceedingly well. However, once the teeth are removed, the process loses its *raison d'être* and, in accordance with Wolff's Law (form follows function), undergoes resorption. Attempts to "restore" function by means of dentures will not retard this process, and in some instances, may accelerate it. Without discussing the biomechanics involved, it is sufficient to point out that dentures merely replace the crowns of the teeth, not the roots. Therefore the denture bases exert pressure on the entire surface of the alveolar process. This force differs in direction and intensity from the tension exerted by the periodontal fibers (ligaments) as they suspend the roots from the socket walls.

The alveolar process is not suited physiologically to the role of denture bearer. Therefore many who are condemned to wear dentures early in life come to the dentist in later years with an alveolar process that is incapable of supporting dentures.

At this point the patient may be referred for some type of heroic surgery, such as a ridge extension, sulcus deepening, or grafts to create a new foundation for the denture base. This foundation is difficult to create and impossible to maintain, for no matter how skilled the preprosthetic surgeon, the results will be unsuitable physiologically for denture bearing. The designation *preprosthetic surgery* is a misnomer; this discipline should be named *postdentistry surgery*. It is a last-ditch effort after the fruitless series of maneuvers perpetrated on patients by themselves with the aid of the dental profession.

TO WHOM IT MAY CONCERN

This chapter is aimed at fulfilling the need of those who deliver prostheses. Dentists can be classified into two groups: those who perform the necessary surgery themselves and those who refer the patient elsewhere. The former are more likely to be in general practice and are probably treating younger, less mutilated patients. It is to this group that the main thrust of this chapter is directed. What they do in their practices may ultimately produce the problems encountered by the latter group.

A revelation of exotic new techniques should not be anticipated. Fortunately, not many are worth discussing, especially if Brewer and Fenton's (1973) procedure criteria are applied: "There are several reasons for using a given procedure. It must be as good as, or better than another procedure. It helps if it is easier—and easier for all concerned. And most important—it should preserve what is left." Whatever procedure is contemplated, its success will be predicated on an appreciation of the tissues available and the best method of conserving them. The minimal surgery required in this overdenture scheme must be performed with delicacy and finesse, with strict adherence to the cardinal rules of surgery, and only after due consideration and assessment of its extent by the use of all available diagnostic aids. This knowledge is as essential to those who refer the surgery (so that they can prescribe and appreciate it) as it is to those who perform it.

THE MANDIBLE

For practically the entire first year of life people are edentulous. However, the jaws are perfectly able to function as jaws, that is, to form the mouth and enable the infant to get nourishment. The mandible can exert great pressure against anything that comes between it and the fixed maxillae, as any mother who has nursed a child will attest, and it does this without benefit of the alveolar process. Infants are considered toothless, whereas in truth they are alveolarless, too. The mandible of the newborn resembles the edentulous one of an adult, and both mandibles are stress-formed and configured to withstand the varied and sizable strains necessary to sustain life. The alveolar process adds little to the integrity of the mandible, inasmuch as the mandible is an articulated bone designed to withstand considerable force perpendicular to its body and symphysis.

The body of the intact dentulous mandible (Fig. 7-1, *A*) appears to be a solid block of bone. When the outer cortical plate is removed (Fig. 7-1, *B*), it can be seen that the roots of the teeth occupy a large percentage of the space and that spongelike cancellous bone surrounds the roots. The trabecular pattern of this bone is not oriented along lines of stress or strain, indicating that the purpose of the alveolar bone is tooth support, not mandibular rigidity. Removing the teeth and the cortical bone surrounding the necks of the teeth (Fig. 7-1, *C*) reveals how little substance there is to the alveolar process. The thin outer and inner cortical plates contact the roots for most of their length, and the tooth sockets occupy most of the space between them. It is not surprising that after removal of the teeth, the body immediately begins to rid itself of bony residue that is useless to the structural integrity of the mandibular body. Therefore the ultimate form of the edentulous mandible will give maximum rigidity and resistance to stress and strain with minimal structure and bulk (Fig. 7-1, *D*). A side-by-side comparison (Fig. 7-1, *E*) of dentulous and edentulous mandibles from the lingual aspect indicates how little the alveolar process contributes to the strength and bulk of the mandibular body.

The apparent individual differences in rate and extent of the resorptive process are understandable in view of the infinite variations in the population. For example, people differ in type of mandible, that is, normal, micrognathic, or prognathic; size of body and index of mandibular use; muscles attached and their tone; presence and extent of periodontal disease during the dentulous state; presence of dentures and their fit after extraction, and other respects. Such a multiplicity of factors times infinite variation equals inability to predict with accuracy the resorptive rate of a particular patient. Although it is impossible to forecast the rate of change, one can predict with certainty that change will occur.

THE MAXILLAE

Embryologically, structurally, and functionally, the maxillae differ from the mandible. The maxillae are membranous rather than cartilaginous, hollow rather than solid, and fixed rather than movable. The maxillae are a pair of hollow bones (maxillary antra), complex in shape, that border on the optic, nasal, and oral cavities, that are sutured to each other and to the zygomatic, nasal, palatal, temporal, lacrimal, and sphenoid bones, and that provide support for the maxillary dentition (Fig. 7-2, *A* and *B*). When the outer cortical plate is removed (Fig. 7-2, *C*), the spongelike cancellous bone surrounding the roots appears to be the same as in the mandible. However, slightly beyond the cortical plate (Fig. 7-2, *D*) there is a highly important difference. The posterior teeth of the maxillae rest not on solid bone, as do the teeth of the mandible, but on a space—the maxil-

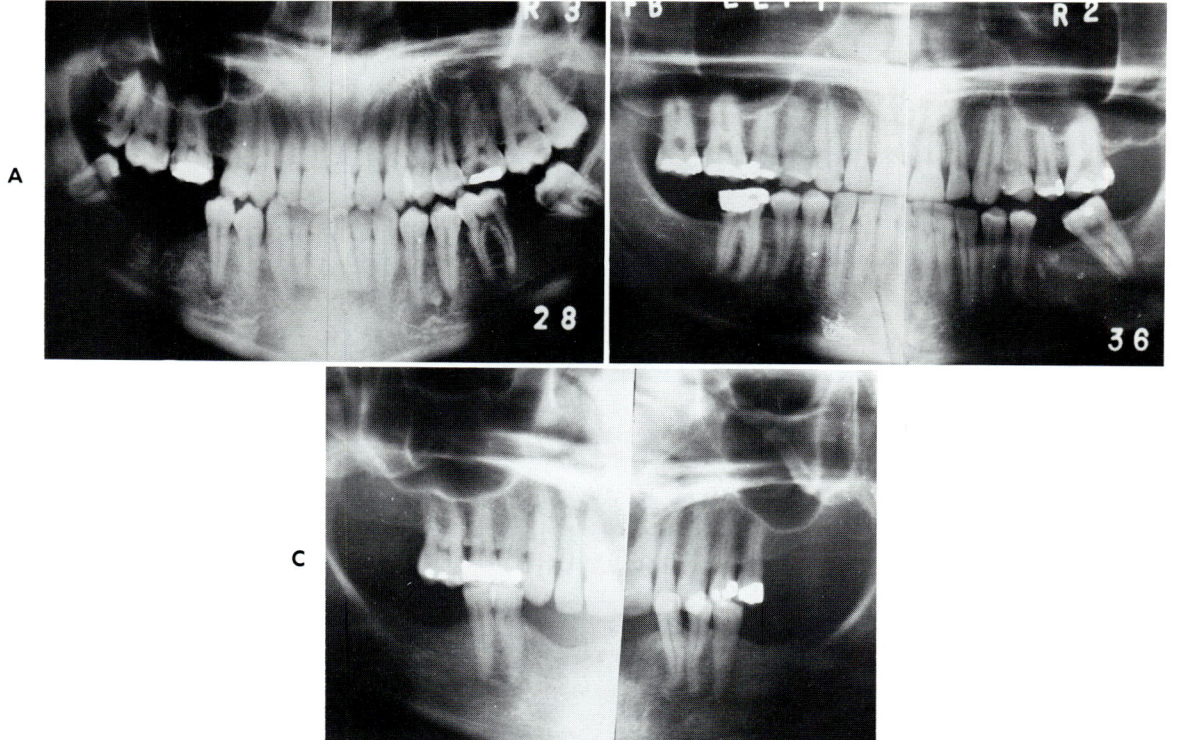

Fig. 7-3. **A,** Panoramic radiograph of 21-year-old patient. Note level of maxillary antra and amount of alveolar bone loss in area of mandibular left first and second molars. Rapidity of bone loss is evident from patient's age and short period of time since extractions, as shown by visible root outlines. **B,** Panoramic radiograph of 22-year-old patient revealing encroachment of antral floors on apices of maxillary posteriors. Note level of antral floor and alveolar crest height in area of missing right second and third molars, and compare with other side. **C,** Panoramic radiograph of 22-year-old patient. Compare alveolar crest heights of edentulous areas of maxillae to those of mandible. Note that apparent loss of crest height of right maxilla primarily lowers antral floor (pneumatization).

and there is maximum strength and rigidity with minimum structure and bulk—are applicable to the maxillae. Whatever there is of the purely tooth-supporting maxillary alveolar process is probably resorbed at the same rate as that of the mandible, but most of this resorption is not visible or measurable during the usual examination. Radiographic studies (Figs. 7-3 and 7-4) have shown that the usual pattern of maxillary restructuring in response to changing stress patterns caused by aging or loss of teeth has been internal. It is apparent from a study of these radiographs that for maximum use of the edentulous maxillae, the physiologic processes of the body find it more advantageous to retain the cortical outline of the maxillary ridge instead of its substance.

THE SURGICAL PRESCRIPTION
Words without thought

It is always a source of amazement to observe men who have been trained to record critical measurements with precision instruments refer their patients to surgery with only the cryptic but carte blanche instructions, "do alveolectomy and create sufficient space." This is a semantic locution that has been fostered by an erroneous thought pattern. One does not create space, for space is nothing bound by something. Surgery removes or destroys tissue and, as a result, leaves a void surrounded by the patient. It is a matter of perspective, but this fact emphasizes the need for modifying one's thinking. Invariably, after surgery, less of the patient remains. If "remove tissue" were written (and

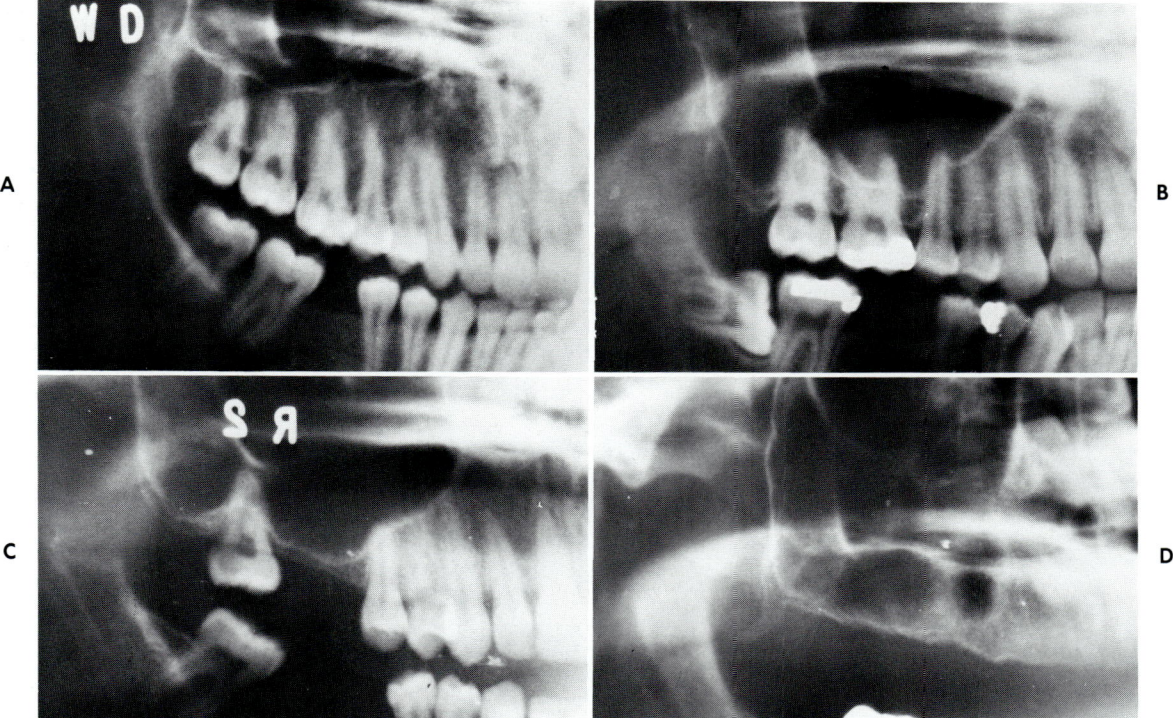

Fig. 7-4. **A,** Radiograph of 19-year-old patient with full complement of maxillary teeth. Note high level of antral floor. **B,** Radiograph of 23-year-old patient with only maxillary third molar missing. Note encroachment of antral floor on apices of posterior teeth. **C,** Radiograph of 22-year-old patient with missing maxillary first and second molars. Remaining molar is literally surrounded by air. **D,** Radiograph of 25-year-old patient with edentulous maxilla. Using crest height of dentulous anterior areas in **A, B,** and **C** as references, note that maxillae show remarkably little loss in alveolar crest height compared to rapid gross loss of alveolar process after mandibular extractions.

thought) instead of "create space," the referring doctor might not be so inclined to indicate "sufficient" in the prescription. Sufficient is an imprecise word, and, unlike beauty, which resides in the eye of the beholder, sufficient has meaning only in the mind of its declarer.

The prosthodontist has articulated casts that give him exact measurements and guidance. The oral surgeon, who has merely a written prescription, can only "eyeball" the patient (Fig. 7-5, *A* and *B*) and cut with the intention of overcutting if he must err in any manner. He has learned that the prosthodontist or the patient or both are prone to take exception to another appointment in the event that too little tissue is removed the first time.

The logical solution

It is apparent how little substance there is to the alveolar process and its relationship to the roots of the teeth. Therefore if teeth or roots or both are to remain in place under denture bases, the current thinking about alveolectomy and ideal ridge form needs reappraisal.

The days of eyeballing should be over. The weak links in denture therapy that requires surgery are a lack of understanding of the other man's discipline and the failure to communicate. For too long, prosthodontists have referred their patients to oral surgeons with only the most vague instructions and have been content to build on whatever is left. Even worse, on innumerable occasions I have received a clear acrylic template

68 PRELIMINARY PROCEDURES

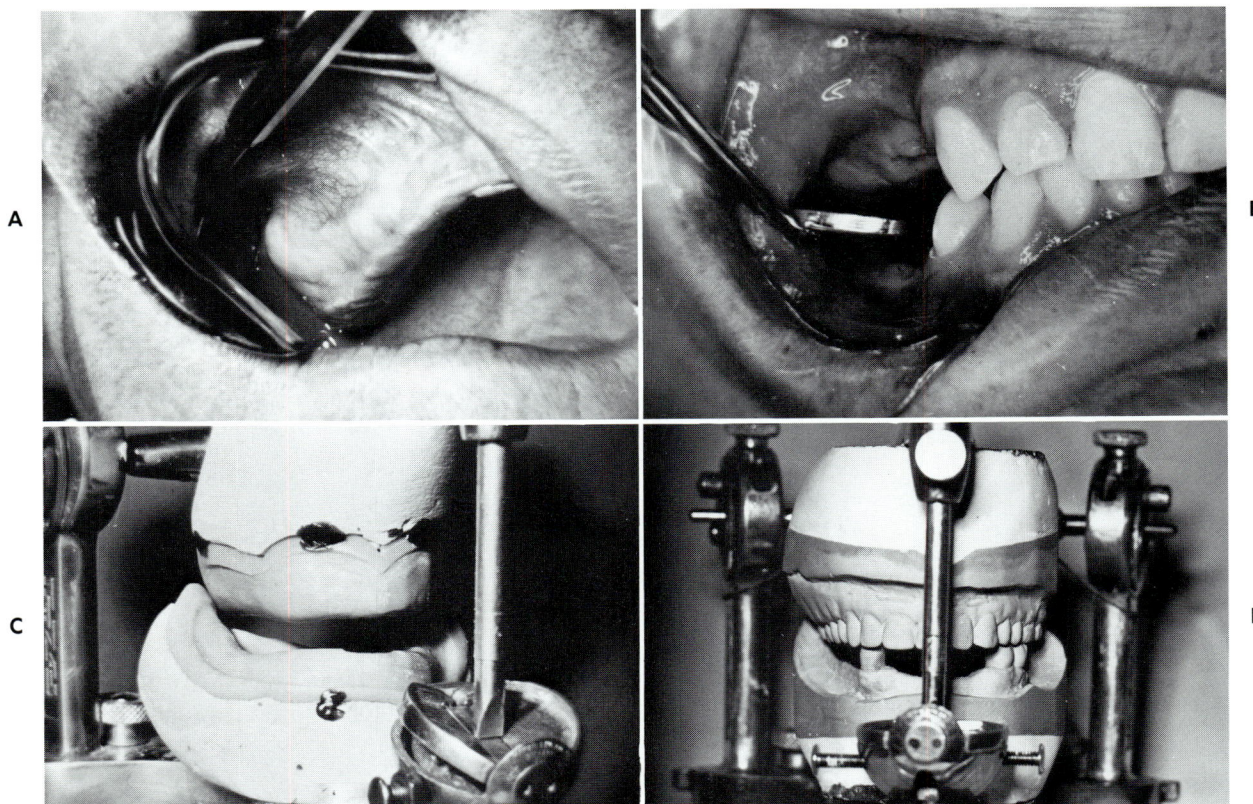

Fig. 7-5. **A,** Edentulous maxillary tuberosity referred to surgery for reduction. With only this view of patient, it is extremely difficult for the surgeon to decide whether to reduce ridge height, undercut, or possibly both, and, of more importance, it is difficult to decide extent of reduction or reductions needed. **B,** Time-honored but ridiculously inadequate method of determining whether interalveolar space is ample. Only information derived from this maneuver is whether patient can wear a dental mirror. **C,** Prosthodontist needs a set of articulated casts to determine configuration of structures to be constructed on denture bases, and surgeon also needs them to determine extent of tissue alteration required beneath bases. Note one type of impingement that is almost impossible to determine accurately without articulated casts. **D,** Articulated casts of patient who is to receive new maxillary complete denture and mandibular overdenture. If surgeon had used these casts to determine accurately adequacy of space available for denture base and if he had used surveyor to determine insertion path of overdenture that would permit minimal sacrifice of alveolar process in undercut areas, chances are excellent that patient would derive maximum benefit from least amount of surgery.

and an immediate denture with instructions to "whittle" on the patient until the patient fits the template or denture. In the majority of these episodes, the templates or dentures were built by a technician after he, the technician, trimmed the casts.

The logical solution is to establish parameters and points of reference that will be common to both disciplines. Casts of the jaws, the articulator, the surveyor, and the radiograph are most important diagnostic aids, but they are only aids when used by the dentist. For a successful overdenture, it is absolutely imperative that these aids be available to all of the dentists concerned (Fig. 7-5, *C* and *D*).

THE MINIMAL SURGERY NECESSARY
Goal of surgery

The overdenture concept is concerned primarily with maintaining as much of the patient's alveolar process as possible, for millions of patients condemned to full dentures are crippled by the loss of the alveolar process. Therefore the maintenance of teeth and roots, even those that are embedded, will prevent resorption of this most important process.

Surgical criteria

Simply stated, surgery for the overdenture depends on the denture base, and the following aspects are of primary consideration:

1. There must be room for the denture base.
2. The base seal is predicated on the removal of undercuts to the extent that it is practical.
3. Alveolar coverage of the roots must be maintained.

To achieve these ends, both the prosthodontist and the oral surgeon require an intimate knowledge of the alveolar process relative to the dental roots, a radiographic survey of the teeth and the alveolar process, and surveyed and articulated casts of the patient's jaws. When these diagnostic aids are used, the oral surgeon's task (like the prosthodontist's) will be apparent in all planes.

Limiting factors

Unlike surgery involving edentulous jaws, in which bone can be removed in any direction and in almost any amount, surgery for the overdenture is exceedingly restrictive. As in removable and fixed partial denture therapy, it is essential to consider insertion paths to maintain adequate alveolar coverage (support) for the teeth or roots to be covered by the denture bases. Therefore, before surgery is initiated, the following must be considered:

1. Maintenance of alveolar coverage of roots
2. Space for denture bases and denture teeth
3. Removal of undercuts, exostoses, and tori consistent with maintenance of alveolar coverage of roots
4. Insertion paths of denture bases
5. Redundant soft tissue
6. Pneumatization of antrum into posterior maxillary alveolar ridge

Surgical procedures

It should be evident by now that only minimal amounts of bone are removed in preparing jaws for the overdenture. Bone is removed easily with bone files or with carefully applied small rotating stones or both. These procedures do not differ from reducing the tooth structure or denture material.

Mucoperiosteal flap

The surgical part of overdenture surgery and, in fact, the foundation of oral surgery is the mucoperiosteal flap. It is simple in concept and logical in design, but it is exceedingly difficult for the uninitiated to execute.

A flap must give access to a definite area, have as its base its widest dimension and be oriented toward the blood supply to assure its viability, have sharp, clean edges that will be supported by solid bone at the end of the procedure, and be truly mucoperiosteal in nature. The problems in execution arise from attempting to cut through an exceptionally tough tissue that adheres tightly to irregularly surfaced bone and then trying to lift the tissue away without shredding or tearing it.

There are two vectors of force in cutting, elevating, and filing, and they are at right angles to each other. It is extremely difficult, if not impossible, to apply both directions of force at the same time with one hand and achieve any degree of control and accuracy. Therefore the first consideration in flap construction is the plane of the surgical field. A vertical field, as when the patient is seated upright, makes it difficult to cut with sufficient force to obtain a continuous through cut (Fig. 7-6). Accuracy and control also are diminished in this position, especially if the one-handed instrument grasp is used.

Adjusting the patient to obtain a horizontal field and using two-handed control of the scalpel permit maximum cutting pressures with maximum control and accuracy (Fig. 7-7). In like manner, the periosteal elevator is positioned and controlled to lift the flap, and the bone files are manipulated to accomplish bone reduction and shaping. A poorly designed or poorly executed flap can negate the entire procedure.

Attempting these procedures on the mandible when the patient's mouth is open for access introduces another hazard, for the patient cannot stabilize his lower jaw. The nature of the temporomandibular joints is such that the mandible moves freely in all planes unless the muscles of mastication are in a contracting state. It is impossible for

70   PRELIMINARY PROCEDURES

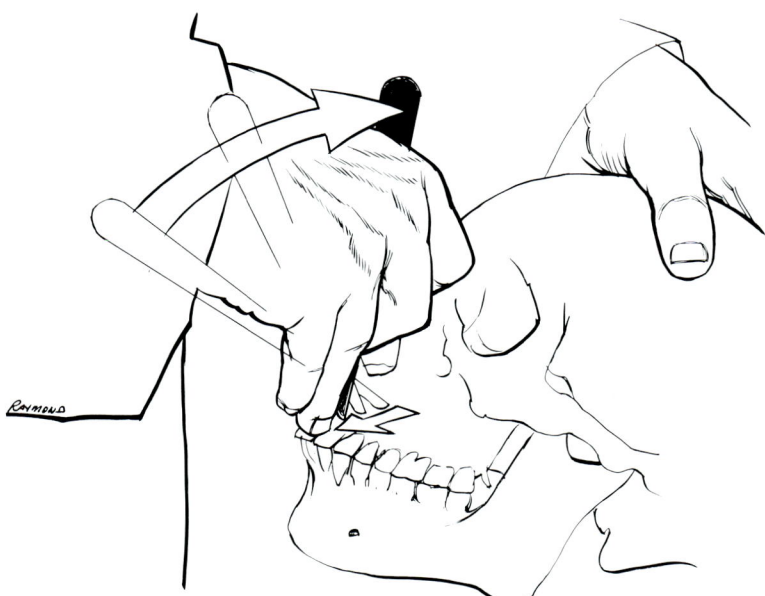

Fig. 7-6. Attempting mucoperiosteal incision for flap construction with patient in upright position and with one-handed control of scalpel. As cut proceeds from top (beginning) to bottom, surgeon's wrist must bend, obscuring view of wound, and guiding and stabilizing fingers of knife-holding hand lose contact with patient. Highly unstable and dangerous condition would exist if surgeon exerted force necessary to cut through exceedingly tough periosteum underlying mucosa and lost control.

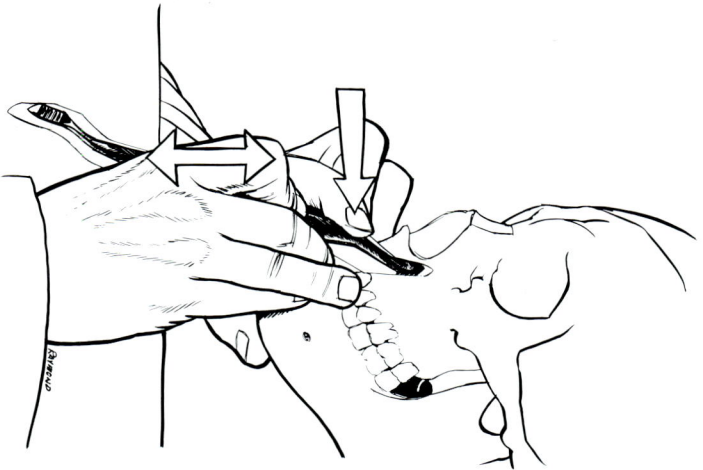

Fig. 7-7. Two-handed control of bone file (knife or periosteal elevator) with operative field in horizontal plane. One hand controls cutting force (downward vector) while other controls instrument direction (to and fro vectors). Stabilizing and guiding fingers of both hands are always in contact with patient, and surgeon has control of instrument. It is unnecessary to bend wrist of instrument-holding hand, and field of view is not obscured.

the patient to hold his mouth open and contract the masticatory muscles at the same time unless an object such as a bite block or a mouth gag is interposed between the mandible and the maxillae (Fig. 7-8). By this simple expedient an accessible and stable field is attained easily. Adjusting the patient to obtain a horizontal field permits flap construction and bone reduction to be effected as in the maxillae, using two-handed manipulation of the instrumentation (Fig. 7-9). Often it may be necessary to approach the mandible on its lingual aspect, for example, when reducing lingual tori or exostoses or both. Use of the proper surgical field orientation, a bite block to stabilize the mandible, and two-handed manipulation of the cutting instruments makes this approach no more difficult than that used for the buccolabial procedures (Fig. 7-10).

Redundant soft tissue

The problem of redundant soft tissue is largely one of interpretation. At one time many prosthodontists insisted that every last vestige of soft tissue that was not a thin layer of tightly adherent mucoperiosteum must be removed. Today, with the welcome trend toward conserving the patient, more and more of this valuable tissue is retained and used. However, in instances when some tissue must be sacrificed, the principles governing bone reduction apply. For example, in earlier times patients were referred to surgery with only the instructions, "remove maxillary fibrous tuberosities," and that is exactly what was done. The prosthodontist built on an alveolar process covered with a

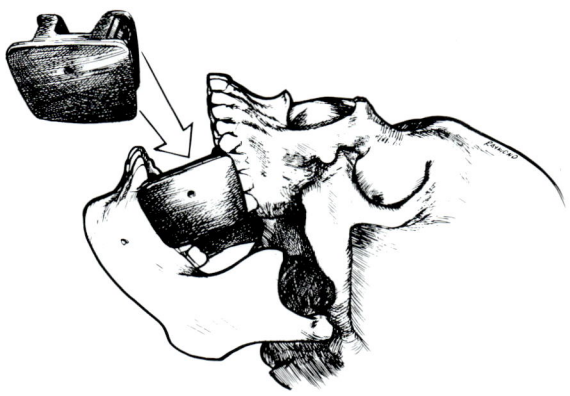

Fig. 7-8. During surgical procedures involving mandible in open position, absolute stability of field is essential. When mouth is open, configuration of temporomandibular joints is such that mandible is freely movable in all planes. Muscles of mastication can "fix" mandible only when they are in contracting state. Therefore only method of assuring stable operating field is to interpose a bite block (mouth gag) between mandible and maxilla and instruct patient to "lock" his mandible against it. Stable operative field is gained, temporomandibular joints are protected from inadvertent strain or trauma or both, and both patient and surgeon feel less vulnerable.

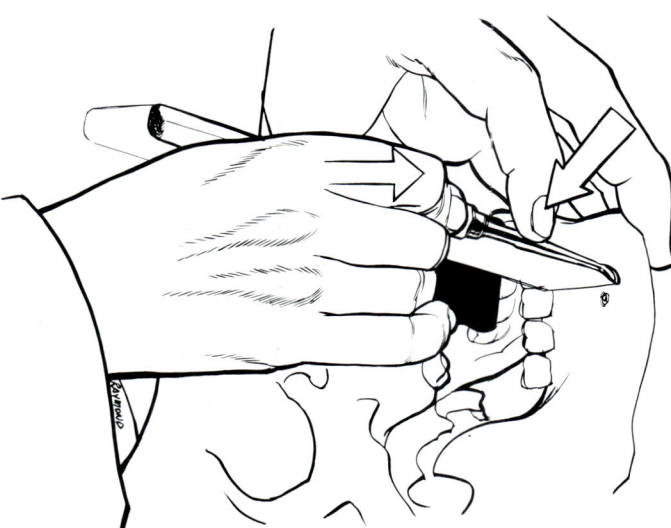

Fig. 7-9. Two-handed use of elevator (knife or bone file) during surgery involving anterior mandible. Note bite block in place, horizontal position of operating field, and absolute control of all aspects of surgery.

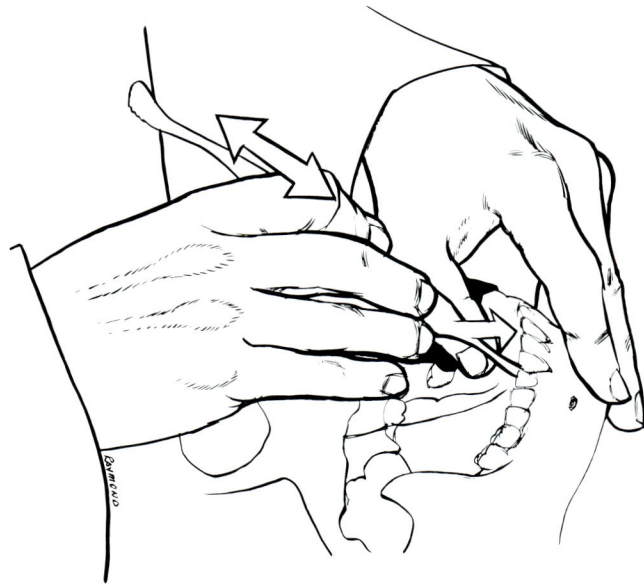

Fig. 7-10. Two-handed use of instrument on lingual side of mandible. Cutting force is delivered to instrument by thumb of left hand while fingers of left hand provide fixation and stability. Instrument-holding hand is stabilized against patient's maxilla and surgeon's left thumb. Note bite block in place.

thin layer of periosteum. Today this patient can be referred to surgery with the articulated and surveyed casts, the radiographic survey, and a detailed prescription indicating the exact dimensions and extent of the tissue to be removed. With these aids, the only tissue removed is that required to provide space for the denture base or to eliminate undercuts. The rest remains to provide the area and bulk needed to improve stability and retention and to provide the elasticity and resilience for shock absorption.

Therefore surgery of the soft tissue similar to that of the hard tissue is based on the principle that as little as possible be done consistent with achieving the desired effect. The actual mechanics of the surgery are identical to those involved in mucoperiosteal flap construction with the exceptions that (1) the wound is designed for removal of tissue, not replacement, and that (2) the area uncovered must be closed (covered) from the sides.

The elliptical V-shaped (watermelon slice) cut is ideal for this procedure, and it should be four times as long as its widest dimension. This 4 to 1 (length to widest point) ratio of the elliptically shaped wound, in addition to careful and thorough undermining of the wound margins, permits the proper wound closure (without tension), which is essential for rapid healing. It may be well to repeat an old surgical axiom at this point: "Wounds heal from side to side, not end to end." Therefore a 10-inch incision properly closed requires the same length of time for healing as a 1-inch incision. Although I preach conservatism in the amount of tissue removed at surgery, I encourage generosity in flap and wound design consistent with obtaining adequate exposure and access.

Pneumatization of maxillary antrum into posterior alveolar ridge

There may be instances when it is necessary to reduce some dimension of the posterior maxillary alveolar process and the radiographic examination shows that the process is filled with the maxillary antrum (Fig. 7-4, *C* and *D*). Although constructing a flap and removing bone could be disastrous, the oral surgeon must find some means of providing room for the denture base.

The solution to this problem is based on the fact that the layer of cortical bone separating the antrum from the oral cavity in these patients is only eggshell thick and is lined on both sides with mucoperiosteum on the outside and schneiderian membrane (antral lining) on the inside. Therefore if a blunt serrated punch approximately 6 mm. in diameter is malleted sharply against the area to be reduced, the extremely thin cortical bone will fracture and telescope inwardly. The tough mucoperiosteum and the antral lining will hold the fragments together, and wiring a previously prepared stent to place over the area allows the healing to be uneventful.

THE FUTURE

I have removed thousands of root tips and entire embedded roots at the request of prosthodontists to prepare mouths for prostheses. I cannot remember one fragment that was symptomatic. In fact, I can recall only a few that appeared suspicious radiographically other than being a root without a crown. Invariably, the patients asked whether it was really necessary to remove these fragments, especially when they had nonsymptomatic history for as long as 50 years in some instances.

Perhaps we are overtreating, and the odds of cyst formation, foci of infection, and fistulae are so small and the sequelae would be of such minor consequence that the sizable effort and cost of protection are not warranted. Goska and Vandrak (1972) reported a case in which the roots were submerged intentionally to preserve alveolar bone. An evaluation of this patient 2 years later indicated the following:

1. Oral mucosa proliferated over the roots that were contoured to the crest of the alveolar bone.
2. A prosthesis was worn over the submerged roots without pain or discomfort.
3. There was no evidence of either eruption or systemic rejection of the submerged roots.
4. The ridge in the area of the submerged roots was relatively broader.

It is hoped that definitive animal research can be funded to determine the feasibility of merely cutting the crowns off at a point low enough on the root to permit complete soft tissue coverage rather than resorting to endodontics when the pulp appears to be vital. It is necessary to ascertain the following information:

1. The ultimate fate of submerged roots
2. The fate of alveolar bone surrounding roots
3. Which teeth lend themselves best for submergence and subsequent denture support
4. Whether endodontic therapy is necessary

SUMMARY

If it is possible to give a needed service that is better, easier for all concerned, and cheaper, it follows that we can provide it for more of those who need it. Certainly there are patients who need it. This is what it's all about.

REFERENCES

Atwood, D. A.: Reduction of residual ridge: a major oral disease entity, J. Prosthet. Dent. **26:**266-277, 1971.

Brewer, A. A., and Fenton, A. H.: The overdenture, Dent. Clin. North Am. **17:**723-746, 1973.

Goska, F. A., and Vandrak, R. F.: Roots submerged to preserve alveolar bone: a case report, Milit. Med. **137:**446-447, 1972.

PART THREE
METHODS

8

OVERDENTURES FOR CONGENITAL AND ACQUIRED DEFECTS

ALLEN A. BREWER

Many patients present with congenital and acquired defects that cannot be treated successfully by orthodontic therapy or by surgical intervention. Nor can they be successfully treated with conventional procedures, either fixed or removable.

I have enjoyed a high degree of success in treating these patients by providing them with complete dentures over their existing teeth (Brewer and Fenton, 1973). Since the existing teeth are not altered, the procedure is completely reversible.

INDICATIONS
Congenital defects

The congenital dental defects that we most frequently treat with the overdenture are associated with the following:
1. The cleft palate
2. Oligodontia (Fig. 8-1)
3. Microdontia
4. Cleidocranial dysostosis
5. Class III patients—the prognathic mandible (Fig. 8-2)

Acquired defects

The acquired defects that we most frequently treat in this manner usually result from accidents, disease, or misuse.

We have patients whose teeth are so misaligned after accidents that the overdenture becomes the preferred method for obtaining an adequate result.

In many patients with teeth badly eroded or abraded, the overdenture provides the most acceptable result. It is sometimes necessary to shorten the flanges in the areas where there are large soft tissue or bony protuberances (Fig. 8-3).

The objective with this treatment is the same as with any other type of prosthesis, to preserve what remains and to improve the function and esthetics. In addition, needed support of the lips and other soft tissues can be provided for many patients. This is done in the simplest way possible, provided that it is as good as or better than alternative methods of treatment. It is seldom necessary to alter the existing teeth.

PROCEDURES

Complete mouth radiographs (Fig. 8-4) and diagnostic casts (Fig. 8-5) are made. These are aids to making a complete examination and subsequent treatment plan. All carious teeth are restored, and necessary extractions and periodontal therapy are accomplished. The patient is trained to properly accomplish oral hygiene procedures. Plaque control for the overdenture patient is a must. The patient must be made to realize that this is his responsibility. Impressions are made of both arches using stock trays and irreversible hydrocolloid. These are cast in stone. For some patients the tray must be altered with impression compound, and rarely an individual or custom tray must be made. The

Text continued on p. 82.

78 METHODS

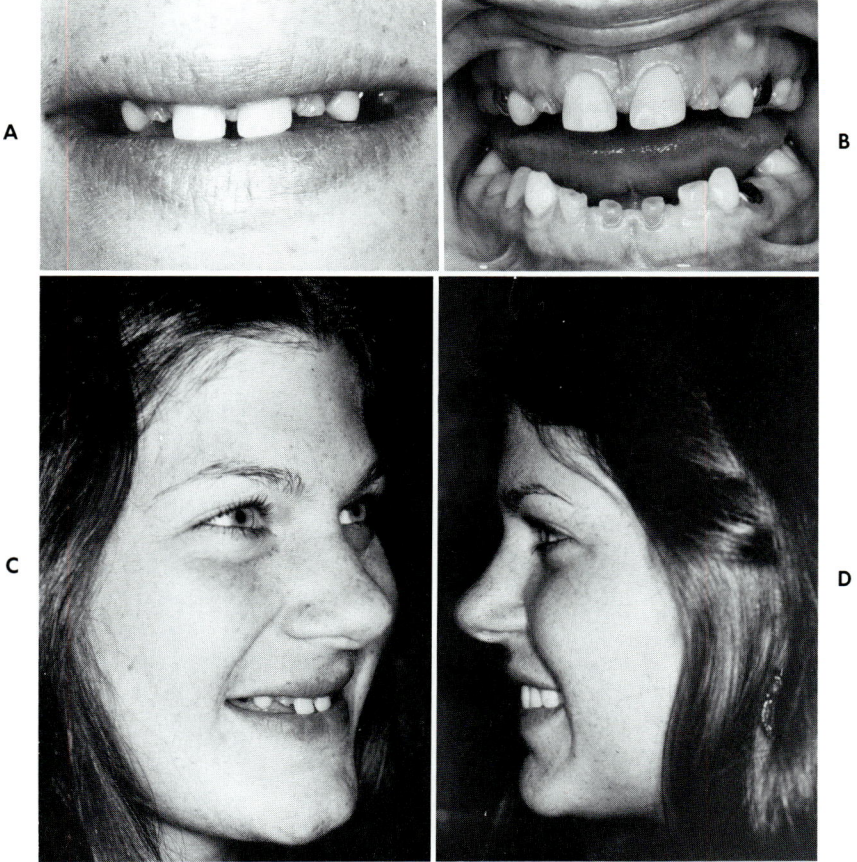

Fig. 8-1. A, Oligodontia; patient's smile. **B,** Intraoral view. **C,** Profile without overdenture. **D,** Profile with overdenture.

OVERDENTURES FOR CONGENITAL AND ACQUIRED DEFECTS 79

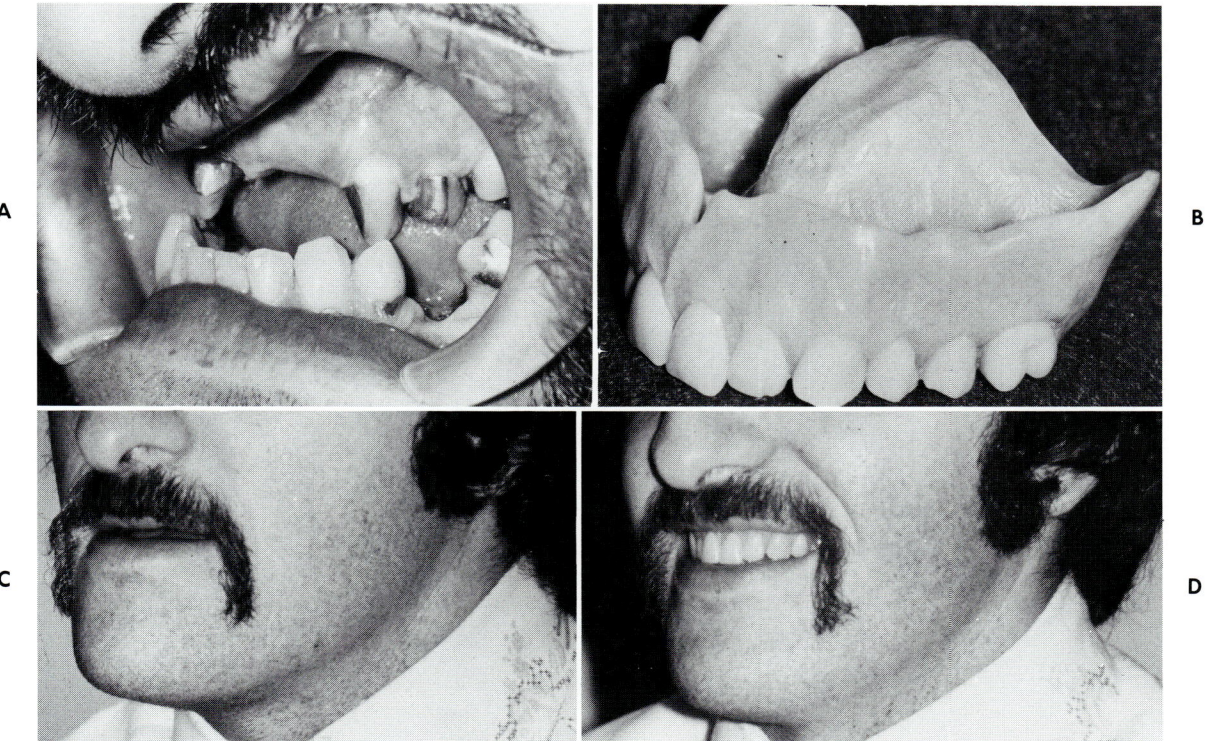

Fig. 8-2. **A,** Class III patient, intraoral view. **B,** Overdenture as completed. **C,** Before denture was inserted. **D,** After denture was inserted. (From Brewer, A. A., and Fenton, A. H.: Dent. Clin. N. Amer. **17:**723-746, 1973.)

80   METHODS

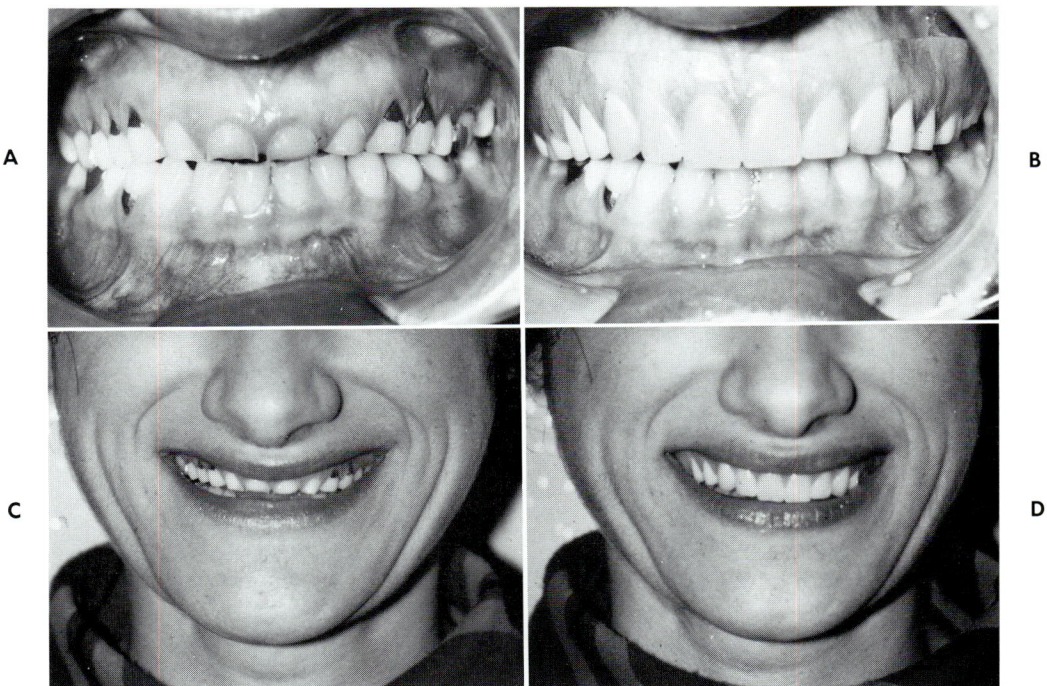

Fig. 8-3. **A,** Eroded teeth, intraoral view. **B,** Intraoral view of short flange overdenture. **C,** Full-face view without overdenture. **D,** Full-face view with overdenture. (From Brewer, A. A., and Fenton, A. H.: Dent. Clin. N. Amer. **17:**723-746, 1973.)

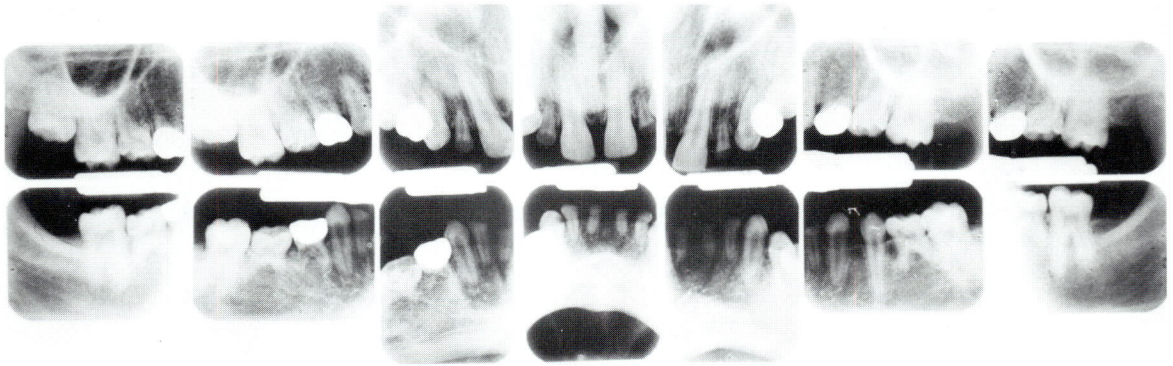

Fig. 8-4. Complete mouth radiographs of oligodontia patient.

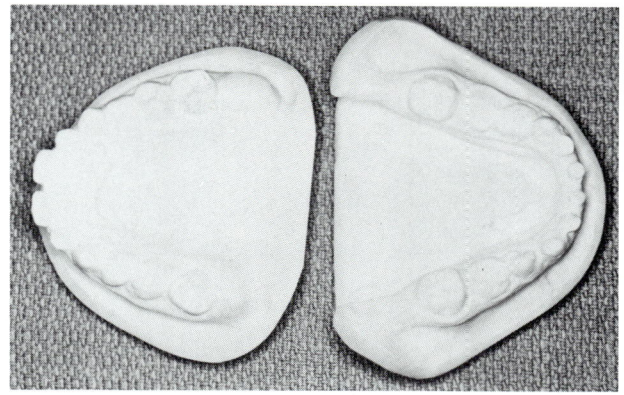

Fig. 8-5. Diagnostic casts of patient with oligodontia.

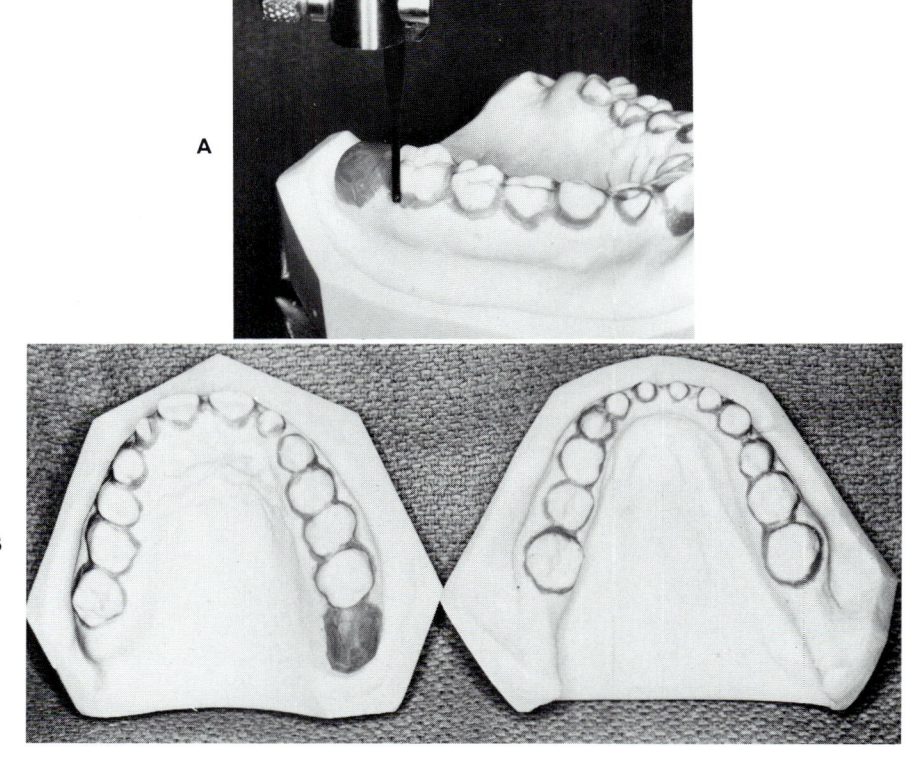

Fig. 8-6. A, Surveying procedure. **B,** Blockout procedure.

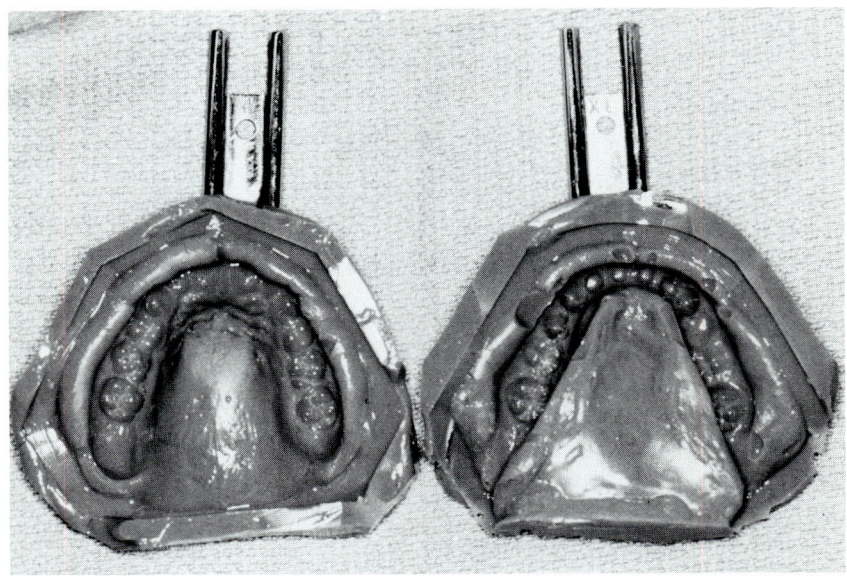

Fig. 8-7. Reversible hydrocolloid impressions of master casts prepared for duplication.

casts are positioned on a surveyor to determine the most desirable path of insertion. Undesirable undercuts are waxed out, and blockout wax is placed around the free margin of the gingiva on each tooth (Fig. 8-6). These casts are duplicated using reversible hydrocolloid (Fig. 8-7). The maxillary cast is coated with sodium alginate, and a base plate is made using autopolymerizing resin by the sprinkle method (Fig. 8-8). Great care must be taken not to chip the teeth on the cast. A face bow transfer is made, and the maxillary cast is attached to the instrument of choice with quick-setting stone (Fig. 8-9). A maxillomandibular relationship record is made in wax using the tactile method (Fig. 8-10). Every attempt is made to accomplish this at the selected vertical dimension of occlusion. This is then checked with centric check points as described in Chapter 14. Teeth of proper mold and shade are selected and ground on the lingual aspect to overlay the existing teeth (Fig. 8-11). These are sometimes almost paper thin. The posterior teeth are hollow ground and reduced so that they may be fitted into the available space. The dentures are waxed and processed in the conventional manner. A gel is made by placing ⅛ inch of methyl methacrylate polymer in a 6 oz. bottle and filling the bottle with monomer. After this sets for 2 weeks, it may be used to paint the surfaces of the

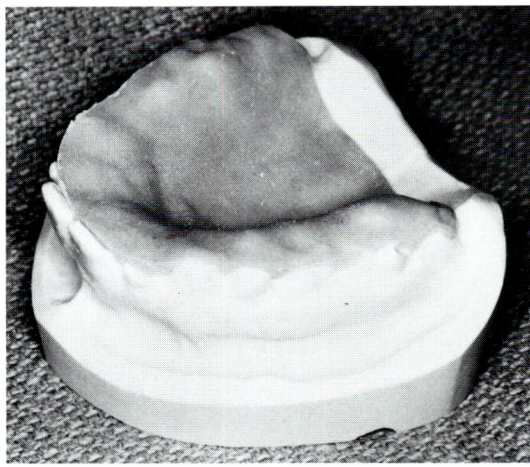

Fig. 8-8. Baseplate formed of autopolymer resin, sprinkle technique.

OVERDENTURES FOR CONGENITAL AND ACQUIRED DEFECTS 83

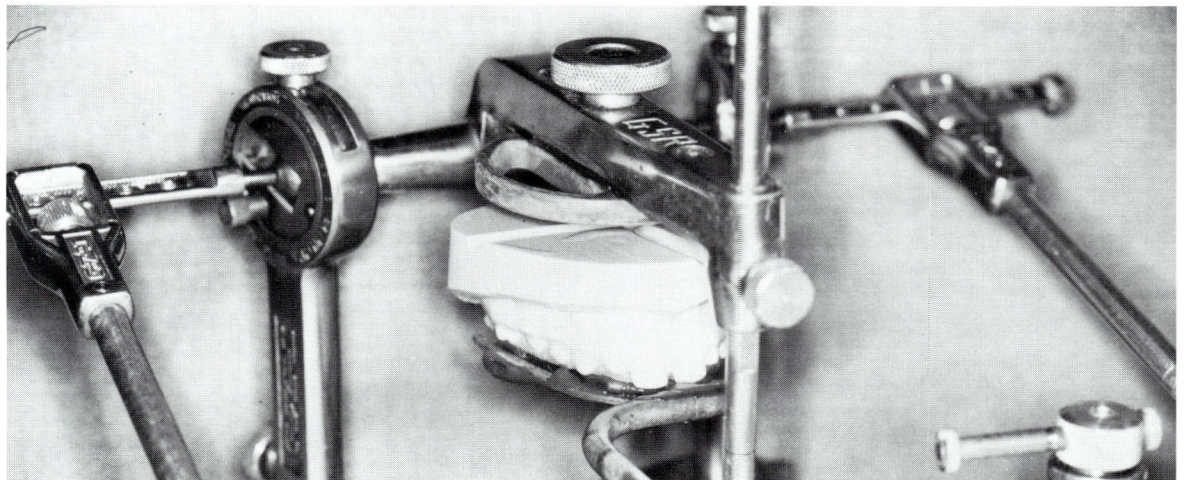

Fig. 8-9. Face-bow transfer of maxillary cast to articulator.

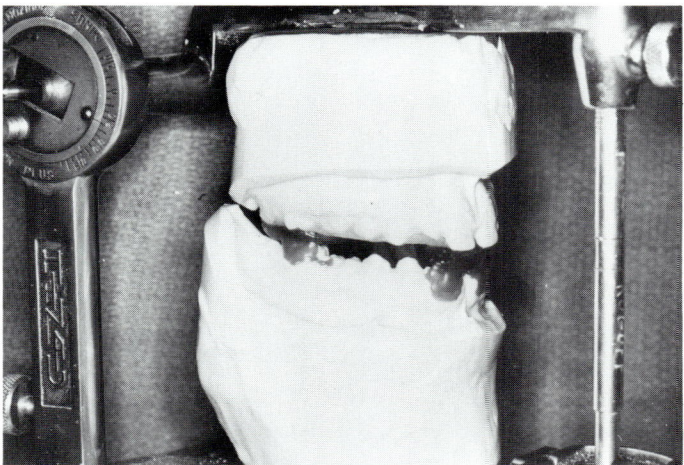

Fig. 8-10. Mandibular cast related to maxillary cast on articulator by wax registration.

84 METHODS

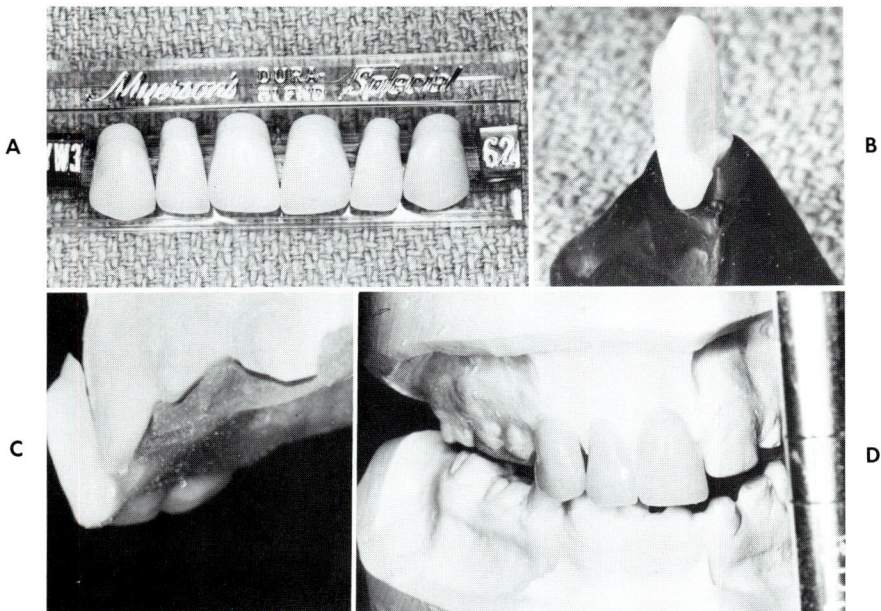

Fig. 8-11. A, Teeth selected. **B,** Teeth hollow ground. **C** and **D,** Teeth arranged for try-in.

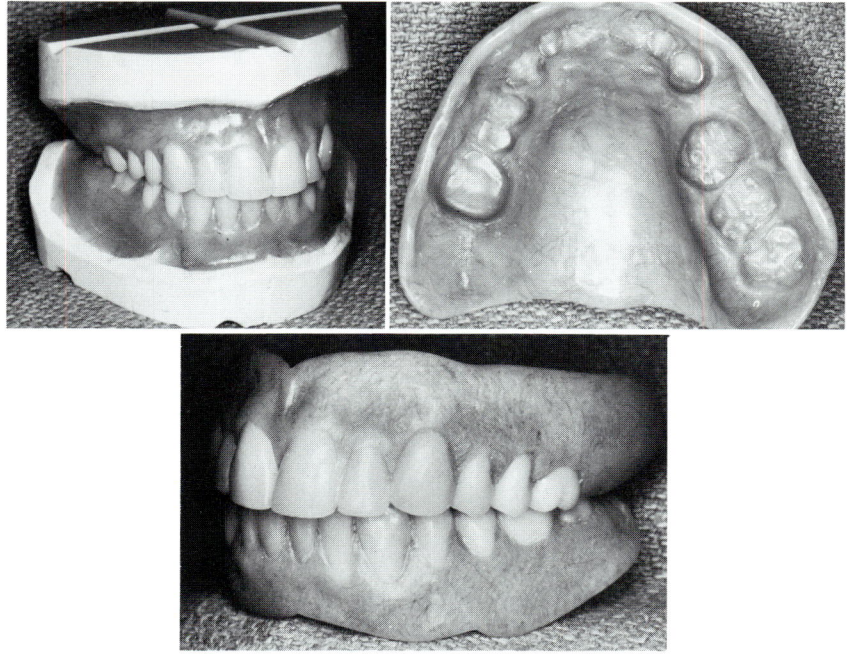

Fig. 8-12. Overdentures processed, finished, and polished.

OVERDENTURES FOR CONGENITAL AND ACQUIRED DEFECTS 85

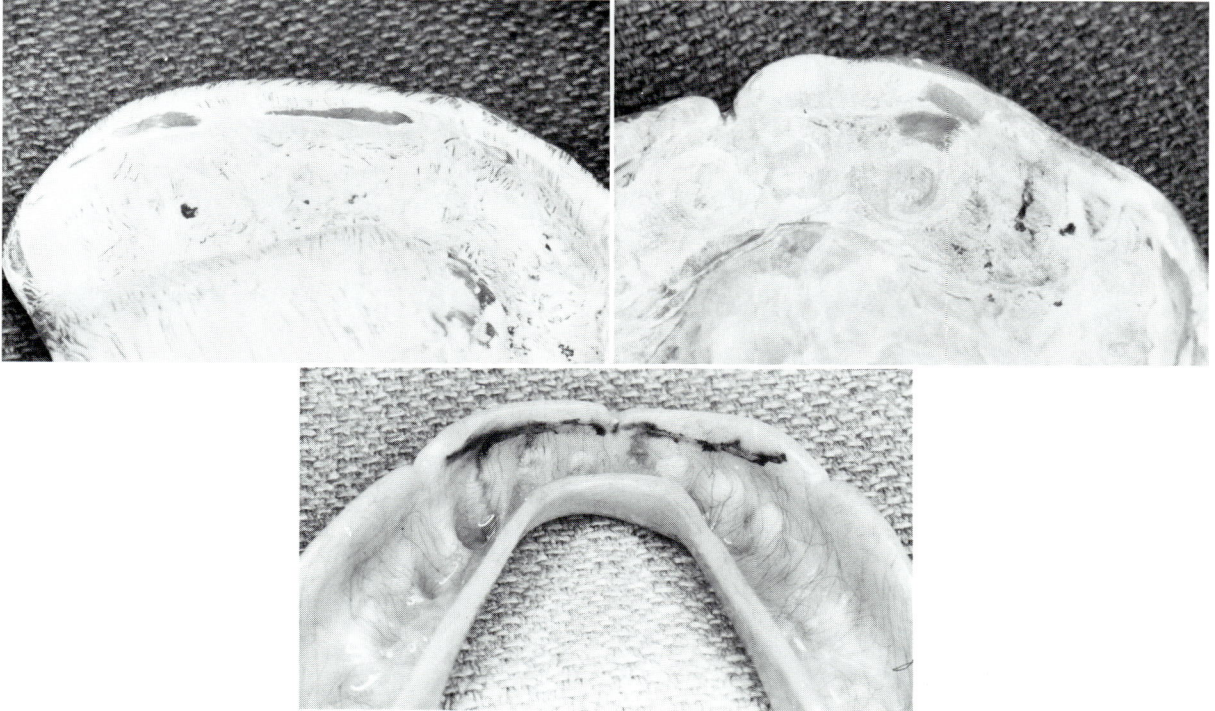

Fig. 8-13. Overdentures fitted to mouth with disclosing wax. Areas of impingement are defined.

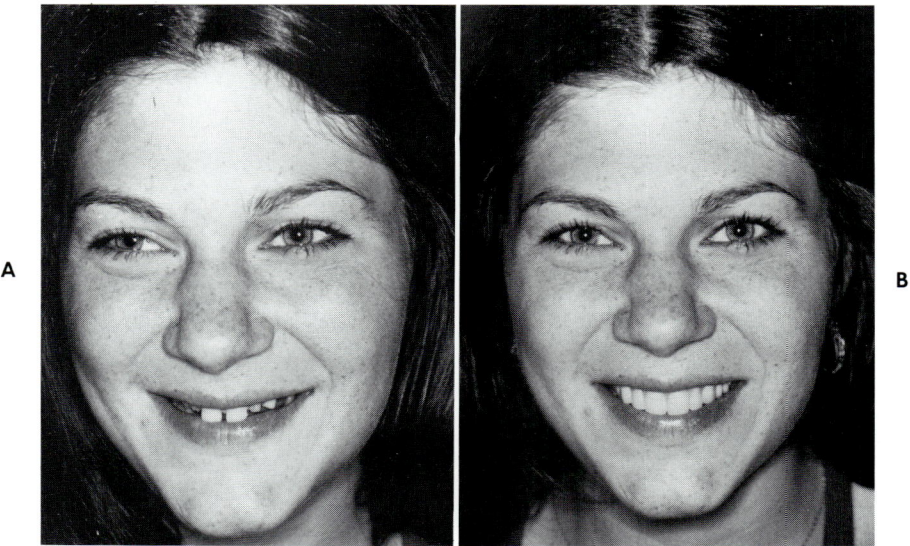

Fig. 8-14. **A,** Without overdenture. **B,** With overdenture.

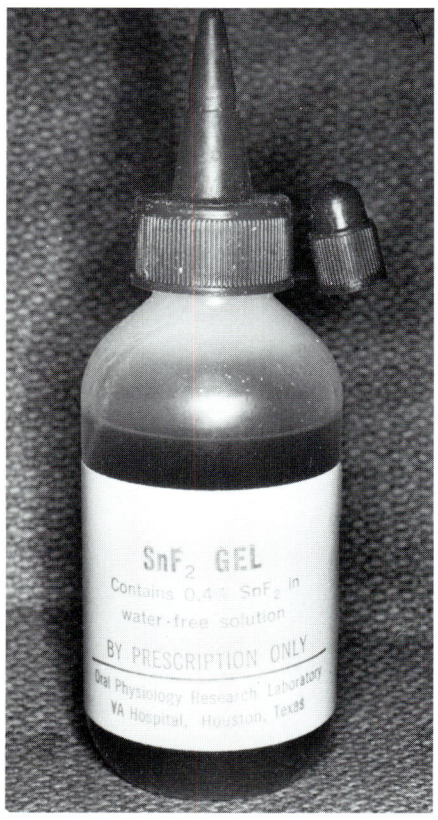

Fig. 8-15. Stannous fluoride gel for protection of tooth surfaces.

acrylic denture teeth that will be contacted by the denture base material. This softens these surfaces of the teeth and provides a good bond with the denture base. We have yet to have one of these teeth, no matter how thin, separate from the denture when using this method.

The dentures are remounted on the articulator after processing but before release from the casts. Processing changes are corrected, and the occlusion is perfected. After recovery from the casts, the flash is removed, and the peripheral borders are established. As a border molded impression was not made, this becomes an important step that should be accomplished by the dentist. Finishing and polishing are accomplished in the conventional manner as described in Chapter 11 (Fig. 8-12). At the time of insertion, disclosing wax is employed to detect areas of impingement (Fig. 8-13). These are corrected, and the completed overdenture is delivered (Fig. 8-14). At this time, the patient is again instructed in oral hygiene procedures.

The teeth are treated with acidulated phosphate fluoride (APF) and sequential treatment with stannous fluoride gel as explained in Chapter 15. The daily use of this gel (Fig. 8-15) is explained to the patient. Subsequent visits will reveal any areas of impingement, and these are corrected (Fig. 8-16).

The question is often asked, "What happens to the teeth and tissues under these overdentures?" Fig. 8-17 shows the tissues of a 21-year-old woman

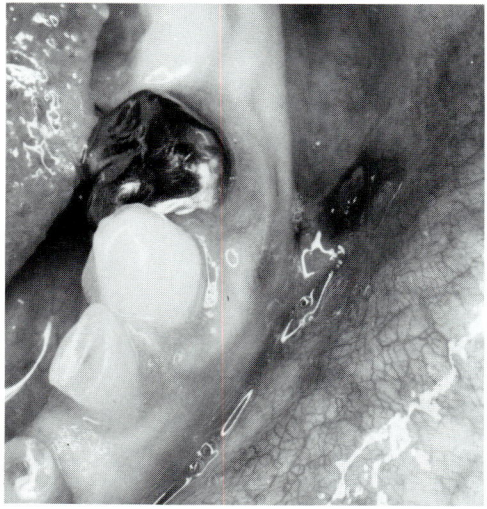

Fig. 8-16. Irritation from overdenture 1 week after insertion. This was the only correction necessary in a 6-month period.

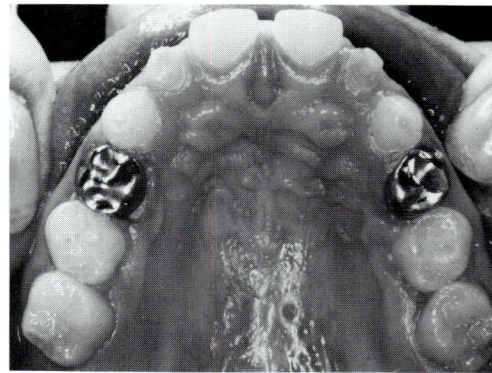

Fig. 8-17. Intraoral view of hard and soft tissues 5 years after insertion.

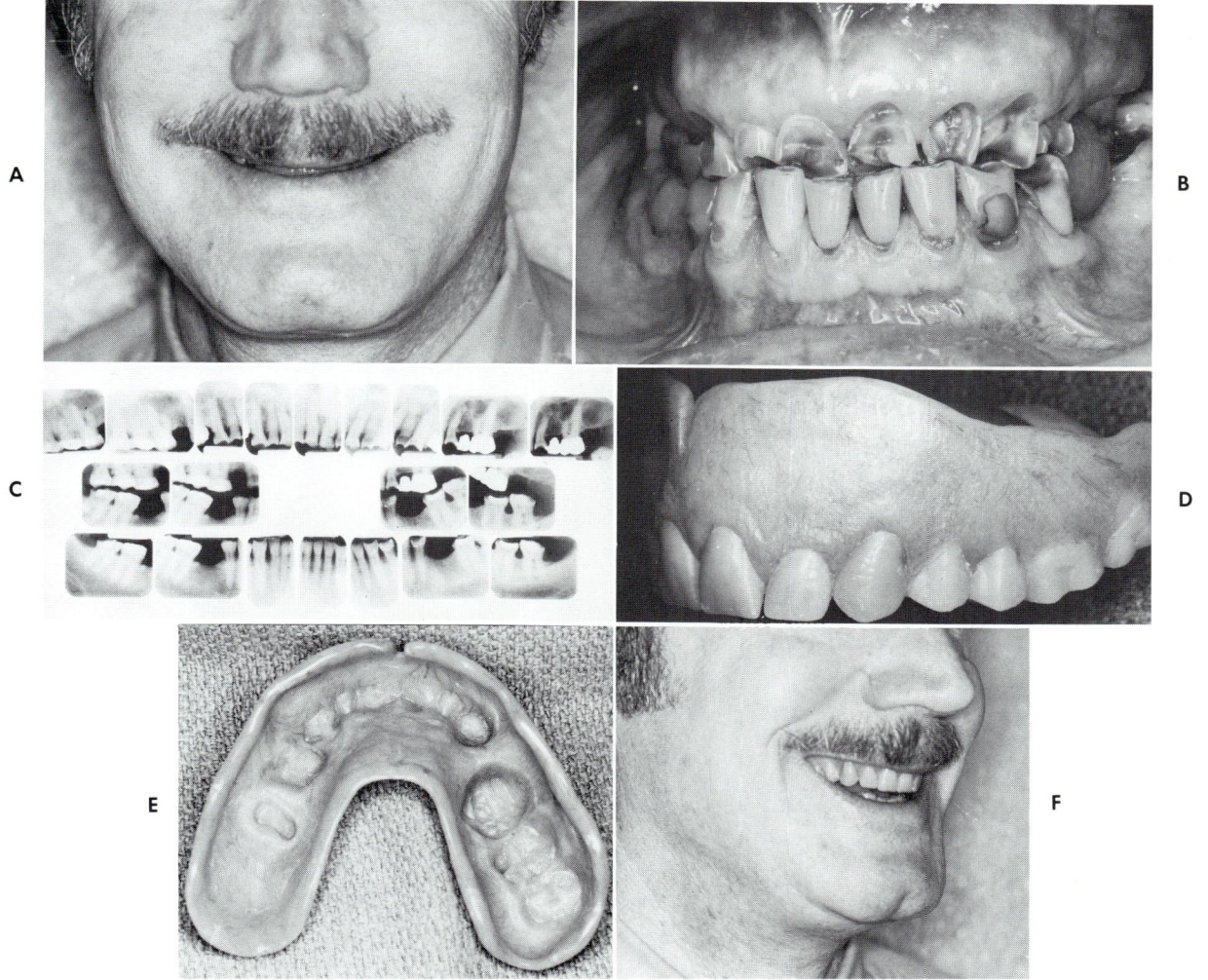

Fig. 8-18. **A**, Full-face view of patient with eroded teeth. **B**, Intraoral view of same patient. **C**, Complete mouth radiographs of same patient. **D**, Completed overdenture. **E**, Palate of overdenture has been cut out. **F**, Patient with completed overdenture in place.

after wearing an overdenture for 5 years. They are as healthy as they were when the denture was placed. No caries has developed nor has the periodontal condition deteriorated.

Fig. 8-18 shows a maxillary overdenture made for a 50-year-old man with teeth badly eroded by unknown causes. Here a roofless overdenture was made. A great deal was accomplished for this patient in a relatively simple and inexpensive manner.

REFERENCE

Brewer, A. A., and Fenton, A. H.: The overdenture, Dent. Clin. North Am. **17:**723-746, 1973.

9
TRANSITIONAL OVERDENTURES

ALLEN A. BREWER
ROBERT M. MORROW

A transitional overdenture, also known as an interim overdenture, is made from an existing removable partial denture, the patient's own teeth, or both. Stock teeth also can be used for the purpose. Frequently, the entire procedure can be accomplished while the patient waits, or part of it can be done before the extraction visit. The objective of this type of treatment is to do the most for the patient with the least trauma to all concerned: patient, dentist, and technician.

ADVANTAGES

Converting an existing prosthesis into an overdenture is less costly than constructing a conventional overdenture. In addition, the patient's previous experience with the partial denture usually permits a smooth transition to overdenture status and minimal interference with function and appearance.

DISADVANTAGES

Border extension, esthetics, occlusion, support, and stability of the removable partial denture often are inadequate, particularly after use for many years, and make satisfactory conversion difficult. Use of autopolymer resin frequently results in an overdenture that is weaker and more apt to break than one that has been processed. Therefore the converted prosthesis is considered as

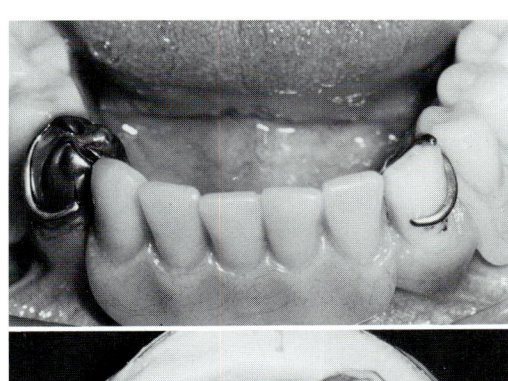

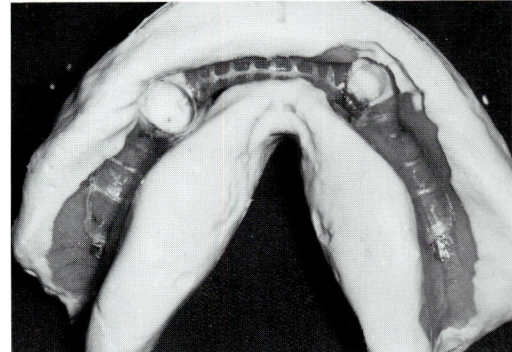

Fig. 9-1. **A,** Removable partial denture to be converted into transitional overdenture. Remaining teeth will be abutments for overdenture. **B,** Alginate irreversible hydrocolloid impression with partial denture.

a temporary or an interim overdenture, to be replaced after a suitable transition period.

CONVERSION USING DENTURE TEETH

Conversion usually necessitates the addition of teeth to the partial denture in increments before removal of the corresponding hopeless natural teeth.

Intermediate modifications

If numerous hopeless teeth remain, conversion can require several intermediate modifications. In this instance, resin denture teeth are added to the partial denture before the hopeless teeth are removed. The partial denture functions as an immediate prosthesis that can be converted into a transitional overdenture after adequate healing and endodontic treatment of abutments.

Conversion to a transitional overdenture

A removable partial denture is converted into an overdenture after endodontic treatment of the abutments (Fig. 9-1, A). An alginate impression is made of the arch with the partial denture in place.

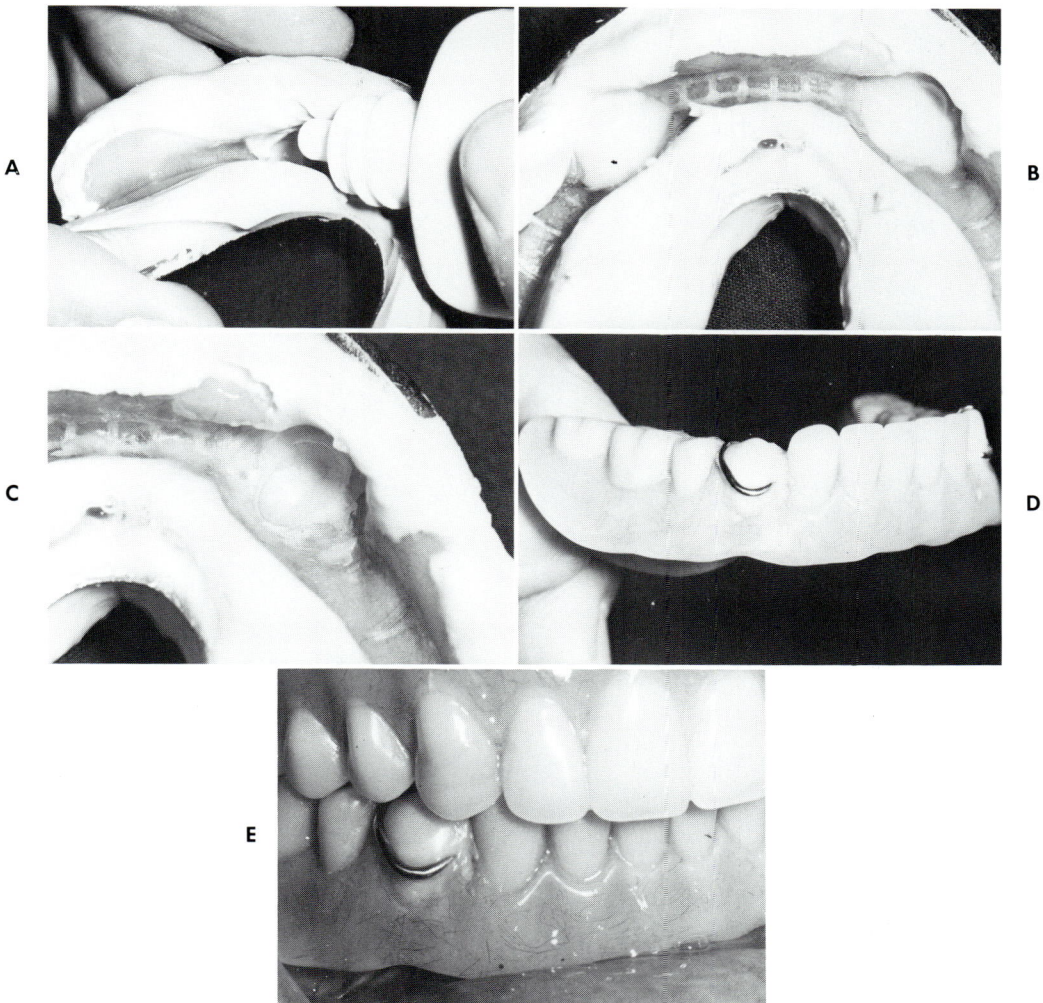

Fig. 9-2. **A,** Autopolymerizing resin of appropriate shade being sifted into abutment indentations. **B,** Autopolymerizing resin is saturated with monomer before reseating in mouth. **C,** Indentation of abutment in cured autopolymerizing resin. **D,** Flanges added to increase strength and retention of transitional overdenture. **E,** Occlusion being checked with transitional overdenture inserted.

After setting, the impression with the partial denture in it is removed (Fig. 9-1, *B*). The impression is placed in a humidor to prevent unnecessary drying and attendant dimensional changes during preparation of the abutment teeth.

The abutment teeth are prepared in the manner described for immediate overdentures, and incisal or occlusal amalgam restorations are placed if needed. Then the abutments are treated with a fluoride anticaries solution. Autopolymer resin* of

---
*Neopar, Miner Dental Products, Emeryville, Calif.

the proper shade is sifted into the abutment indentations of the alginate impression (Fig. 9-2, *A*). After saturation with monomer, the impression with the partial denture in place is seated in the mouth (Fig. 9-2, *B*). Before the resin is completely set, the impression is removed and placed in a water bath at 130° F. until curing of the resin is completed (Fig. 9-2, *C*). A stone cast is poured into the impression with the partial denture in place, and flanges are added with autopolymer resin (Fig. 9-2, *D*). The transitional overdenture is removed from the cast, polished, and tried in

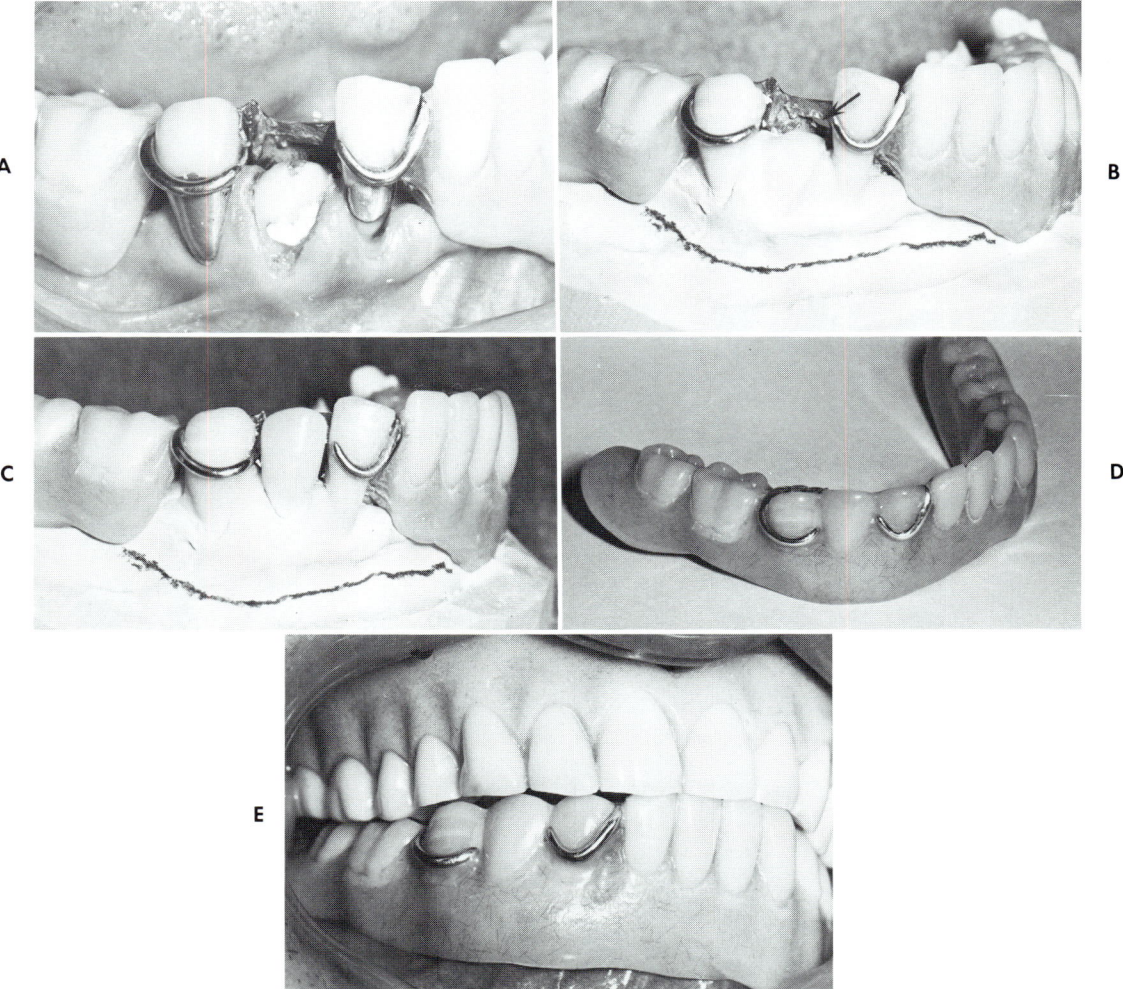

Fig. 9-3. **A**, Abutment tooth is prepared before making impression with alginate irreversible hydrocolloid. **B**, Removable partial denture on cast. A hole (arrow) is made in lingual plate of partial denture framework when additional retention for resin tooth is required. Clasped teeth are of autopolymerizing resin. **C**, Resin denture tooth is adapted to cast and attached with autopolymerizing resin. Line on cast indicates proposed extension of flange. **D**, Transitional overdenture ready for placement. **E**, Completed modification in place.

the mouth. The occlusion is checked, and necessary adjustments are made (Fig. 9-2, *E*).

Other modifications

Conversion procedures can be modified to meet existing requirements. One modification requires preparation of the abutment tooth before making an alginate impression of the arch (Fig. 9-3, *A*). Then the impression is made, and the partial denture is left in the impression. Indentations in the impression made by the teeth to be removed are filled with autopolymer resin of the correct shade, and a cast is poured into the impression (Fig. 9-3, *B*). Resin denture teeth are selected, hollowed, and adapted to the abutment teeth (Fig. 9-3, *C*). The cast is coated with tinfoil substitute, and flanges are added with autopolymer resin (Fig. 9-3, *D*). The remaining hopeless teeth are removed, and the transitional overdenture is inserted and subjected to the usual checks (Fig. 9-3, *E*).

TRANSITIONAL OVERDENTURE USING THE PATIENT'S TEETH

The patient derives a tremendous psychologic boost when he can enter the office and have his teeth removed, but leave 2 hours later with them still in his mouth, even though they are in an overdenture. This method is more economical than one requiring a conventional immediate denture.

Removable partial denture not present

A typical situation is one in which the six maxillary or mandibular anteriors are present (Fig. 9-4). The cuspids are treated endodontically, and the posteriors are extracted. An impression is made in a stock impression tray using irreversible hydrocolloid, and a cast is poured in stone. An occlusion rim is constructed over a resin sprinkle base. Care is taken to extend the rim to the necks of the remaining teeth to stabilize the baseplate adequately. The registration of maxillomandibular relativity is made and transferred to the articulator of choice with the opposing cast or denture. The posterior teeth are arranged and the teeth to be retained prepared on the cast. Resin teeth are hollow ground to cover these preparations (Fig. 9-5). The posterior teeth and the cuspids are secured to the base with autopolymer resin using the sprinkle method (Fig. 9-6). A matrix is formed over the remaining teeth to relate them to the temporary denture (Fig. 9-7).

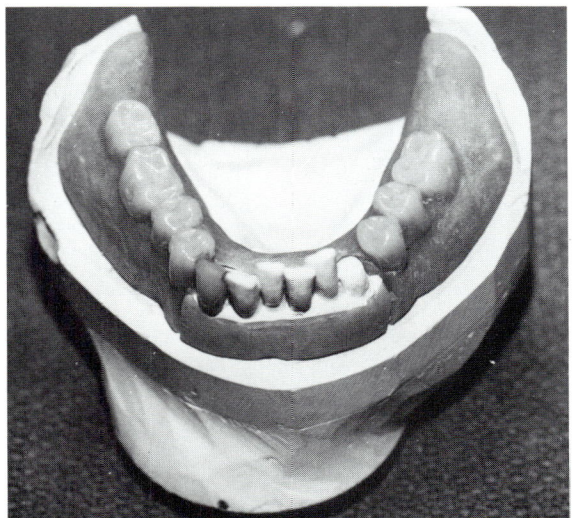

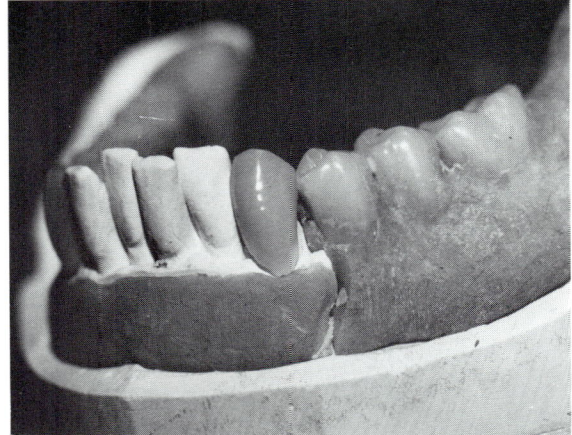

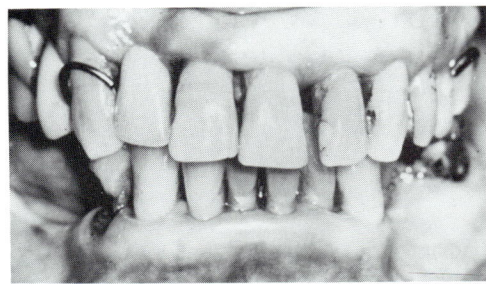

Fig. 9-4. Preoperative view of patient to receive transitional overdentures.

Fig. 9-5. Posterior teeth arranged and teeth to be retained being prepared on cast. Resin teeth are hollow ground to cover these preparations.

92 METHODS

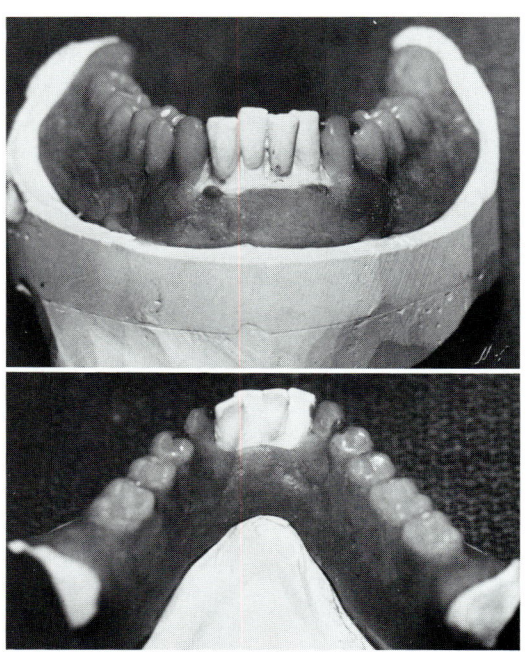

Fig. 9-6. Hollow-ground cuspids positioned and posterior teeth attached to base with autopolymerizing resin.

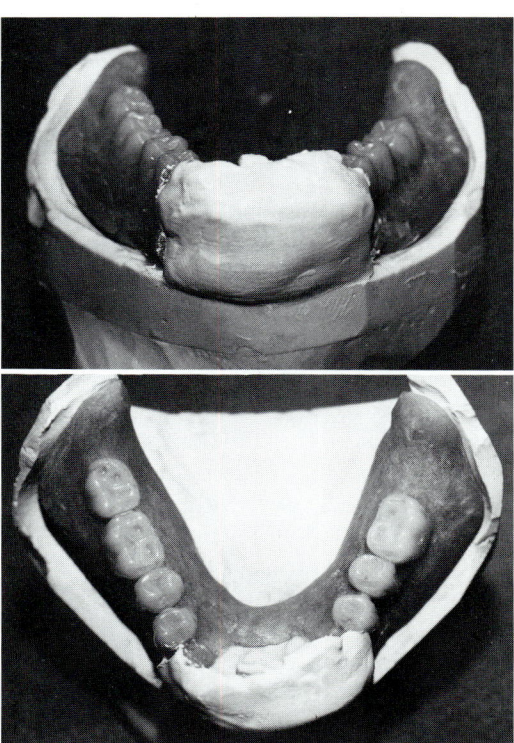

Fig. 9-7. Stone matrix formed to relate patient's teeth to denture.

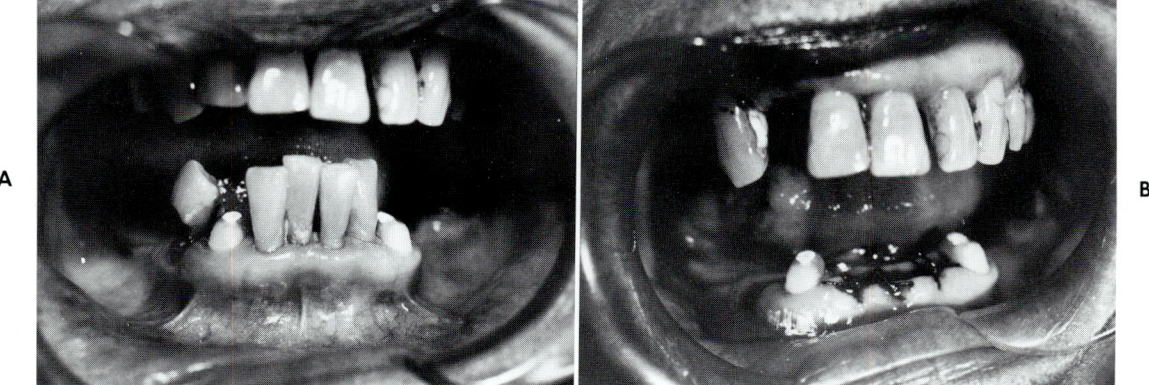

Fig. 9-8. A, Patient's cuspids have been reduced. **B,** Incisors are extracted after reduction of cuspids.

TRANSITIONAL OVERDENTURES 93

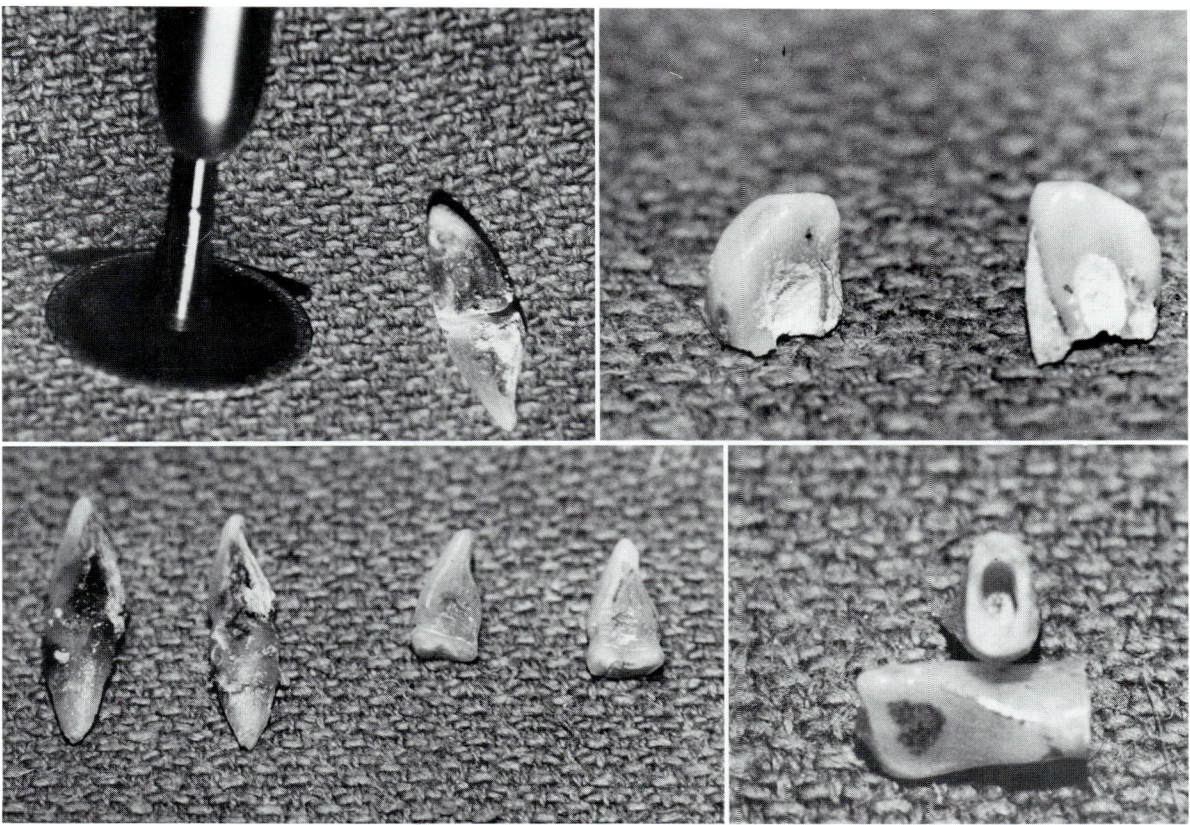

Fig. 9-9. Roots are cut off remaining teeth, and diatorics are cut in crowns.

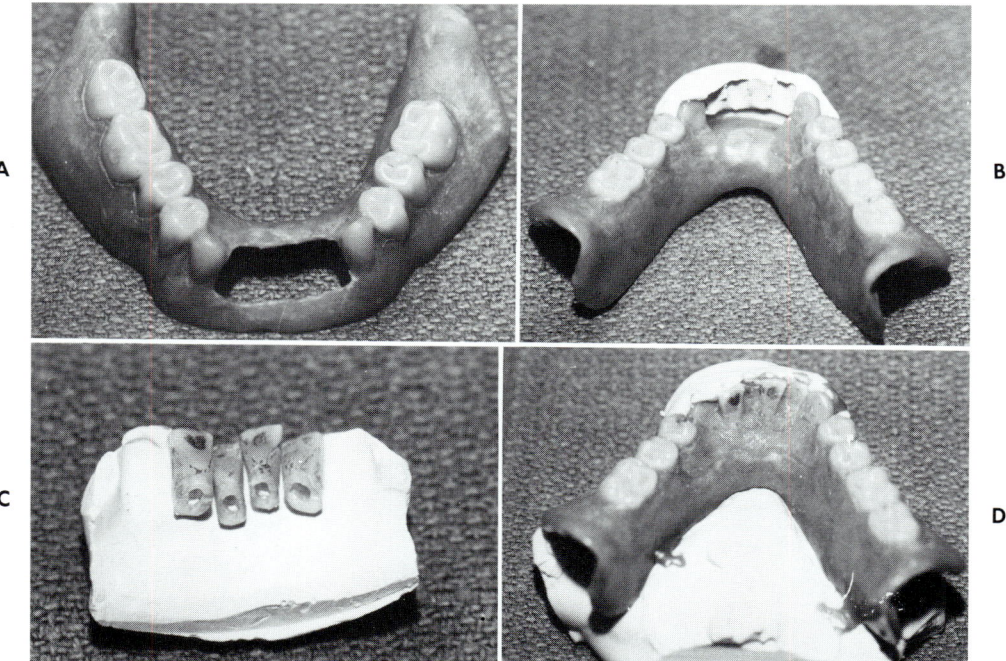

Fig. 9-10. A, Denture base is ready for placement in mouth after extraction. Impression is made over extraction site. **B,** Stone matrix is in position. **C,** Prepared extracted teeth are related to cast and denture base through matrix. **D,** Prepared extracted teeth are joined to base with autopolymerizing resin.

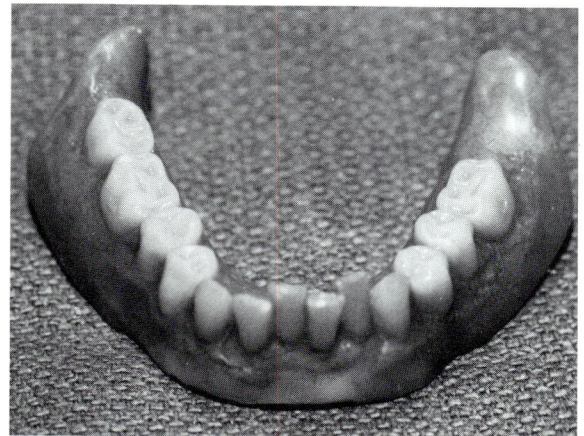

Fig. 9-11. Completed transitional overdenture after polishing.

During the extraction sitting, the teeth to be lost are removed after preparing the cuspids in the same manner as on the cast (Fig. 9-8). An impression of this area is made in irreversible hydrocolloid with the temporary denture in place, and then the area is cast in stone. The roots of the extracted teeth are cut off, and the diatorics are cut into the pulp chamber (Fig. 9-9). These teeth are related to the denture through the matrix and attached with autopolymer resin using the sprinkle technique (Fig. 9-10). The transitional overdenture is finished, polished, and fitted to the mouth with disclosing wax (Fig. 9-11). The patient leaves the office with his own teeth in the same position as before except that they are in the overdenture (Fig. 9-12).

Removable partial denture present

At the first visit an impression is made of the arch in a stock tray using irreversible hydrocolloid. If the tray does not fit properly, it is modified with impression compound. Wax is not recommended

TRANSITIONAL OVERDENTURES 95

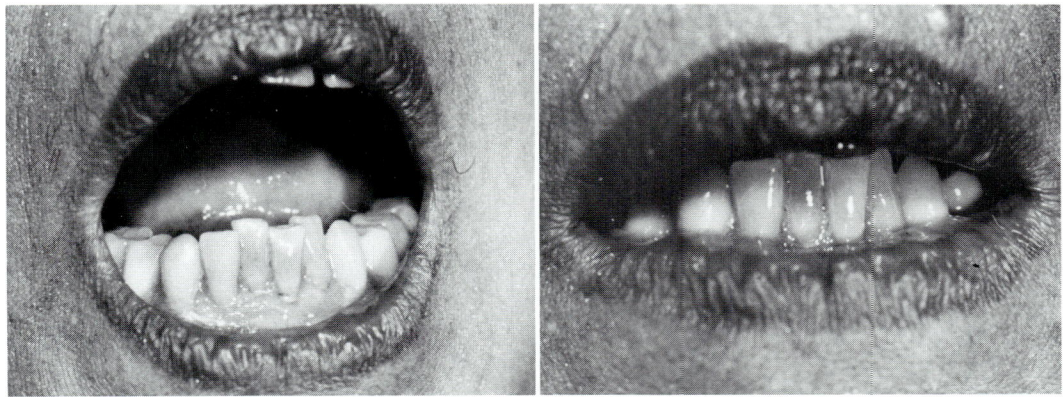

Fig. 9-12. Completed transitional overdenture after insertion.

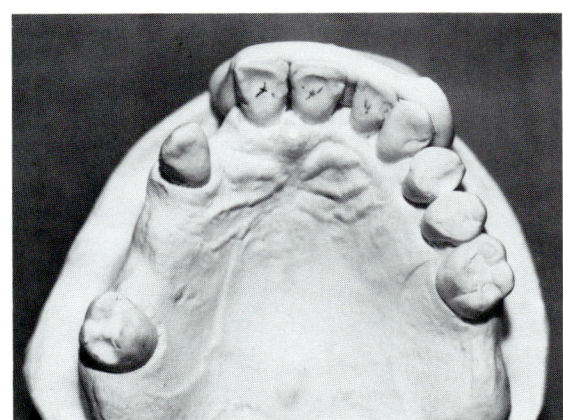

Fig. 9-13. Stone matrix on cast.

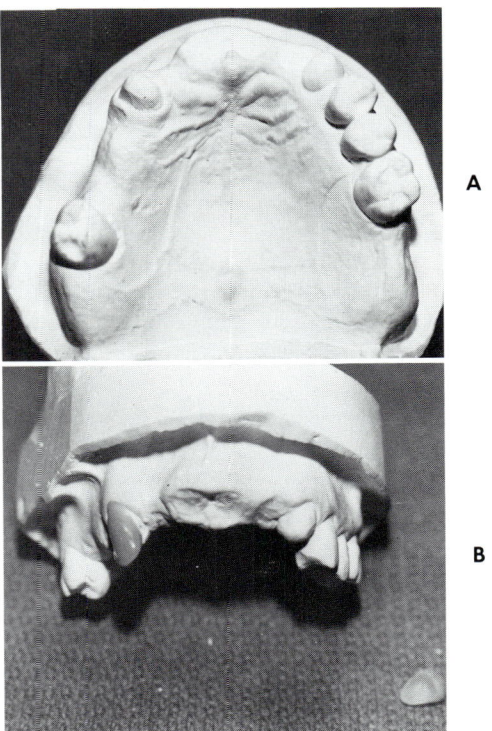

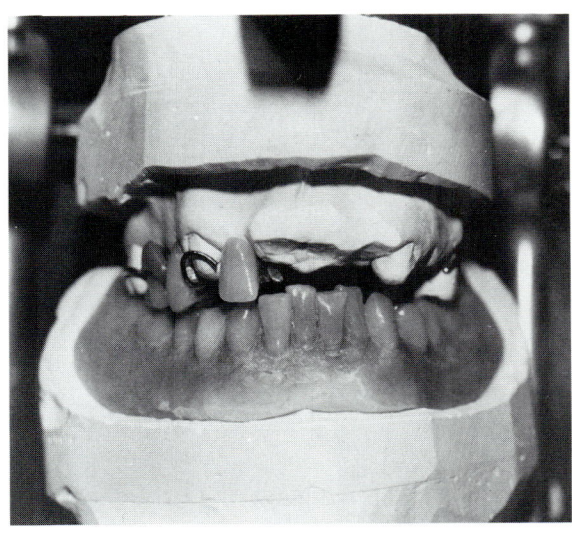

Fig. 9-14. Existing removable partial denture seated on cast.

Fig. 9-15. A, Teeth to be retained are prepared on cast. B, Resin teeth are hollow ground to fit over preparations.

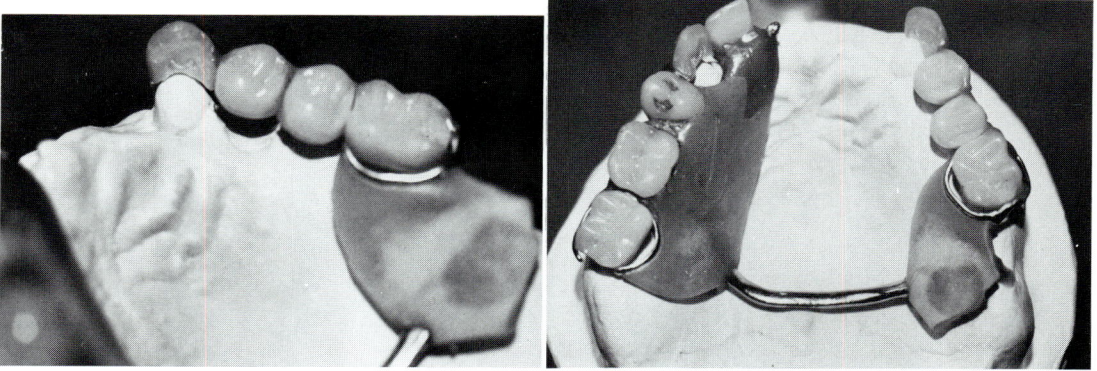

Fig. 9-16. Denture teeth adapted over prepared teeth and extraction sites.

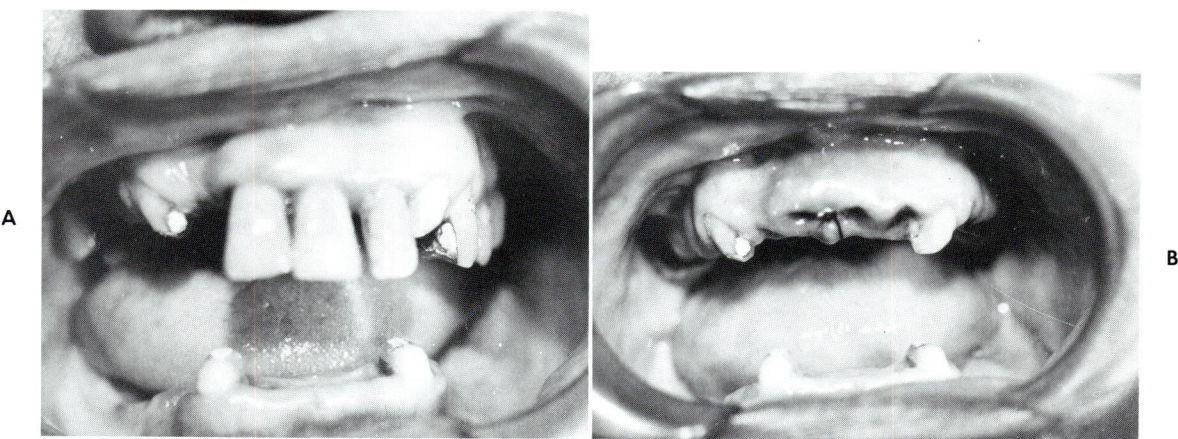

Fig. 9-17. Teeth to be retained are reduced prior to extractions. **A,** Before extraction. **B,** After extraction.

for this alteration because of possible separation of the alginate from the wax. A stone cast is poured, and a stone matrix is formed to relate the existing teeth to the cast (Fig. 9-13). Then the existing removable partial denture is seated on the cast (Fig. 9-14). The teeth to be extracted are cut from the cast; those to be retained are prepared on the cast, and resin teeth are hollow ground to fit over these preparations (Fig. 9-15). Stock resin teeth are used to replace the posterior teeth that will be extracted (Fig. 9-16).

At the second sitting the teeth to be retained are reduced as they were on the cast, and the rest of the teeth are extracted (Fig. 9-17). Those extracted are prepared as described earlier in the procedures for making a transitional immediate overdenture in the absence of an existing removable partial denture. Then these teeth are related to the partial and the cast through the matrix. The cast is coated with tinfoil substitute. The teeth are attached with autopolymer resin using the sprinkle method. Border extensions for the overdenture are formed in the same manner (Fig. 9-18). The overdenture is cured in a pressure pot, released from the cast, finished, and polished (Fig. 9-19). On insertion, disclosing wax is used to locate areas of impingement needing correction. If the discrepancy is too great, the denture can be refitted immediately with a tissue-conditioning material, such as Coe Comfort* or Hydrocast† tissue conditioner, or relined with a self-curing reliner material.

---

*Coe Laboratories, Chicago.
†Kay See Dental Manufacturing Co., Kansas City, Mo.

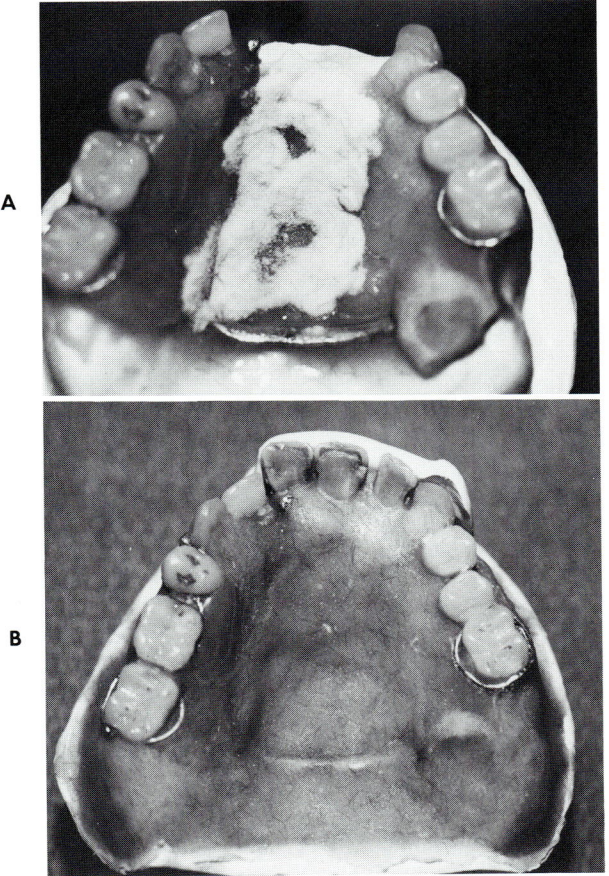

Fig. 9-18. **A**, Units are joined by autopolymerizing resin with sprinkle method. **B**, Balance of denture base is formed in same manner.

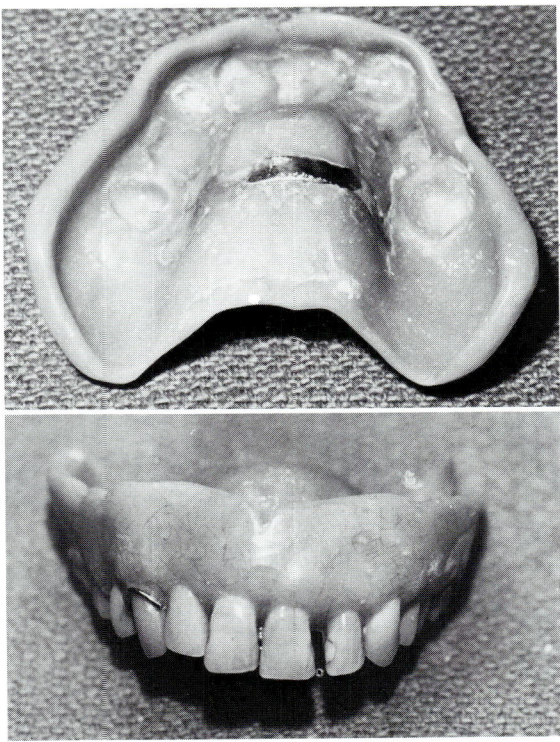

Fig. 9-19. Completed transitional overdenture after polishing.

The natural teeth in these transitional overdentures may change color, become brittle, and be subject to fracture. However, some of our patients wear them for as long as a year before remote overdentures are made. Transitional overdentures can be retained for emergency use.

POSTINSERTION CARE

The majority of patients experience minimal postinsertion difficulty with the transitional overdentures. Some miss the positive retention afforded by clasps, although it is seldom a serious problem. Oral hygiene instructions are provided, and a series of postinsertion visits is scheduled for regular maintenance and service throughout the transitional overdenture period. Usually the transitional prosthesis is replaced by a more definitive overdenture after 8 months to a year. At this time gold copings can be placed on the abutments if desired, and the transitional overdenture can be adapted to the new contours of the abutment teeth with autopolymer resin. Use of the transitional overdenture by the patient during construction of a new overdenture enables the dentist to initiate this type of treatment at minimal cost and with the least interference with function.

10

IMMEDIATE OVERDENTURES

ROBERT M. MORROW

An overdenture is a complete denture fabricated over retained teeth or roots and the residual ridge (Lord and Teel, 1969). An immediate overdenture is an overdenture constructed for insertion immediately after the removal of natural teeth. It may be used as an interim prosthesis.

The majority of overdenture techniques include most of the following procedures: (1) selection of teeth to serve as abutments, (2) removal of hopeless teeth, (3) periodontic treatment of abutments, (4) endodontic treatment of abutments, (5) placement of an immediate interim prosthesis, (6) preparation and cementation of cast gold copings or attachments or both on abutments, and (7) construction of an overdenture, sometimes requiring special attachments or castings over restored abutments. These procedures, which lengthen the period of treatment and significantly increase the cost, can discourage the use of overdentures, particularly when the prognosis is equivocal. Therefore removal of the few retainable teeth and construction of conventional complete dentures may be preferable to avoid possible early failure of an overdenture after such extensive preparatory treatment. The immediate overdenture may be a more conservative approach in this situation, for it enables a dentist to use a simplified construction technique that allows flexibility in planning treatment as requirements change. In many instances, especially in the presence of good oral hygiene practices and regular professional supervision, an immediate overdenture may have a long service life. At other times an immediate overdenture can be an interim prosthesis that serves as a prognostic aid before a more comprehensive overdenture procedure. However, if response to the treatment is poor and failure of the abutments is imminent, an immediate overdenture can be converted to a serviceable complete denture.

ADVANTAGES OF IMMEDIATE OVERDENTURES

Overdentures demonstrate increased support and stability afforded by natural teeth retained as abutments, preserve residual ridges by retention of natural teeth, and usually receive favorable response from the patient. Immediate overdentures have additional advantages, since minimal discomfort and interference with function usually characterize the postoperative course, the construction technique is relatively simple, and modification to permit relining or other adjustments is comparatively easy. A major advantage of the immediate overdenture when it is used as an interim prosthesis is that it allows the dentist ample opportunity to evaluate the response of the abutments and supporting tissues to an overdenture and to observe the effect of corrective oral hygiene procedures. Therefore the immediate overdenture, which is made with ease and which uses no specialized castings in the denture or on the abutments, is a reliable prognostic aid and a prerequisite to the more sophisticated overdenture techniques.

DISADVANTAGES OF IMMEDIATE OVERDENTURES

Immediate overdentures, being made of conventional denture base resins, are not as strong as those reinforced with metal castings and are more prone to breakage. However, improved construction techniques and better materials (discussed later) can compensate for these disadvantages to some extent.

CLINICAL PROCEDURES
Examination and diagnosis

The patient with numerous hopeless teeth should be examined carefully to select the teeth to be retained as abutments for the immediate overdenture. Patient and abutment selection are discussed in Chapter 4.

Pretreatment records

When a proposed immediate overdenture is opposed by a natural dentition or by another overdenture, pretreatment measurements between selected index points are recorded. One measurement is made from the gingival margin of an abutment or tooth to an opposing abutment or tooth with the patient's teeth in the closed position (Fig. 10-1, *A*). The information is entered in the patient's dental record for later use after the last vertical stops are removed during abutment preparation (Fig. 10-1, *B* and *C*). Although some gingival retraction can occur after preparation, pretreatment measurements between retained teeth are effective guides in reestablishing the vertical dimension of occlusion during later appointments. Diagnostic casts are obtained and can be supplemented with photographs and profile registrations.

Treatment planning

When planning treatment, achieving the most effective use of time and materials is a primary aim. Careful planning and scheduling reduce undesirable delays between various phases of treat-

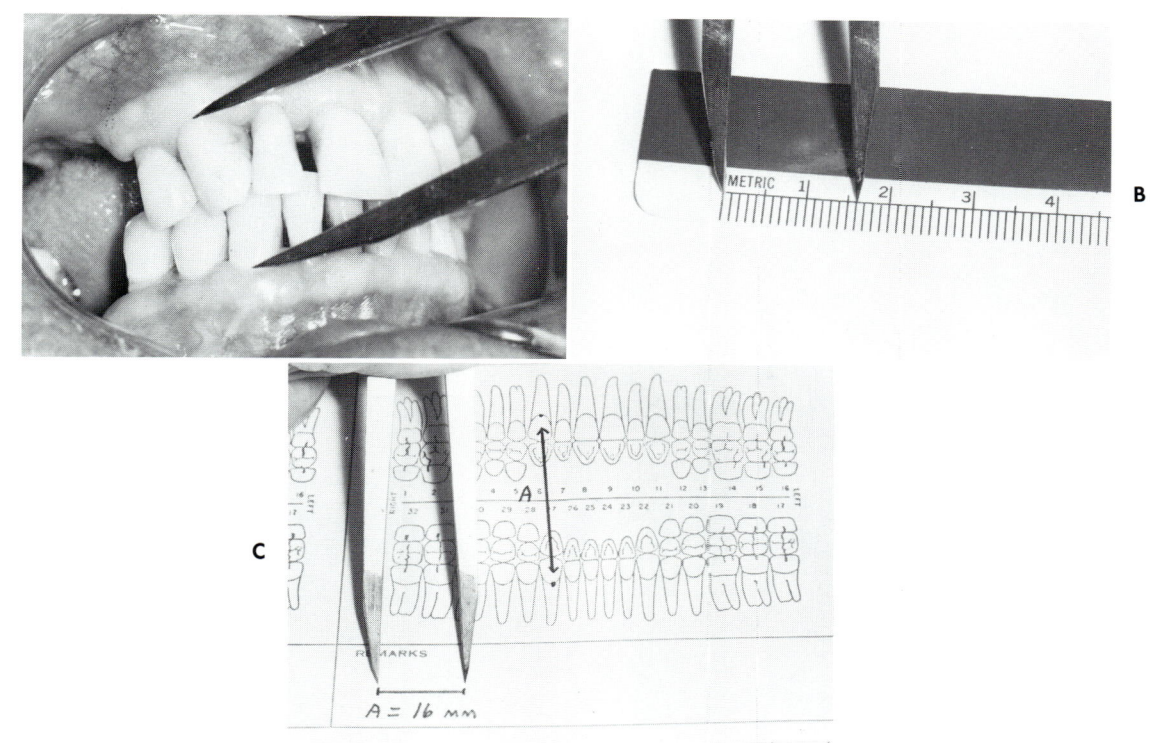

Fig. 10-1. **A,** Dividers are used to record distance between an abutment tooth and an opposing tooth that is to be retained. **B,** Measurement is made with a millimeter ruler. **C,** Measurement is recorded in patient's file for future use.

102 METHODS

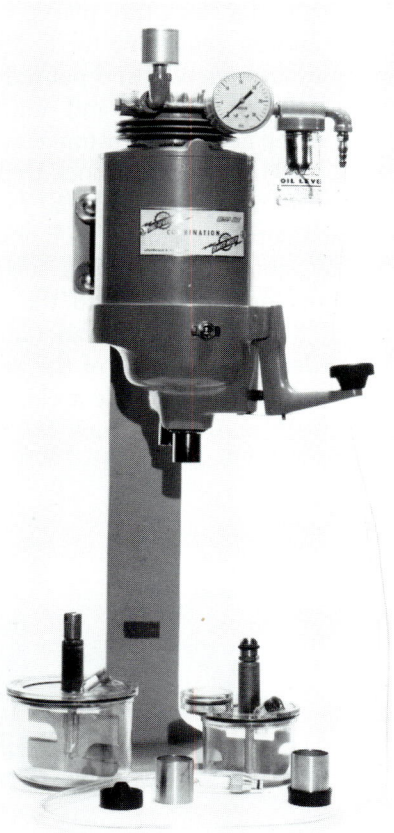

Fig. 10-5. Combination Vac-U-Vestor and power mixer aids in producing smooth, bubble-free mixes of stone and alginate impression materials. (Courtesy Whip-Mix Corp., Louisville.)

loid is used to make the final impression. An adhesive* prevents separation of the alginate impression material from the impression compound. Cotton fibers embedded in the warmed surface of the impression compound serve the same purpose (Fig. 10-4, *C*). The embedded fibers are flamed to produce a stubble for retention (Fig. 10-4, *D*).

Alginate impression material is proportioned by weight and mixed with the recommended volume of distilled water. The combination Vac-U-Vestor and power mixer, a mechanical spatulator, combines the impression material with the water under reduced atmospheric pressure, thus producing a smooth, bubble-free mix (Fig. 10-5). The tray is loaded, and, to minimize voids, alginate is applied to the teeth with a finger before the tray is seated. After setting, the impression is removed, examined, and, if acceptable, poured in artificial stone (Fig. 10-6). Cast surfaces are improved by using compatible alginate impression material and artificial stone combinations (Morrow and co-workers, 1971).

Pouring the cast. A two-stage procedure is used in pouring the impression. The first pour includes the anatomic portions of the impression (Fig. 10-7). The impression with the stone is placed in a tray holder, allowed to set, then immersed in clear slurry water† for a few minutes. Then a second

---
*Hold, William Getz Dental Products, Inc., Long Island City, N. Y.
†Tap water to which stone chips or particles are added and allowed to set for 48 hours. The resultant solution does not affect the surface of the casts adversely.

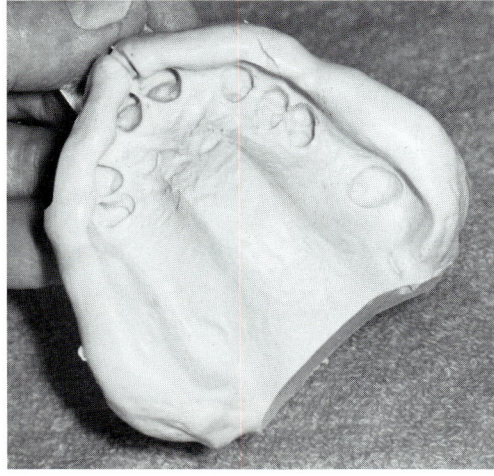

Fig. 10-6. Impression is examined carefully to determine acceptability.

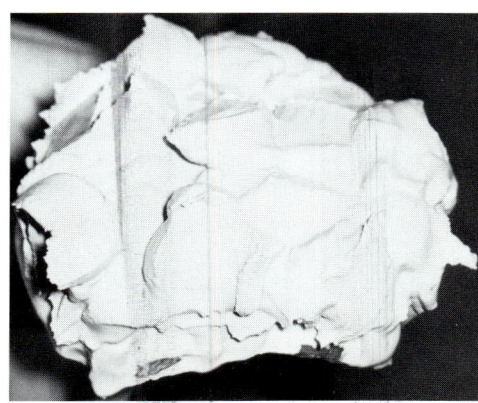

Fig. 10-7. First pour of stone should have undercuts to prevent separation of base.

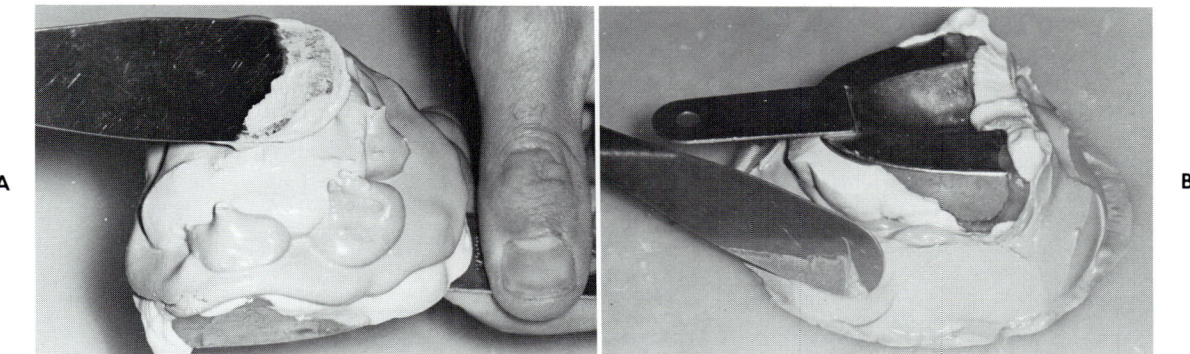

Fig. 10-8. A, Base is added to first pour, and spatula is used to place stone in undercut areas. **B,** Tray is inverted into stone and allowed to set. Impression should be separated from cast within an hour.

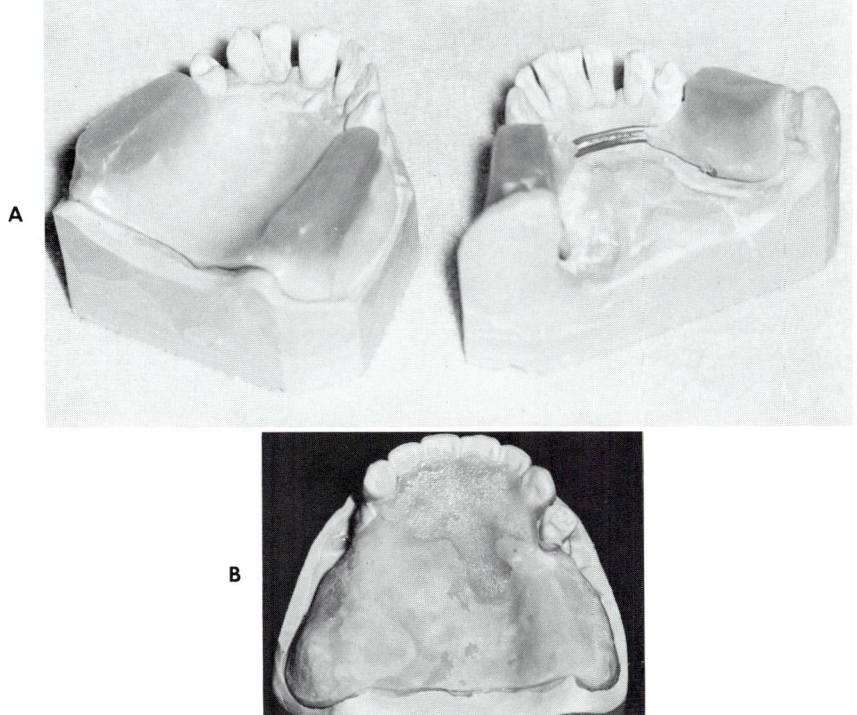

Fig. 10-9. A, Baseplates and occlusion rims are essential when too few teeth remain to assemble casts accurately. **B,** When space permits, maxillary baseplate should be extended onto lingual surfaces of remaining anterior teeth. This procedure improves stability and support of baseplate and results in accurate jaw relation records.

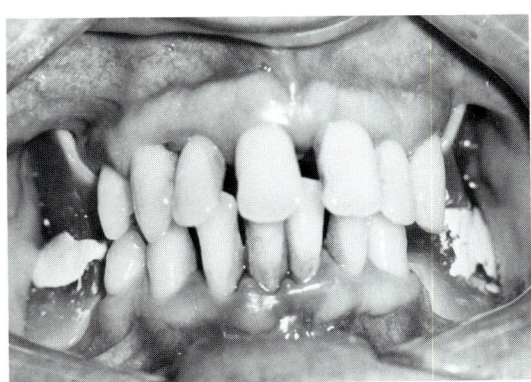 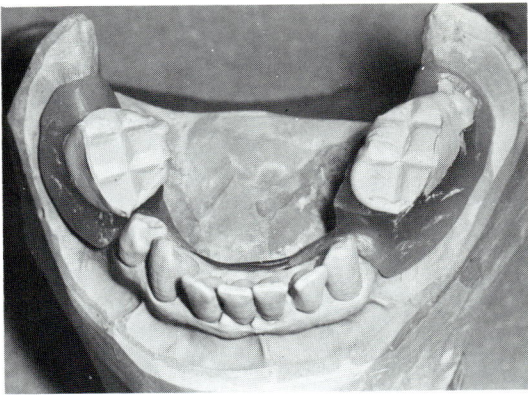

Fig. 10-10. Zinc oxide impression paste gives a firm, sharp record and facilitates accurate cast relation.

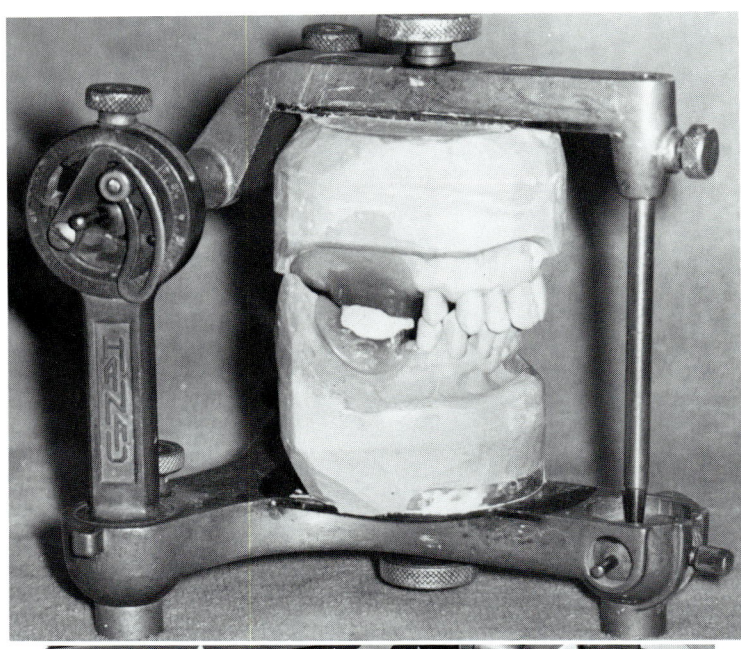

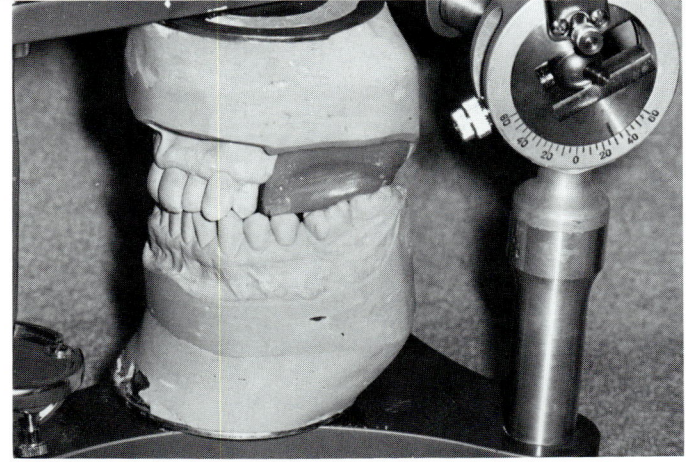

Fig. 10-11. Casts are mounted in suitable articulator.

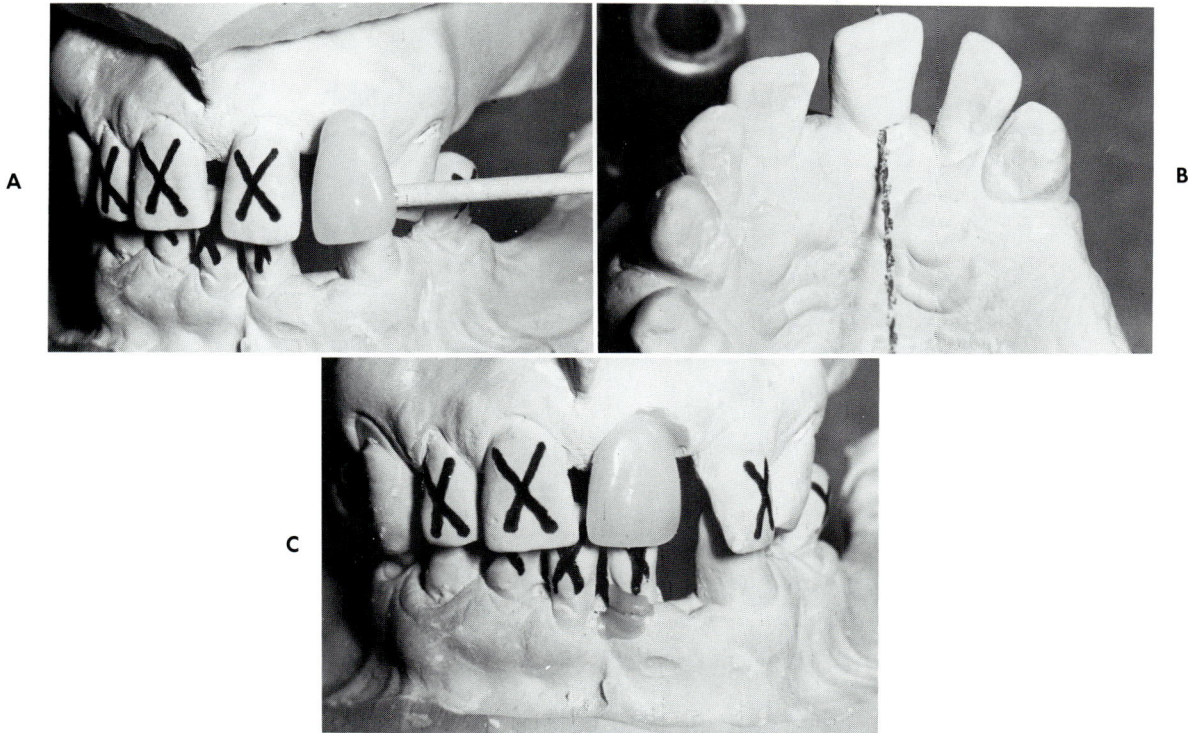

Fig. 10-12. **A,** Resin denture teeth of apppropriate shade and mold are selected by using cast as a guide. **B,** Tooth is removed from cast with a saw in same manner as conventional immediate dentures. **C,** Replacement tooth is waxed into position.

mix of artificial stone is poured for the base (Fig. 10-8). The impression is separated from the cast within an hour.

Jaw relation records

The cast is indexed and, when not enough teeth are present for orienting the casts, baseplates are fabricated to facilitate recording jaw relationships (Fig. 10-9). Interocclusal records can be made with wax, zinc oxide impression paste, or slurry-activated artificial stone* (Fig. 10-10). It is essential that jaw relation records obtained in this manner be checked for accuracy before mounting casts. The casts are mounted in an articulator with slurry-activated artificial stone. A face-bow transfer facilitates the mounting of the maxillary cast in the articulator. A semiadjustable articulator is adequate for constructing interim overdentures (Fig. 10-11).

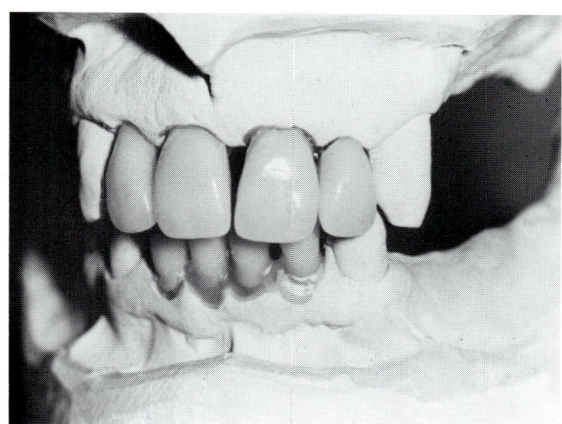

Fig. 10-13. All anterior teeth except abutments are replaced.

---

*Artificial stone mixed with stone slurry, a thick liquid made by grinding stone casts on a cast trimmer.

CONSTRUCTING THE OVERDENTURE
Selecting and positioning teeth

The technique for constructing the immediate overdenture is a modification of the methods described by Lord and Teel (1969), Brewer and Fenton (1973), and Morrow and co-workers (1973). Denture teeth of the appropriate mold and shade are selected and positioned by removing one tooth on the cast and substituting the corresponding replacement for comparison (Fig. 10-12). Resin teeth are used over each abutment and in areas adjacent to abutments to minimize breakage of the denture in service; porcelain teeth can be used elsewhere if desired. All teeth except those serving as abutments are replaced by denture teeth (Fig. 10-13). Anatomic or nonanatomic posterior occlusal schemes can be used to complete the setup as the situation requires. Next the abutment teeth on the cast are prepared. Each abutment tooth is shortened to a height of 3 to 4 mm., and the axial surfaces are tapered to remove undercuts and create space for the denture tooth replacement (Fig. 10-14); the reduction should be sufficient to make the resin thick enough. Reduction of the abutment on the cast should be less than anticipated for the natural tooth, which is prepared at the time of insertion. Resin denture teeth of the proper size and shade are hollowed with a No. 8 bur, positioned over the cast preparation, and waxed to place (Fig. 10-15). The posterior palatal seal is placed on the cast prior to completion of the setup.

Waxing and flasking

The denture is waxed and flasked in a conventional manner, and the wax is eliminated with boiling water to which a detergent is added. A final flushing with clean boiling water removes all traces of wax and detergent. Careful flasking and pack-

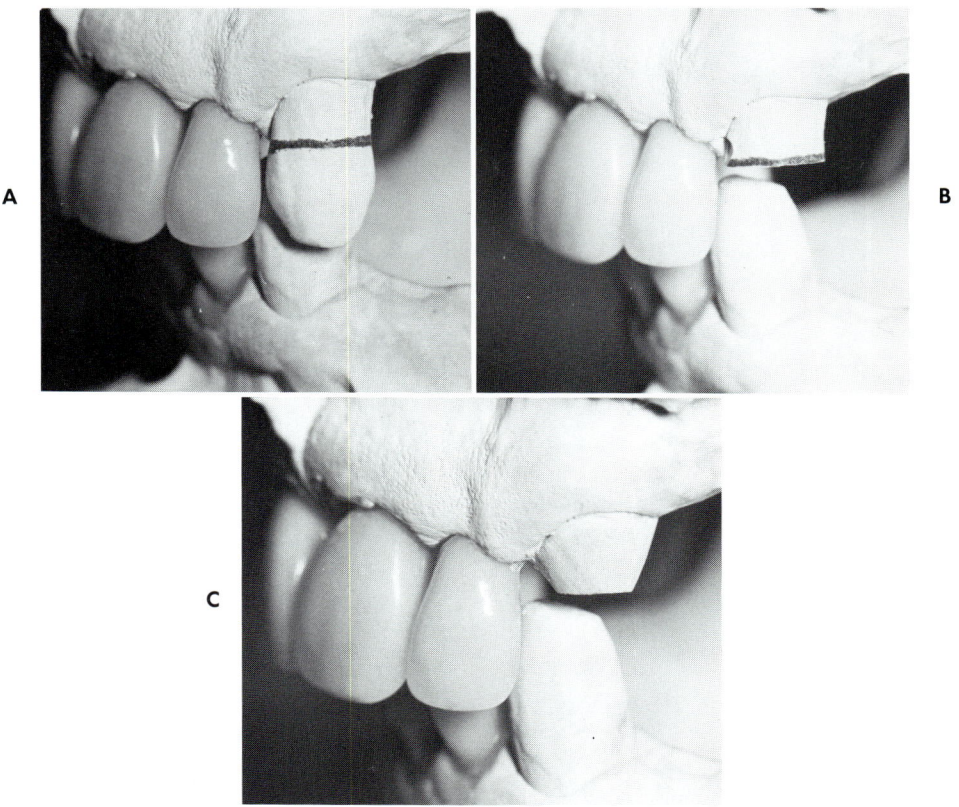

Fig. 10-14. **A,** Line indicates how much abutment tooth on cast should be shortened. **B,** Abutment on casts is shortened with a bur or saw. **C,** Abutment preparation on cast.

IMMEDIATE OVERDENTURES 107

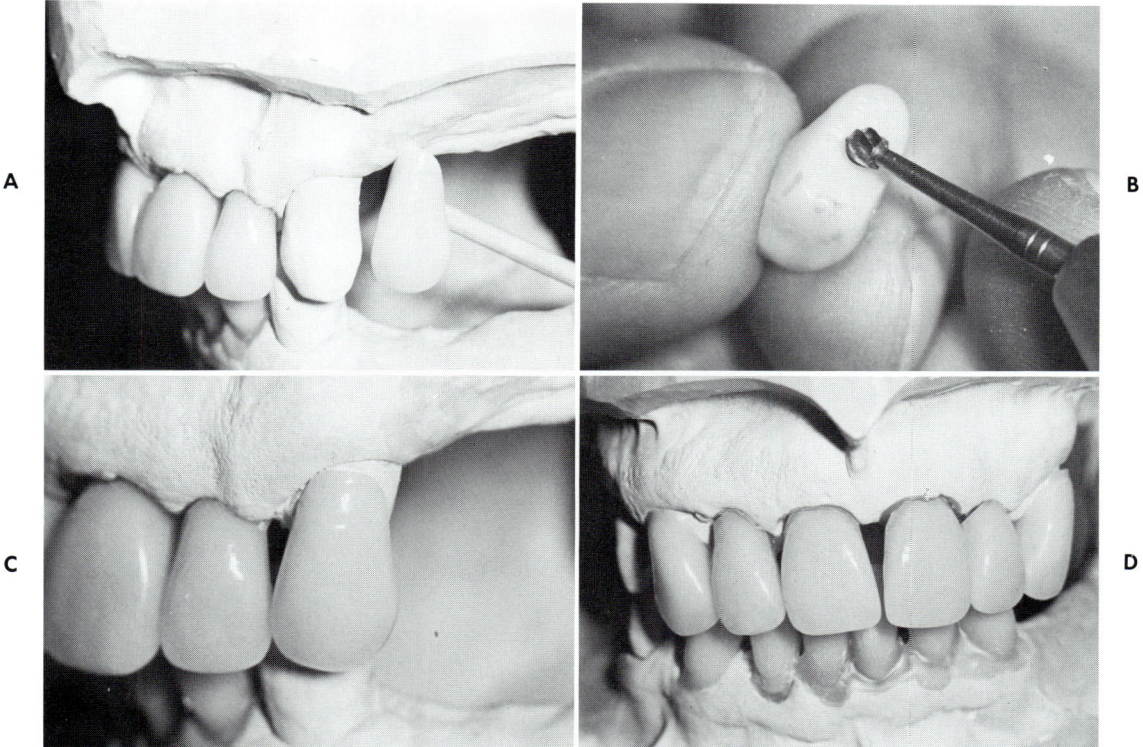

Fig. 10-15. **A,** Resin denture tooth is selected for positioning over cast preparation. **B,** Resin denture tooth is hollowed with a No. 8 bur. **C,** Resin denture tooth waxed into position on cast. **D,** Completed anterior setup.

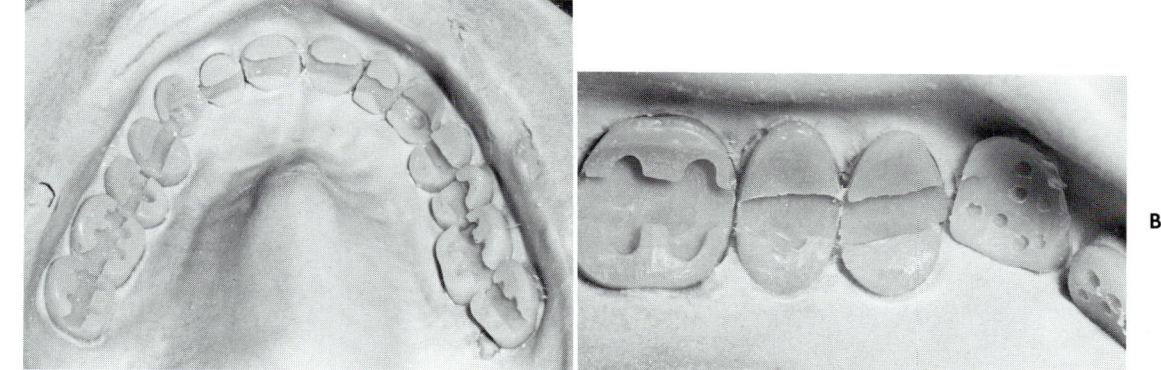

Fig. 10-16. **A,** Ridge laps of resin denture teeth are indexed to improve bonding of teeth to denture base. **B,** Retention grooves in posterior teeth are 1 to 2 mm. deep.

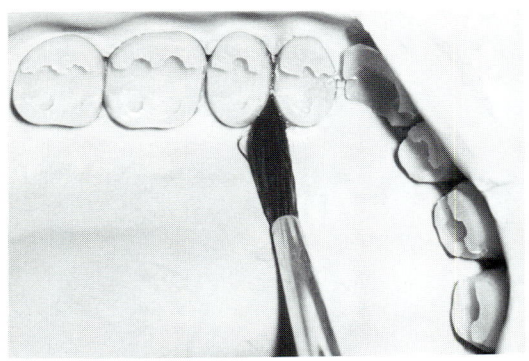

Fig. 10-17. Care should be taken to prevent placing tinfoil substitute on denture teeth ridge laps.

ing procedures significantly reduce "processing error" in the cured overdenture (Rudd, 1964).

Packing the overdenture

Retentive grooves placed in the ridge laps of the denture teeth increase the area available for physical and chemical bonding and secure the teeth to the base more firmly (Fig. 10-16). The "glaze" should also be removed from the ridge lap surface of plastic denture teeth. Treatment of these surfaces by painting with a gel made from denture base resin monomer and polymer also contributes to retention of denture teeth. The gel is made by placing ⅛ inch of polymer in a 6 oz. bottle and filling the bottle with monomer. This is allowed to set for two weeks, after which the resultant gel is ready for use. A thin coat of the gel is painted on the ridge lap of the denture teeth before packing. The stone surfaces are coated with

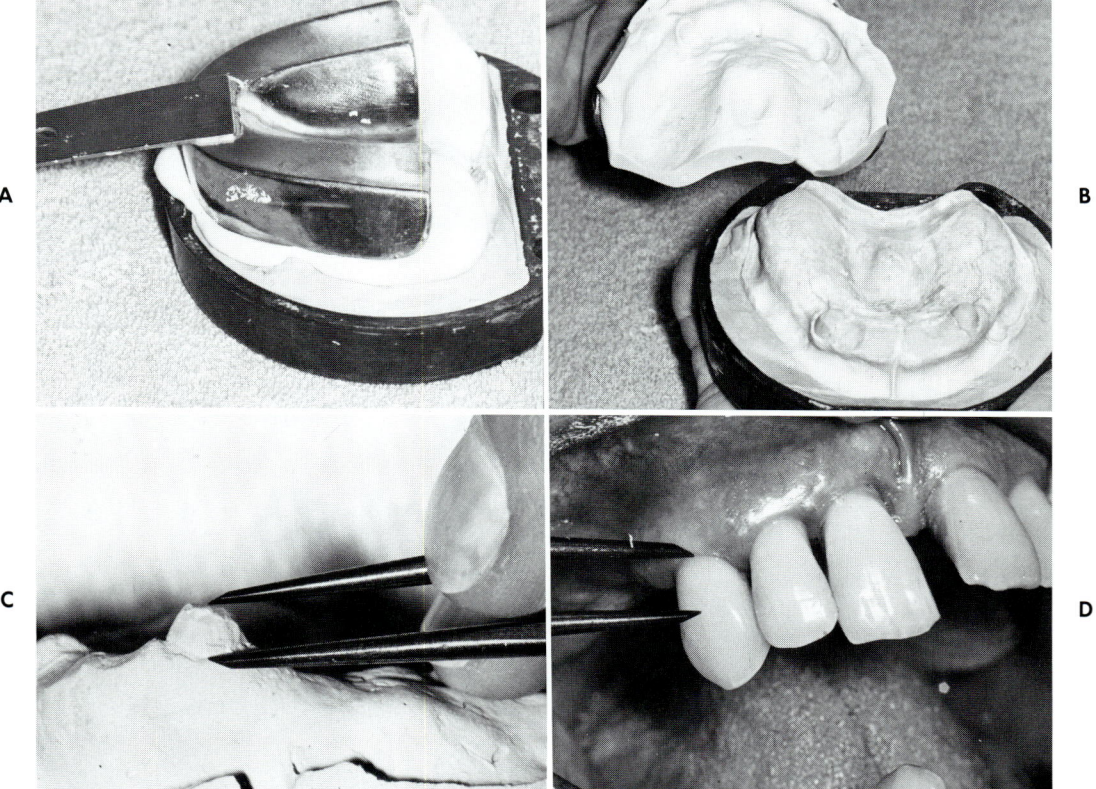

Fig. 10-18. **A,** Alginate impression is made of cast in flask. **B,** Impression is separated. **C,** Abutment height is measured on cast and used as guide during preparation of abutment for patient. **D,** Measurement indicates how much abutment should be shortened.

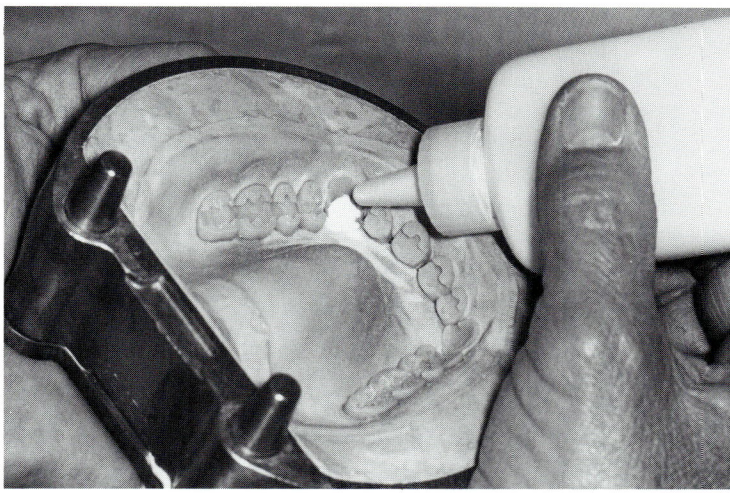

Fig. 10-19. Tooth-colored heat-curing resin of appropriate shade is sifted into hollowed-out abutment tooth in flask.

a tinfoil substitute, and care is taken to avoid putting the tinfoil substitute on the ridge laps of the teeth (Fig. 10-17); this procedure is important to prevent dislodging denture teeth after processing. An impression of the flasked cast is made from alginate in a stock tray, and it is poured in stone. The resultant cast is used as a reference guide in preparing the patient's abutment teeth before insertion of the denture (Fig. 10-18). At this time the overdenture bases can be tinted to give a better esthetic effect. Tooth-colored heat-curing resin is sifted into the hollowed-out denture teeth over the abutments and saturated with monomer (Fig. 10-19).

Conventional heat-curing denture base resins can be used for the overdenture; however, newer "high-impact" resins* with their improved physical properties can result in stronger, breakage-resistant dentures. The resin is proportioned and mixed according to the manufacturer's recommendations, and plastic gloves are used while packing to prevent contamination of the resin (Fig. 10-20). Plastic film or cellophane sheets are placed, and the filled flasks are closed slowly during the initial closure to give the resin ample time to flow throughout the mold. Trial packing is repeated until metal-to-metal contact of the flask halves is ob-

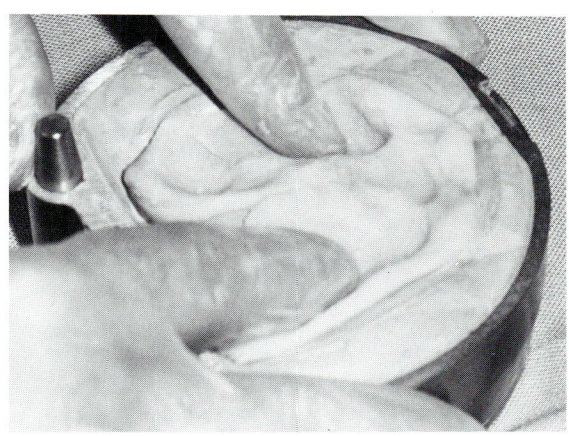

Fig. 10-20. Plastic gloves are used to pack denture base resin to prevent contamination.

tained. The overdenture is cured for the cycle appropriate for the resin selected. Then the overdentures are bench cooled, removed from the flask, and remounted on the articulator (Fig. 10-21). After any processing change has been corrected, the overdentures are removed and polished.

Finishing and polishing

Of the many techniques for finishing and polishing dentures, we have found one that is both simple and effective for overdentures. When the overdenture is taken from the cast, it is placed in the

---

*Hircoe, Coe Laboratories, Inc., Chicago, or Lucitone 199, The L. D. Caulk Co., Milford, Del.

appropriate solution in an ultrasonic cleaner to remove any plaster or stone still present. Usually the denture will be plaster-free in 3 or 4 minutes. The overdenture borders are trimmed with a lathe-mounted arbor band to the desired thickness (Fig. 10-22). If the immediate overdenture is made on a cast from an alginate impression without border molding, the flanges generally require recontouring.

A slurry of flour of pumice and a lathe-mounted rag wheel are used to polish the borders and other accessible areas of the overdenture. A handpiece with a rubber cup is used with flour of pumice in less accessible areas of the denture (Fig. 10-23). In this manner, the surface is polished without obliterating the carefully carved anatomic features of the denture base. A stippled surface can be created by etching the denture surface lightly with a finishing bur* (Fig. 10-24). A high polish is obtained with a clean fluffy lathe-mounted rag wheel

---

*Finishing bur No. 200, S. S. White Co., Philadelphia.

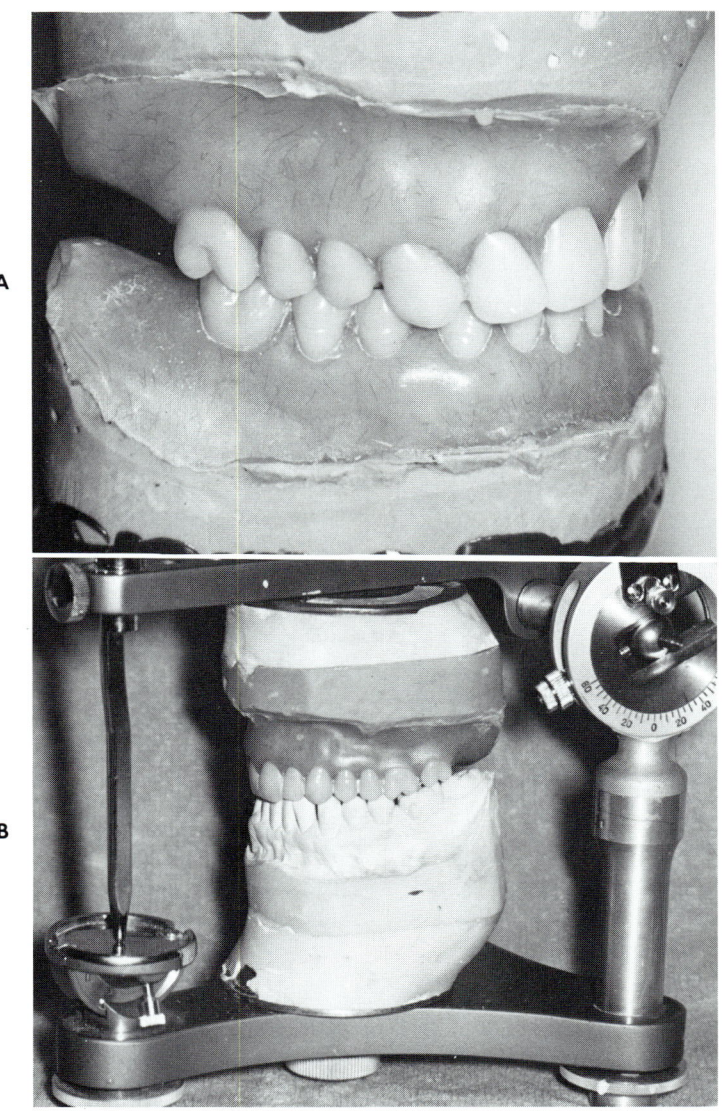

Fig. 10-21. Cured overdentures are remounted in articulator. **A,** Maxillary and mandibular overdentures. **B,** Maxillary overdenture only.

and polishing compound* (Fig. 10-25). The polished overdentures are cleaned with soap and water, and the interior of the interim overdenture is carefully checked for nodules or defects. If porcelain denture teeth were used, the occlusal surfaces of teeth modified by grinding are restored to a high polish before the denture is placed (Morrow and associates, 1973). The margin around each abutment indentation is smoothed to minimize gingival irritation (Fig. 10-26). The completed overdentures are stored in water until insertion. Duplicate overdentures can be made at this time to serve as back-up or replacement prostheses. A simplified method of duplicating overdentures is described in Chapter 14.

PLACING THE OVERDENTURE

Abutment teeth are prepared immediately before removal of the last hopeless teeth and placement of the immediate overdenture.

Abutment preparation

The abutments are reduced in a manner similar to that used on the cast, but they are made smaller to allow placement of the overdenture without in-

---
*No. 341 Ti-Gleam, Ticonium Co., Albany, N. Y.

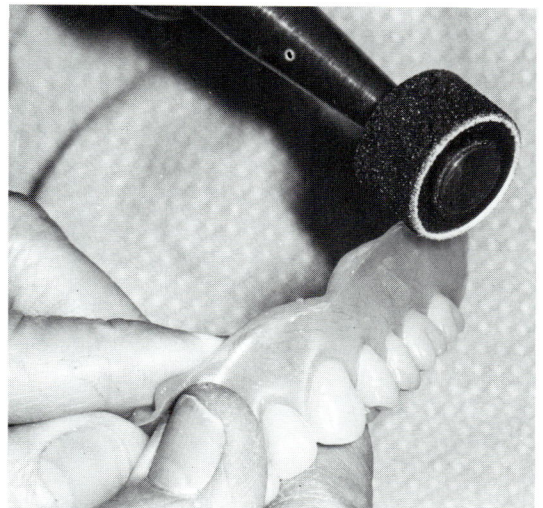

Fig. 10-22. Overdenture borders are trimmed with a lathe-mounted arbor band.

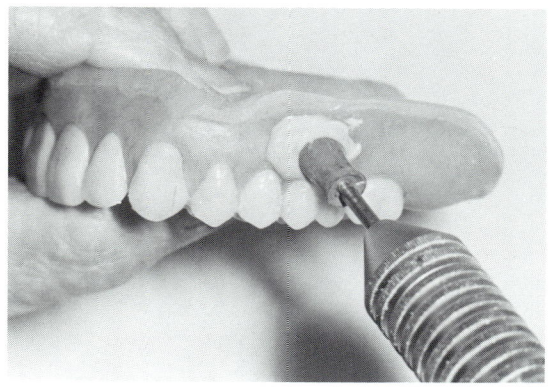

Fig. 10-23. Rubber cup mounted in a handpiece and flour of pumice are used to polish contours of overdenture.

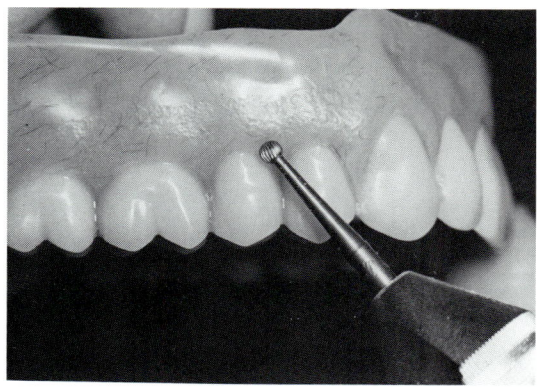

Fig. 10-24. Stippled surface can be obtained by etching denture surface lightly with a finishing bur rotated slowly in a handpiece.

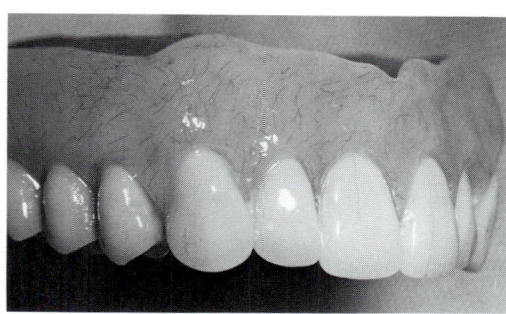

Fig. 10-25. Polished overdenture.

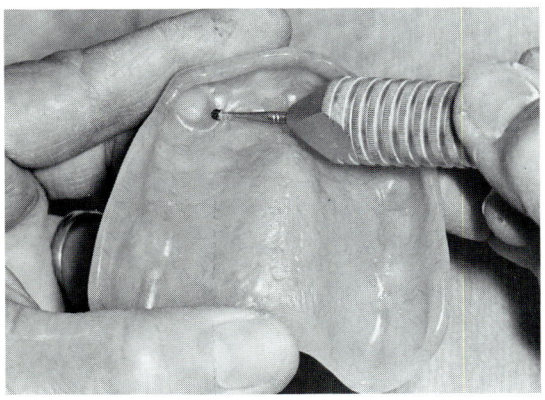

Fig. 10-26. Margin around each abutment tooth indentation should be smooth before insertion.

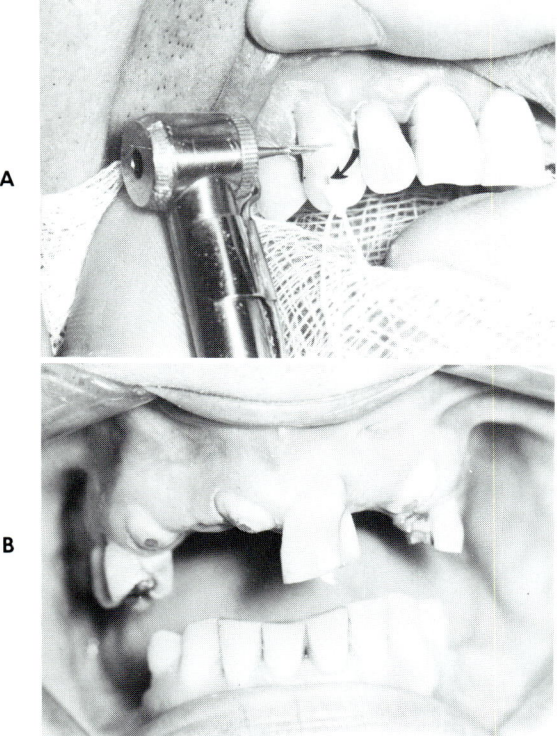

Fig. 10-27. **A,** To prevent swallowing or aspiration of crown, a hole (arrow) can be made in portion of endodontically treated abutment tooth that is to be removed, a piece of dental floss threaded through hole, and the ends tied in a knot. A piece of 4- × 4-inch gauze is used to catch tooth particles. **B,** Abutments should be 2 to 3 mm. high and tapered axially.

terference (Fig. 10-27, *A*). The reference cast, obtained earlier, is used as a guide during preparation. The abutments should be 2 to 3 mm. high, and the axial surfaces should be tapered (Fig. 10-27, *B*). The abutment surfaces are smoothed, and amalgam restorations are placed in the occlusal or incisal surface to seal the root canal (Fig. 10-28). The prepared teeth are treated with fluoride anticaries solution. First, a 2-minute application of APF gel is used, which is followed by a 2-minute application of 0.4% stannous fluoride as described in Chapter 19.

Surgical procedures*

Consultation with an oral surgeon to jointly plan the surgical phase of overdenture treatment is often indicated. The sequence of tooth removal and, where indicated, undercut correction, tuberosity reduction, and frenectomy should be discussed and a treatment plan formulated. A thorough patient history is taken, abnormalities are noted, and proposed surgical procedures are modified accordingly. Radiographs are carefully reviewed, and a decision is made as to the best method for tooth removal. Aseptic techniques are observed in all surgical procedures.

Usually, hopeless maxillary and mandibular posterior teeth are removed from one side to minimize interference with function. After a suitable healing period the remaining hopeless posterior teeth on the opposite side are removed. Good sur-

---

*This section was contributed by Hampton Green, Jr.

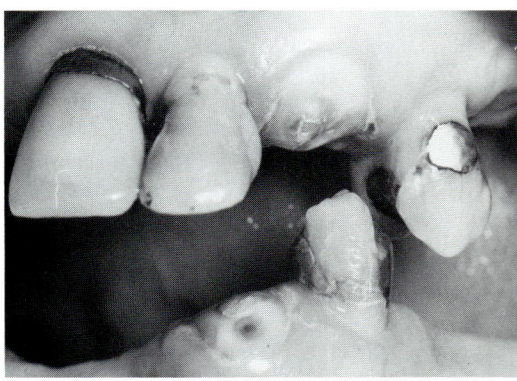

Fig. 10-28. Amalgam restorations are placed in abutment to seal root canal.

gical technique requires careful handling of tissues to minimize trauma and facilitate a smooth postoperative course. One effective technique involves an incision made along the crest of the alveolar ridge and around the necks of the teeth. The tissue is carefully reflected on the buccal and lingual aspects, and the teeth are luxated with straight exolevers and removed with the appropriate forceps. Sharp bony spicules are rounded with rongeurs and smoothed with a bone file. The area is debrided to remove any bone particles, and soft tissue margins are trimmed, approximated, and sutured with 3-0 silk. Gauze pressure dressings are placed over the operative sites. The patient is then given postoperative instructions and dismissed. Sutures are removed approximately 4 to 5 days after the operation.

Where indicated, tuberosity reduction can contribute significantly to overdenture success. This is particularly true when large tuberosities compromise available denture space. Removal of excess tissue provides for greater interridge space and a more stable foundation for the overdenture base. Correction of this abnormality can often be accomplished by making an elliptoid incision over the tuberosity. Beginning at the most distal aspect of the tuberosity, the incisions are joined on the crest of the alveolar ridge approximately 1 cm. anterior to the tissue to be removed. A curette or periosteal elevator can be used to undermine the wedge of tissue for easy removal. After removal of the tissue, the margins are contoured, repositioned, and sutured. If the patient is wearing a prosthesis that covers the area, a tissue conditioner can be placed in the prosthesis. The prosthesis can then serve as a surgical stent.

Inserting the overdenture. Anterior teeth are removed when the overdentures are ready for insertion. If gingival tissues are inflamed and there is noticeable bone loss, a tissue flap is raised. An incision is made through the interdental papillae, and the mucoperiosteum is reflected. Care is taken to prevent tearing or lacerating the tissue. The teeth are removed as atraumatically as possible, and bone irregularities are smoothed with a bone file. Every effort is made to preserve bone, and alveolectomy is seldom required. Granulation tissue is dissected and curetted. The labial and lingual alveolar ridges are compressed gently with finger pressure. Excess tissue is trimmed from the margins with tissue scissors, and the tissues are approximated. Sutures are placed between the sockets.

If severe periodontal defects are not present, only the tissue around the necks of the teeth is reflected before removal. Sutures, in this case, are usually not necessary (Fig. 10-29, *A*). The over-

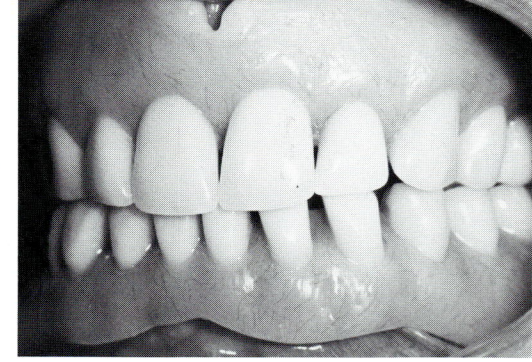

Fig. 10-29. **A,** Remaining hopeless teeth are removed. **B,** Immediate overdenture is inserted.

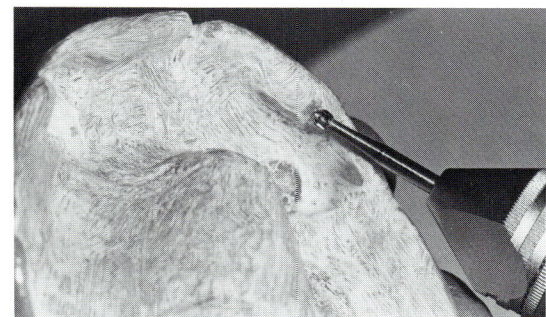

Fig. 10-30. Indicator paste is used to disclose areas requiring adjustment.

denture is inserted, and occlusion is checked (Fig. 10-29, *B*). The patient is instructed to not remove the overdenture until the first postoperative visit, which is scheduled for the next day. At that time the overdenture is removed and cleaned, and indicated corrections are made. The overdenture provides excellent protection for the surgery site. Sutures are removed in 3 to 5 days.

If, in the opinion of the prosthodontist, a frenum attachment may compromise overdenture retention, correction may be accomplished at the time of tooth removal. The immediate overdenture then serves as a surgical stent throughout the healing period.

If indicated, adjunctive periodontal surgical procedures can be used to reduce pocket depths of abutment teeth or to improve supporting tissue contour at the time of removal of the hopeless teeth. Interfering undercut areas can be located with indicating paste, and the overdenture can be adjusted (Fig. 10-30). Root eminences within the denture are reduced to avoid scuffing during insertion or removal. Interferences occasionally exist between the overdenture and abutments, and their removal is essential. Kerr disclosing wax is used in locating them, and either the overdenture or abutment is reduced to allow seating of the denture (Fig. 10-31). Adaptation of the overdenture to the

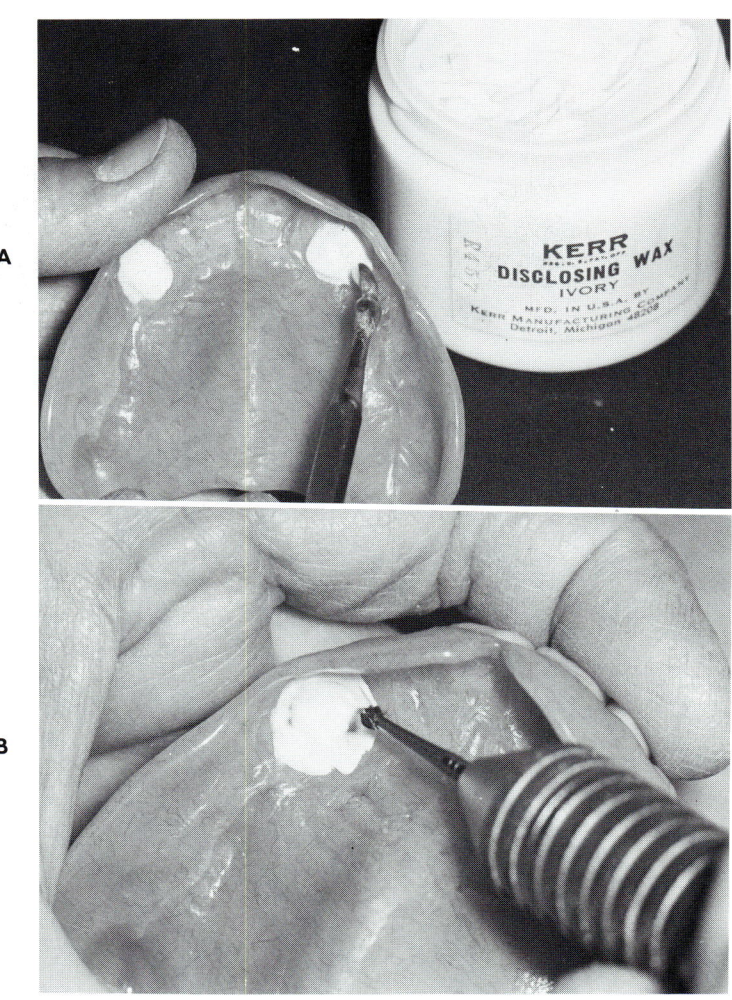

Fig. 10-31. **A,** Disclosing wax is flowed into abutment indentations to locate interferences. **B,** Interfering areas are reduced with bur.

abutment teeth with autopolymerizing resin is deferred until the first postinsertion appointment to prevent contamination of the resin with blood. Occlusion, border extensions, tissue undercuts, and adaptation are checked at this same appointment.

POSTINSERTION CARE

The postoperative course of the immediate overdenture patient is usually uneventful, and the patient has minimal discomfort and uninterrupted function. The overdenture is not removed until the patient is seen on the day after surgery, when the necessary adjustments are made.

Adapting overdentures to abutments

Abutment teeth should be polished before adapting the overdenture. Abutments are smoothed with a fine grit sandpaper disk and polished with a rubber cup and flour of pumice. Amalgloss can be used to place a high gloss on the amalgam restoration and abutment surfaces.

The overdenture is adapted to the abutment teeth by adding tooth colored autopolymerizing resin to the abutment indentations of the denture. A definite circumferential margin is made around each indentation, and a small hole is placed in the depths of the indentation to vent the excess resin (Fig. 10-32). Abutment teeth can be lubricated lightly with Masque* before seating the overdenture to prevent sticking. Tooth-colored autopolymerizing resin is sifted into the indentations and saturated with monomer, and the overdenture is inserted (Fig. 10-33). Before complete hardening of the resin, the overdenture is removed and placed in a water bath at 130° F. to accelerate setting of the resin. Excess resin is removed and the

*Harry J. Bosworth Co., Chicago.

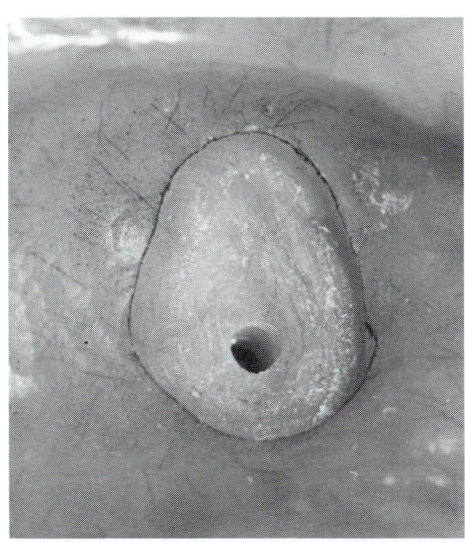

Fig. 10-32. Definite margin is created around abutment indentation and hole is made to vent excess resin.

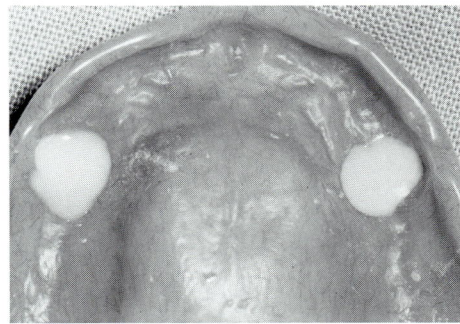

Fig. 10-33. Tooth-colored autopolymerizing resin is sifted into indentation and saturated with monomer.

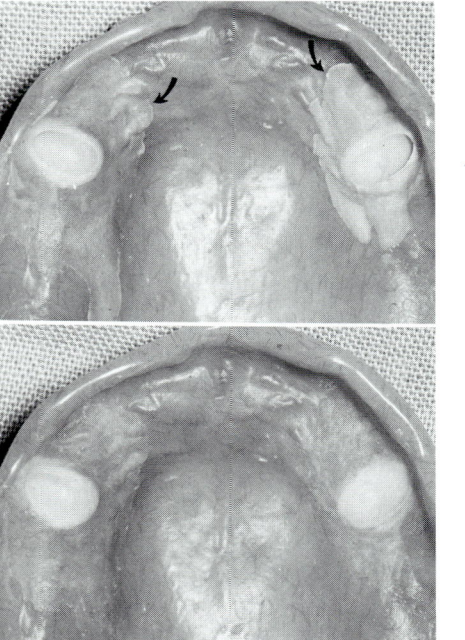

Fig. 10-34. A, Excess resin "flash" must be removed. B, Margins of abutment indentations are smoothed to minimize gingival irritation.

indentation margins are smoothed before the overdenture is reinserted (Fig. 10-34). Usually sutures are removed on the fourth postoperative day, and careful abutment hygiene is instituted.

Oral hygiene instructions

Each patient is instructed how to clean the abutment teeth and the denture. Soft-bristle toothbrushes, disclosing tablets, dental floss, and bubble gum therapy are used to maintain gingival health. Bubble gum therapy is effective for conditioning tissues when used properly, and the patient can be placed on bubble gum massage after a week. However, this massage can be delayed in the event of slow healing or unusual tenderness. Often four to six cakes of bubble gum are required; it is softened initially by kneading in warm water before chewing. The overdentures are removed, and the bubble gum is chewed for 30 to 60 minutes a day, this period of massage being increased gradually. To prevent unnecessary addition of sugar to the diet, sugarless bubble gum is used, or the gum is rinsed in water and soaked in water until it is reused. Mouthwash can be used to flavor the water.

Overdenture hygiene

The patient is instructed to keep the overdenture clean by removing it after each meal and brushing with a soft bristle toothbrush and ordinary hand soap. He is cautioned against using harsh abrasives to clean overdentures. At the end of the first postoperative week, the patient is instructed to remove the overdenture on retiring for the night. The overdenture should be brushed and then soaked overnight in a suitable vessel containing a satisfactory denture cleansing solution. Small ultrasonic denture cleaners for home use also seem to be effective. Disclosing tablets can be used periodically to determine the effectiveness of the patient's denture cleansing regimen.

The interim overdenture is a ready-made fluoride gel carrier, and 2-minute applications of acidulated phosphate fluoride gel followed by 2-minute applications of 0.4% stannous fluoride gel are repeated throughout the postinsertion period (Fig. 10-35). Oral hygiene measures are stressed throughout the healing period; otherwise, the service life of the overdenture can be affected adversely by the patient's relapse into previous habits of oral neglect.

Relining the immediate overdenture

As healing progresses, relining of the interim overdenture usually becomes necessary to main-

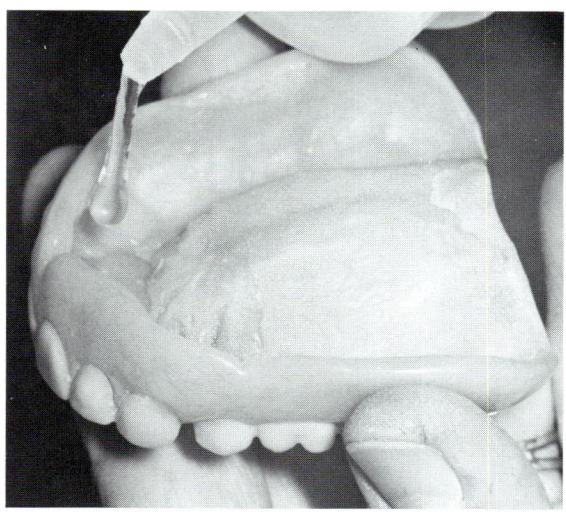

Fig. 10-35. Overdenture is an excellent fluoride gel tray.

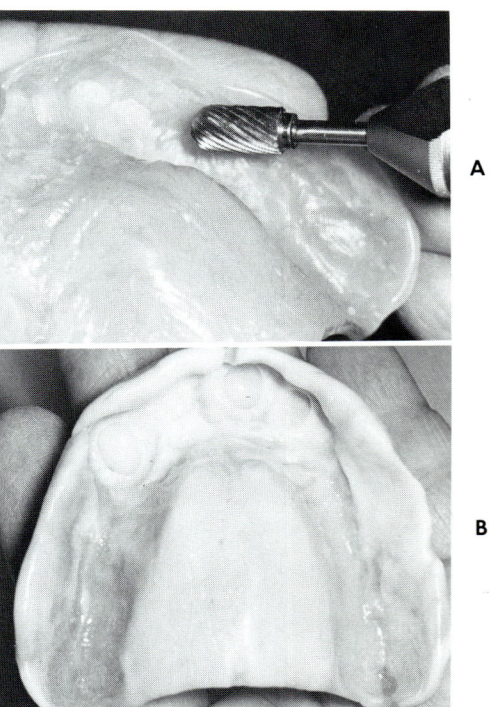

Fig. 10-36. **A**, Undercuts are removed in overdenture before addition of tissue treatment material. **B**, Tissue treatment material impression in overdenture.

tain adequate tissue adaptation. This relining is accomplished in a conventional manner. The undercuts are then removed from the overdenture, and an impression is made with a tissue treatment material* (Fig. 10-36). Generally, it is desirable to have the patient wear the overdenture with the tissue treatment material in it for 24 hours before examination. In some instances it is necessary to repeat tissue treatment, particularly in the presence of abused tissue, which may require additional time for healing. Abutment teeth serve as guides when inserting the overdenture with tissue treatment material and thereby minimize the possibility of anterior displacement of the denture. When the functionally molded impression is deemed adequate, the occlusion is verified and the overdenture is removed for relining. A cast is poured into the impression, and the overdenture and cast are mounted in a relining jig (Fig. 10-37). All traces of the tissue treatment material are removed from the overdenture before the autopolymerizing relining resin is added (Fig. 10-38). The overdenture, mounted in the relining jig, is placed in a pressure container and cured for 30 minutes at 30 p.s.i. After curing, the overdenture is removed from the cast, finished, and polished. At insertion the usual checks are completed; disclosing paste is used to indicate pressure areas and to verify abutment-overdenture contact. The margins of abutment indentations are smoothed to prevent irritation of gingival tissues.

Follow-up care

In my practice, the patient usually wears the immediate overdenture several months when used as an interim prosthesis, but several years when used as a more definitive prosthesis. Throughout the period the patient's response to overdenture treatment and oral hygiene efforts should be monitored periodically. Patients discharged from treatment soon after placement of an overdenture or those seen infrequently after placement invariably experience more relapses into poor oral hygiene practices than those seen regularly for postinsertion examinations. Regular scheduling of postinsertion examinations prevent cyclical recrudescences of poor oral hygiene practice, with their attendant unfavorable influence on the overdenture service life. If the response is poor and oral hygiene inadequate, it is prudent to avoid initiating more definitive prostheses because of the prognosis forecasted by the immediate overdenture. If abut-

---

*Coe Comfort or Hydrocast tissue conditioner or equivalent.

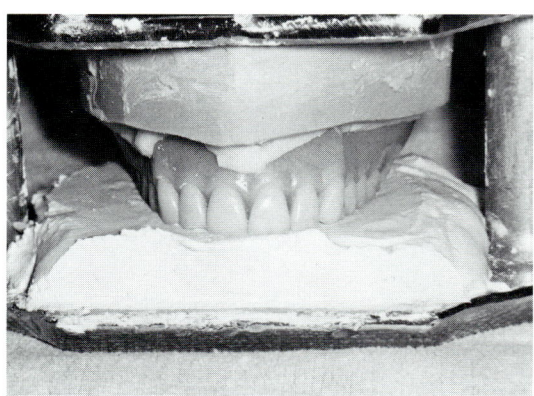

Fig. 10-37. Overdenture with tissue treatment material is mounted in relining jig.

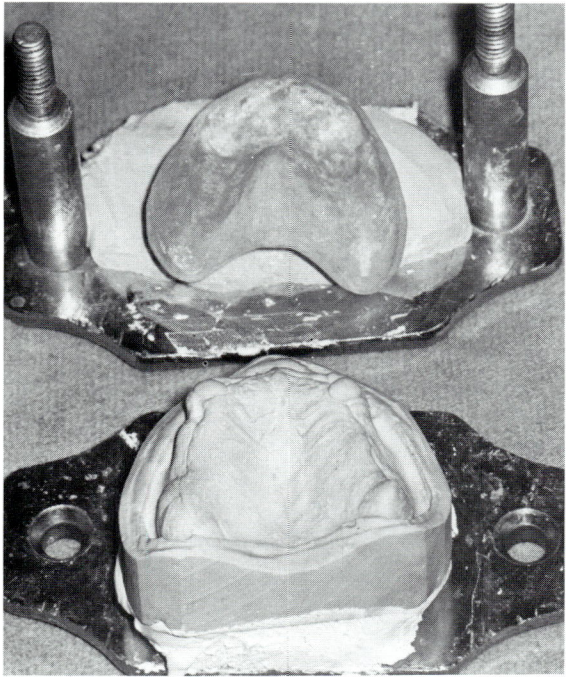

Fig. 10-38. Overdenture is separated from cast and all traces of tissue treatment material are removed before completion of relining.

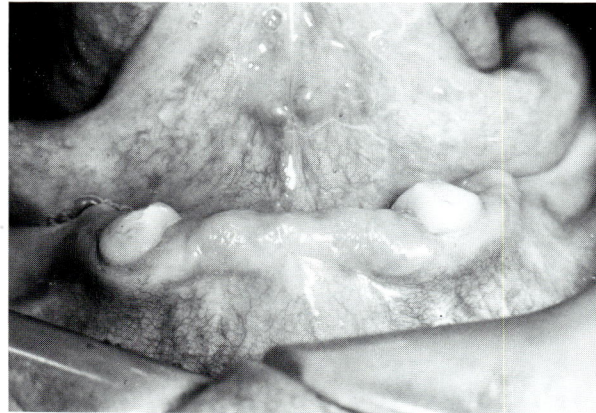

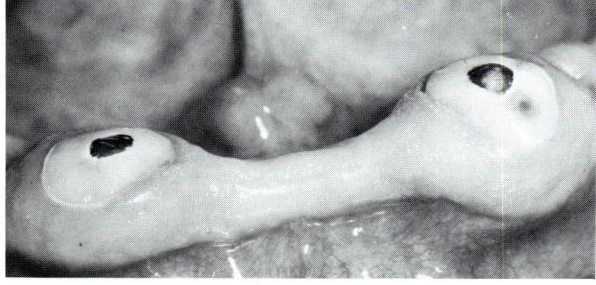

Fig. 10-39. A, Excellent tissue tone and color as well as absence of plaque indicate a favorable prognosis. **B,** Good oral hygiene practices are a significant factor in achieving success with overdentures.

ment failure appears imminent, the overdenture can be converted into a conventional complete denture by relining after loss of the abutment. However, if the prognosis appears equivocal because of the oral hygiene status, the interim immediate overdenture can be maintained, and additional efforts can be made to increase patient motivation. If response to the immediate interim overdenture is good, as manifested by excellent oral hygiene demonstrated consistently throughout the evaluation period, more sophisticated overdenture procedures can be considered and success can be anticipated.

Excellent tissue color and tone, minimal crevicular depths, absence of plaque on abutments and on the overdenture, and minimal mobility are the favorable signs related to good oral hygiene practices (Fig. 10-39). In their presence a more definitive prosthesis can be considered, and a favorable prognosis can be realized. The immediate overdenture then assumes its principal role as an economical means of instituting overdenture treatment, with all the advantages of this preventive prosthodontic concept.

REFERENCES

Brewer, A., and Fenton, A. H.: The overdenture, Dent. Clin. North Am. **17**:723-746, 1973.

Lord, J. L., and Teel, S.: The overdenture, Dent. Clin. North Am. **13**:871-881, 1969.

Morrow, R. M., Rudd, K. D., Birmingham, F. D., and Larkin, J. D.: Immediate interim tooth-supported complete dentures, J. Prosthet. Dent. **30**:695-700, 1973.

Morrow, R. M., Brown, C. E., Larkin, J. D., Bernui, R., and Rudd, K. D.: Evaluation of methods for polishing porcelain denture teeth, J. Prosthet. Dent. **30**:222-226, 1973.

Morrow, R. M., Brown, C. E., Stansbury, B. E., deLorimier, J. A., Powell, J. M., and Rudd, K. D.: Compatibility of alginate impression materials and dental stones, J. Prosthet. Dent. **25**:556-565, 1971.

Rudd, K. D.: Processing complete dentures without tooth movement, Dent. Clin. North Am., pp. 675-691, Nov., 1964.

Rudd, K. D., Morrow, R. M., and Strunk, R. R.: Accurate alginate impressions, J. Prosthet. Dent. **22**:294-300, 1969.

11

REMOTE OVERDENTURES

ROBERT M. MORROW

A remote overdenture is an overdenture other than transitional or immediate. It is usually constructed for insertion at some time "remote" from the removal of hopeless natural teeth. It is implied, then, that the remote overdenture is placed over well-healed residual ridges, usually after a period of satisfactory experience with an interim overdenture, which can be an immediate or transitional overdenture. Although remote overdentures can be constructed entirely of resin, metal bases are frequently used.

METAL BASE OVERDENTURE

The metal base overdenture is a complete denture with a cast metal base that is supported and stabilized by selected natural teeth whose contours are modified for the purpose by the preparation and placement of copings (Fig. 11-1).

Advantages

Overdentures reinforced with a metal base have several advantages. First, the reinforced denture, being inherently stronger, is less subject to breakage, which is a problem sometimes with those made of conventional base resins (Rantanen and associates, 1971). Second, metal base overdentures, which are more rigid, resist the dimensional changes associated with polymerization of denture base resins and the functional forces of mastication. Third, denture-supporting tissues seem to respond more favorably to metal bases (McCracken, 1953). Clinical observations have shown that critical gingival areas immediately adjacent to abutments frequently improve in color and tone after replacement of a resin overdenture with a metal base overdenture. This improvement may be related to greater ease in maintaining cleanliness of the metal base and to effective transmission of thermal changes through the metal base (Applegate, 1955). Fourth, the metal base is excellent for jaw relation recording procedures. Stabilized and effectively supported by abutments, the metal base

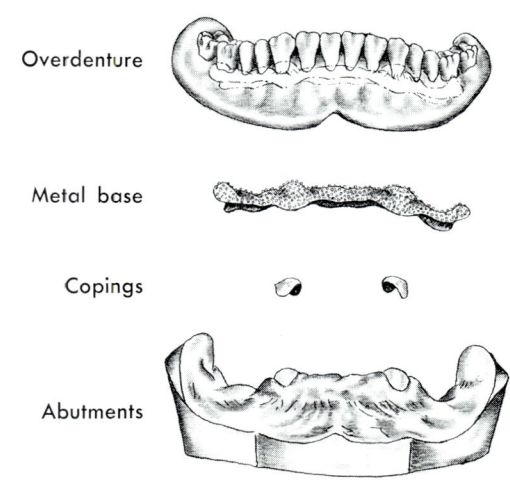

Fig. 11-1. Metal base overdenture. Metal base reinforcement significantly increases strength of overdenture and minimizes breakage.

permits accurate jaw relation records and subsequent success of the denture. Reinforcement of the overdenture by a rigid cast metal base contributes to a more definitive prosthesis.

Disadvantages

Disadvantages of the metal base overdenture are primarily economic, for the additional clinical and laboratory procedures required increase both the time and cost of treatment. Relining presents more technical problems for a metal base overdenture than for one constructed of resin, but it is feasible. Adequate healing of residual ridges before construction of the metal base significantly postpones the need for relining, as does retention of teeth for abutments. Usually the results are better when the patient wears an interim overdenture for 8 to 12 months after removal of the last hopeless teeth. This healing period favors development of a more stable residual ridge topography and postpones the need for relining. Metal base overdentures can be relined if necessary; one method is described in the section on maintenance (Chapter 14). Modifications of metal bases that make relining easier are considered in the section on design requirements (pp. 191 and 192). Since metal bases occupy space, excessively thick castings that interfere with positioning of denture teeth and give poor esthetic effects are a disadvantage.

Indications

Metal base overdentures, being more definitive prostheses, are indicated for patients who respond favorably to an interim overdenture for a minimum of 8 to 12 months. This extensive observation period allows the orderly accumulation of evaluations necessary for patient selection. The interim overdenture is a reliable prognostic indicator, and it is best to defer construction of a metal base overdenture if response to the interim prosthesis is poor. Therefore metal base overdentures are constructed for patients who have the motivation and oral hygiene level necessary for success and for patients who break resin interim overdentures repeatedly.

Contraindications

Contraindications for metal base overdentures are essentially the same as for immediate or transitional overdentures. Poor oral hygiene and lack of motivation are the prime contraindications for overdentures, particularly when the procedures are complex.

Abutment copings

Whether or not to use copings on overdenture abutments is an important consideration for the dentist. In the presence of good oral hygiene, fluoride applications, and regular supervision, many abutment teeth can serve for years without copings. Therefore the decision to use copings should be based on suitable criteria. Preparation of teeth to serve as overdenture abutments usually results in the exposure of considerable dentin surface to the oral environment. Protection of dentin surfaces of abutment teeth with gold copings seems to have several advantages.

Advantages of copings. Properly constructed gold copings cemented with a silicophosphate cement* seem to provide some caries protection for the abutment tooth. Cemented to the tooth, copings effectively reinforce the endodontically treated abutment and make it possible to restore broken-down teeth otherwise unacceptable as abutments. Use of gold copings enables the dentist to produce specific abutment contours and obtain excellent psychologic results.

Disadvantages of copings. The disadvantages include an increase in the time and cost of treatment. Following is a list of the mean numbers of appointments and lengths of time required to complete overdenture treatment, where the period of

---

*Fluoro-thin silicophosphate cement, Type III, S. S. White Dental Products, Philadelphia.

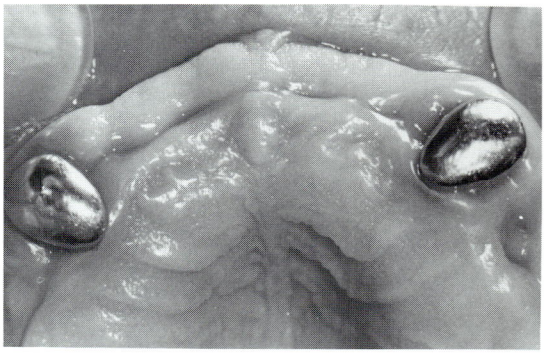

Fig. 11-2. Coping contours are rounded to provide "ball and socket" contact between coping and overdenture.

treatment is defined as beginning with the initial appointment, extending through the placement of remote overdenture, and including both immediate and remote overdenture procedures as well as all prerequisite treatment.

    50 maxillary overdentures
        28 appointments
        13 months
    21 mandibular overdentures
        25 appointments
        11 months
    21 maxillary-mandibular overdentures
        37 appointments
        15 months

Coping margins also can irritate the gingival tissues, and marginal caries can occur, particularly in instances of poor oral hygiene.

Preparation of abutment teeth. The incisal or occlusal surface of the coping for the metal base overdenture is convex (Fig. 11-2). The objective of this design is to form a coping that will provide for a rounded contact between the tooth coping and the metal base of the overdenture, as described by Miller (1958). Normally the indicated periodontal, endodontic, restorative, and surgical procedures are completed before the teeth are prepared for cast gold copings. Gingival sulci measurements should be within normal limits. Sufficient tooth structure is removed from abutment teeth to create a favorable clinical crown-root ratio. The clinical crown should be reduced to a height of 2 or 3 mm. above the gingival margin (Fig. 11-3). Most of the reduction is usually accomplished at the time of insertion of an immediate overdenture when one is used before a metal base overdenture. Sufficient reduction of the abutment allows placement of an artificial tooth similar in size and shape to the natural tooth—an important contribution to the esthetic result. Adequate preparation can often improve unfavorable crown-root ratios from 1:1 to 1:2 or 1:3, and such preparation results in an apparent reduction of horizontal mobility of the abutment. In general, preparation for copings should conform to the basic principles of full crown preparation and include consideration of the (1) occlusogingival reduction of the clinical crown to provide the most favorable mechanical advantage to the existing root and periodontal support and (2) reduction of the axial surfaces to provide sufficient space for esthetic placement of denture teeth of proper size and contour. The abutment can be reduced to the proper height with an S. S. White No. 170L tapered fissure carbide bur or a Densco No. 2½J diamond wheel. Proximal surfaces are tapered and reduced to the level of the gingival margin with a tapered fissure carbide bur or a Densco No. 1 D-T fine grit diamond (Fig. 11-4). A long gingival bevel can be placed in the gingival crevice with a Densco No. ⅛A fine grit flame-shaped diamond, and care should be taken to avoid traumatizing gingival tissues. A short dowel (5 to 7 mm.) in the root canal is used to achieve the desired retention, for the completed overdenture exerts only minimal dislodgment forces on the cemented coping (Fig. 11-5). The canal preparation can be made with a tapered fissure carbide bur if care is taken to avoid under-

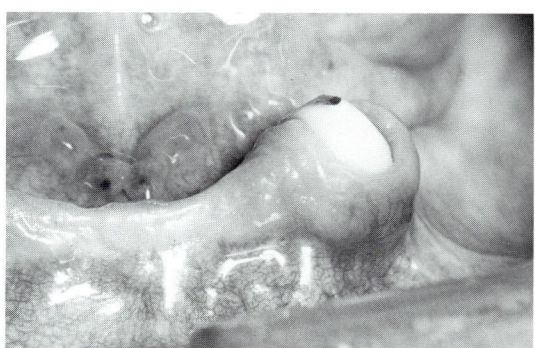

Fig. 11-3. Clinical crown is reduced to height of 2 to 3 mm. above gingival margin. This reduction improves crown-root ratio and contributes to esthetics.

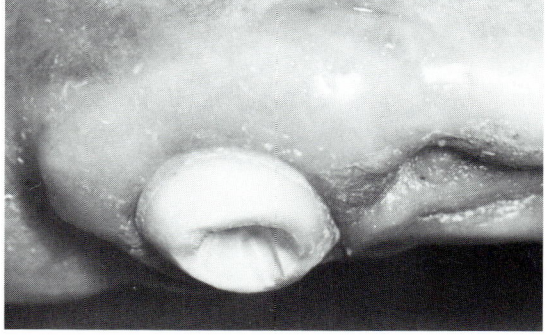

Fig. 11-4. Proximal surfaces are tapered to gingival crest with fine grit diamond or tapered fissure carbide bur.

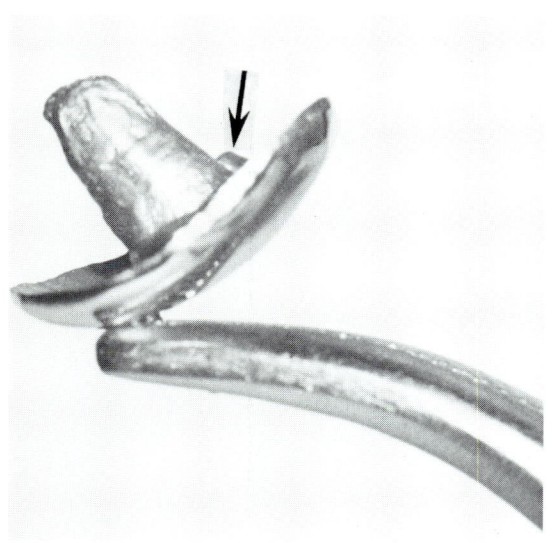

Fig. 11-5. Prepared root canal with short dowel used to achieve retention. Note key (arrow) on post to counteract rotational forces.

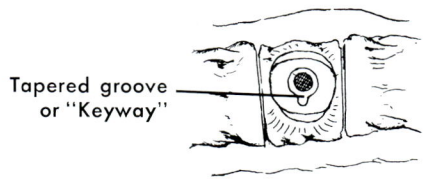

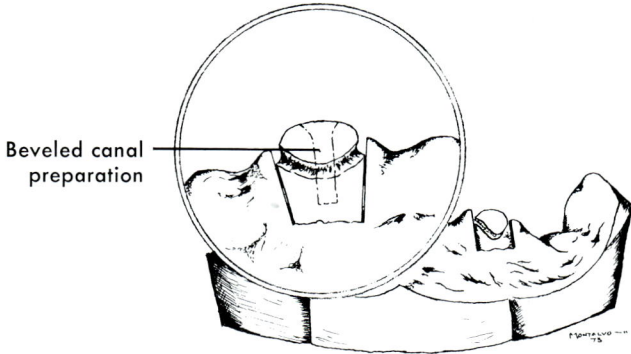

Fig. 11-6. Entrance to canal preparation beveled with fine grit diamond. A parallel tapered groove, placed in buccal or lingual surface of canal preparation, counters rotational forces and aids in identifying the surface during cementation.

cuts and perforations. A parallel tapered groove can be placed in the buccal or lingual surface of the canal preparation to counter rotational forces and to aid in identifying buccal and lingual surfaces of the coping during cementation. The entrance to the canal preparation is beveled with a Densco No. 2 D-T fine grit diamond instrument to eliminate sharp edges and subsequent fitting problems (Fig. 11-6). In some instances pins are used for retention instead of a post (Fig. 11-7). This is true particularly when the root cross-sectional area is small and the teeth used have more than one root. Generally two or three pins 4 or 5 mm. long are adequate.

Making the abutment impression. A full arch impression of the prepared abutment teeth is made by reversible hydrocolloid or rubber base impression techniques. The impression material is injected carefully into the post preparation and over the prepared teeth. When used for retention, plastic pins of appropriate size are placed in the corresponding holes of the preparation before injection of the impression material (Fig. 11-8). After setting, the impression is removed and examined critically to determine its acceptability (Fig. 11-9). Then the abutment teeth are treated with a fluoride solution to inhibit caries, and the canal opening is sealed with gutta percha. The interim overdenture can be worn over the prepared abutments while the copings are being made. It is preferable

REMOTE OVERDENTURES 123

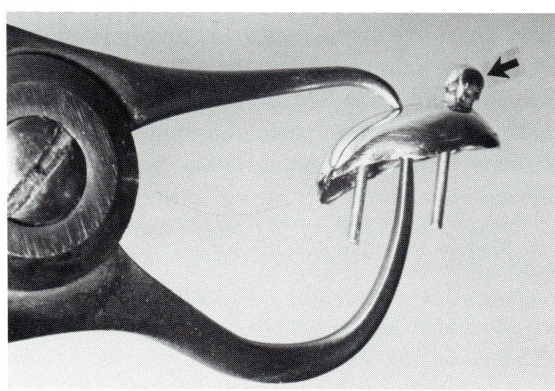

Fig. 11-7. Pin retention used for overdenture copings. Note bead (arrow) on coping, which facilitates placement and removal when checking fit. Copings, at least 1 mm. thick on bearing surface, prevent possible "wear through."

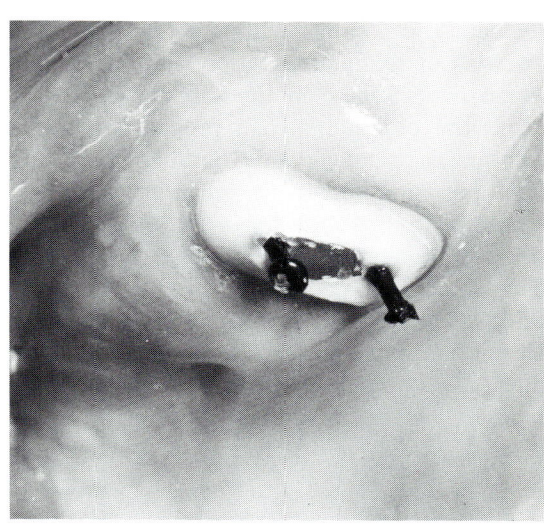

Fig. 11-8. Plastic pins, "mushroomed" on one end with warm wax spatula, lightly lubricated on opposite end, and placed in corresponding holes of abutment. Small dab of rubber base adhesive on projecting ends of pins also aids retention in impression material.

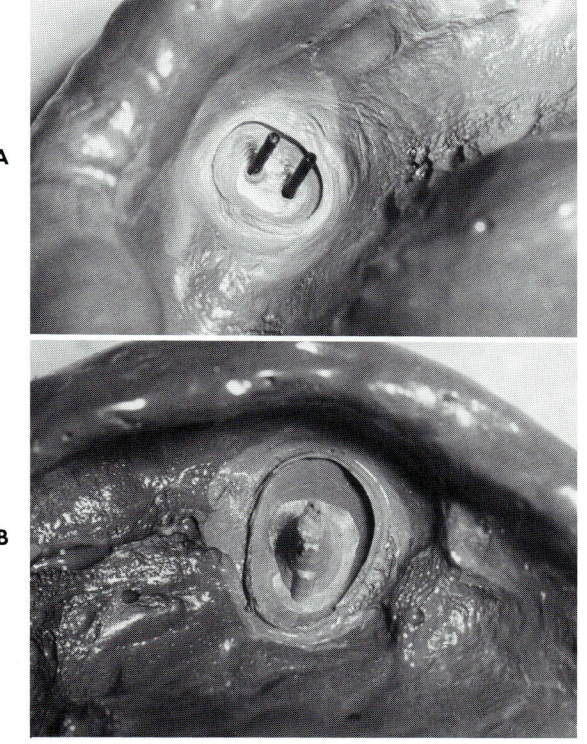

Fig. 11-9. A, Impression should be examined critically to assure that plastic pins pull with impression. B, Impression of canal with no voids. Note sharp impression of tapered groove.

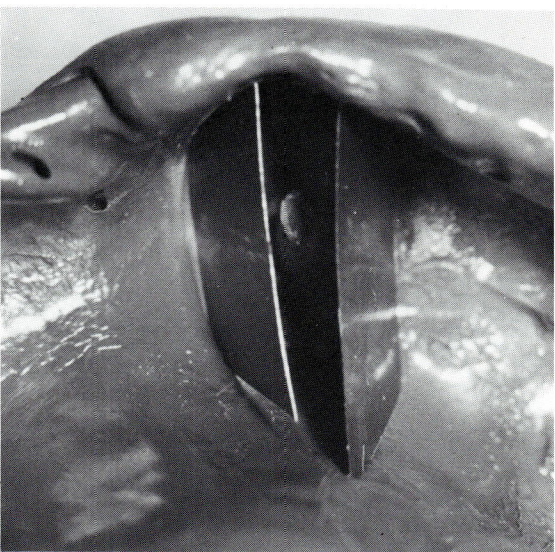

Fig. 11-10. Metal strips placed mesially and distally to abutment impression to facilitate withdrawal of die.

Around each abutment indentation a definite margin is created with a bur to serve as a finish line. Adequate removal of resin can be confirmed with disclosing wax, but care must be taken to remove all traces of the wax before adding the resin. A small hole is made in the depths of the indentations to allow extrusion of the autopolymerizing resin when the denture is seated in the mouth (Fig. 11-18, A). Neopar* autopolymerizing acrylic resin of the proper shade is sifted into the abutment indentations and saturated with monomer (Fig. 11-18, B). It is essential to coat each coping lightly with a silicone lubricant such as Masque† before seating the denture to prevent adherence to the resin. With the interim overdenture seated in the mouth, the occlusion is verified and the denture is allowed to remain in position for 2 minutes. Then it is removed and placed in a warm water bath for 15 minutes to accelerate polymerization of the resin. By using the previously placed finish lines as a guide, excess resin is removed from the interior of the denture (Fig. 11-18, C), and the margins of the abutment indentations are smoothed (Fig. 11-18, D). The interim overdenture, adapted to the contours of the abutment copings, can be used by the patient until the new denture is completed.

Making the impression

An accurate border molded impression is made of the residual ridges and the restored teeth with a rubber-base impression material in an acrylic resin tray. This impression is used to make the master cast on which the metal base and the overdenture are to be constructed.

---
*Neopar, Miner Dental Products, Emeryville, Calif.
†Masque, Harry J. Bosworth Co., Chicago.

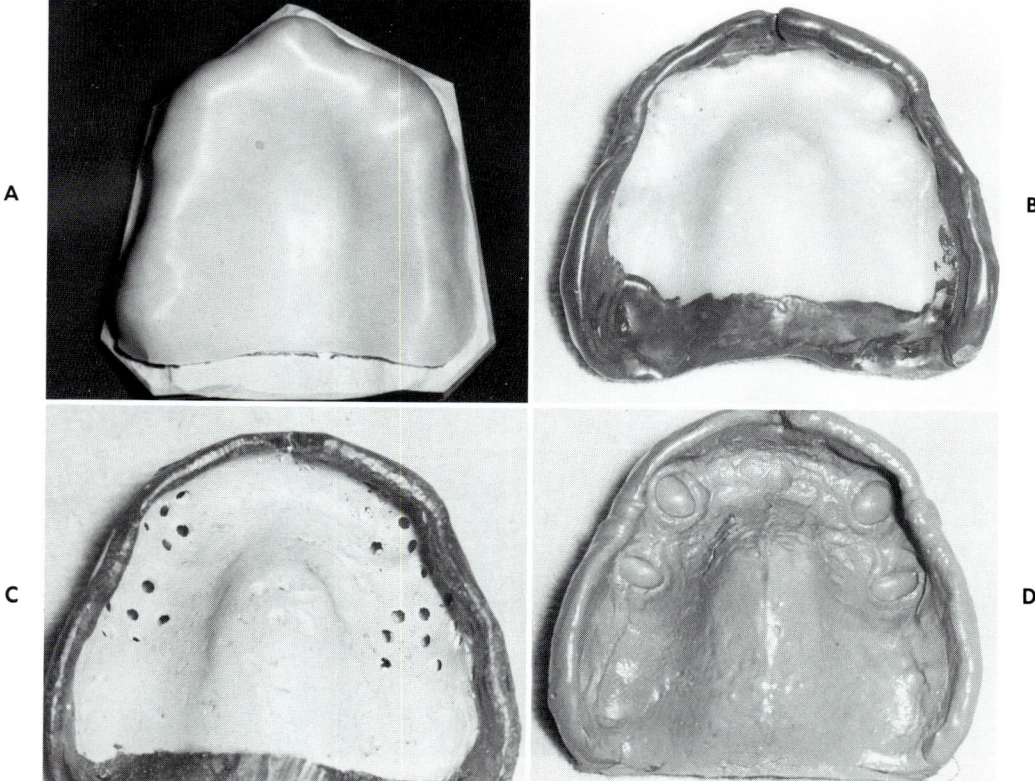

Fig. 11-19. **A,** Baseplate wax adapted to cast to create space for impression material. **B,** Impression compound used to border-mold tray. **C,** Tray (with baseplate wax removed) is perforated to increase retention of impression material with tray and to minimize voids. **D,** Completed impression for maxillary overdenture supported by four abutments.

The outline of the impression tray is drawn on the cast poured into the alginate impression obtained earlier. The borders should be short enough to permit molding with compound. A single layer of baseplate wax is adapted to the cast and trimmed to the indicated border extensions (Fig. 11-19, A). More wax is used over the abutment teeth to add thickness to the impression material and to prevent breakage of the cast on separation. Tinfoil substitute is painted on the wax before adding the tray resin to facilitate removal of the wax from the impression tray. Three relatively small handles added to the resin tray in the anterior area and in the first molar areas on each side are convenient to use during the molding of the border. They are placed so as to not interfere with movement of peripheral tissues during border-molding procedures. The relief wax remains in the tray throughout the border molding and is removed immediately before the corrective wash. A strip of relief wax approximately 2 mm. wide is removed from the entire circumference of the border of the tray and replaced with impression compound. After tempering in a water bath, the compound is used to record the extension and thickness of the borders (Fig. 11-19, B). Functional and simulated function movements of the tongue and associated oral musculature as well as molding of the lips and cheeks through active manipulation by the dentist can be used to develop border thicknesses and extensions compatible with stable and retentive dentures. Particular attention should be directed to the sublingual crescent area, since proper contour is critical for mandibular overdenture retention. On completion of border molding, the remaining relief wax is removed from the impression tray, and the compound border is relieved slightly with a sharp knife. The indentations in the impression tray corresponding to the abutment teeth should be perforated with a No. 8 bur to allow flow of the rubber base impression material through the tray, increasing retention of the rubber base and minimizing voids (Fig. 11-19, C). A coating of rubber-base adhesive is placed on the tray and allowed to dry. Regular body rubber base impression material is proportioned, mixed, and loaded into the impression tray. The copings are lightly lubricated with Masque, and, before the impression tray is seated, a small amount of rubber base material is placed on a finger and wiped over each abutment tooth to minimize voids. Then the impression tray is seated, and border molding movements are reaccomplished. After setting, the impression is removed and examined to determine its acceptability (Fig. 11-19, D).

Pouring the master cast. The cast is more accurate if it is poured soon after the impression is obtained. The impression is boxed readily by using a mixture of plaster of paris and flour of pumice as a support. The pumice is added to weaken the set plaster. The impression is seated into this mix of plaster and pumice using a spatula to create a land area approximately ¼ inch wide and ⅛ inch below the borders of the impression (Fig. 11-20). After setting, the land area can be narrowed on the model trimmer. The plaster surface is coated with separating medium and the impression is boxed with wax. Minimal expansion stone* proportioned by weight and mixed with the recommended volume of water in a mechanical spatulator under reduced atmospheric pressure is used to pour the cast. The resultant bubble-free mix produces a strong, dense cast. Metal mounting plates† can be used in the base of the cast if desired. The

---

*Vel-Mix, Kerr Manufacturing Co., Romulus, Mich., Die Keen, Modern Materials Manufacturing Co., St. Louis, or equivalent.
†Hanau Engineering Co., Inc., Buffalo, N. Y.

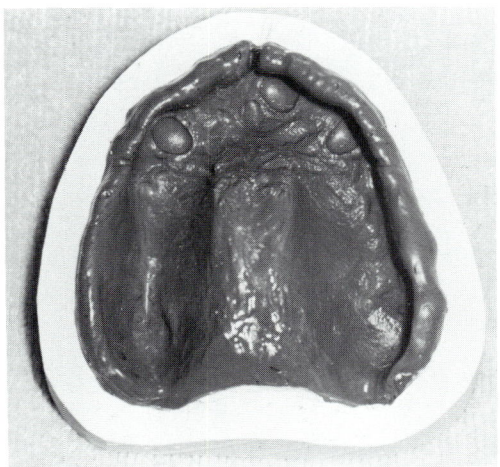

Fig. 11-20. Impression boxed in mixture of plaster of Paris and flour of pumice. Three abutments support this maxillary overdenture.

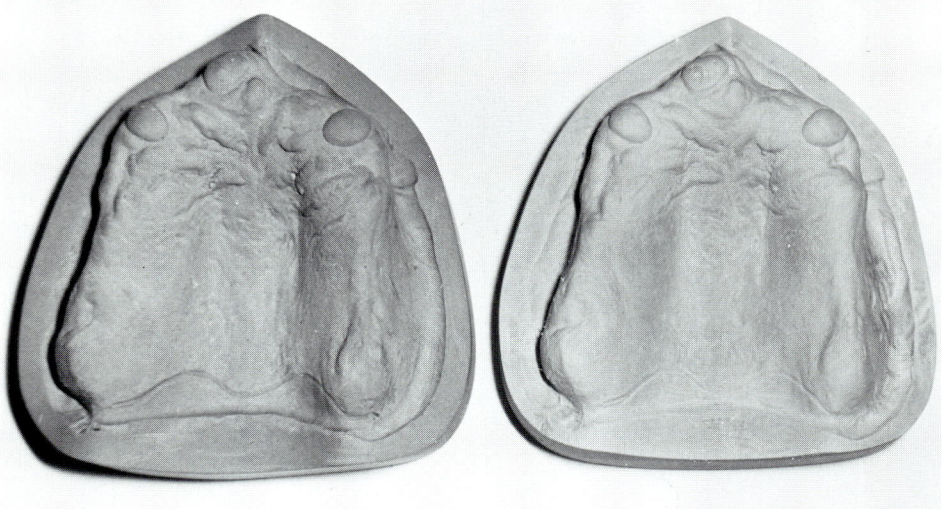

Fig. 11-21. Two casts obtained from impression. Master cast is used for construction of metal base and overdenture, and design for metal base is placed on second or diagnostic cast.

impression is poured twice, the first cast being the master cast and the second being a diagnostic cast on which the design of the metal base is placed (Fig. 11-21).

Duplicate cast. If the impression is damaged at separation of the first cast, it may be necessary to duplicate the master cast rather than rely on an impression that may be inaccurate. The posterior palatal seal is placed in the master cast before duplication. The cast can be duplicated easily by using alginate irreversible hydrocolloid (Morrow and Rudd, 1971). The diagnostic cast can be made of less expensive stone.

Design considerations for the metal base

The diagnostic cast is surveyed to determine the location and extent of tissue undercuts (Fig. 11-22). After the "tilt" is selected for design purposes, the cast is tripoded. The metal base should not extend into pronounced tissue undercuts, since this would interfere with seating the base on the master cast. A slight posterior tilt minimizes anterior undercuts and facilitates extension of the base into this area.

Mandibular metal base design considerations

Extension of metal base. Unless specifically contraindicated, the metal base should extend sufficiently to allow it to be used for jaw relation re-

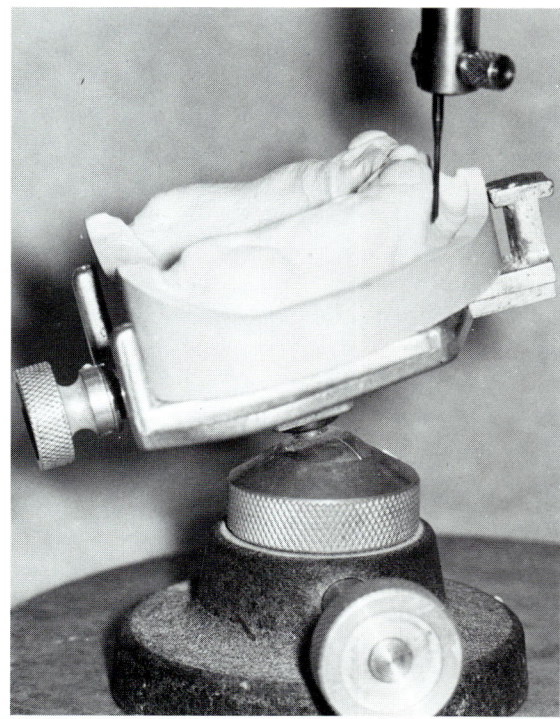

Fig. 11-22. Diagnostic cast showing slight posterior tilt required in this case to minimize significant, undesirable undercuts.

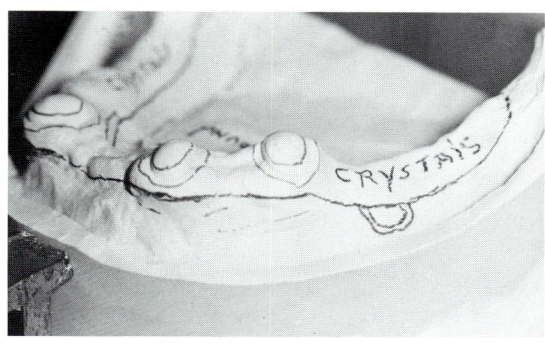

Fig. 11-23. Design for metal base extending over copings and residual ridge, and approximating area covered by attached gingiva. Note indication of "crystal" retention and placement of handle. Lines on abutment teeth and adjacent gingiva indicate area of proposed relief.

cording. Freely displaceable residual ridge tissues and undercut areas may require modifications in base extension, usually a reduction in the area covered. The design for the metal base should extend over the ridge portion of the cast and the copings far enough to approximate the area covered by the attached gingiva (Fig. 11-23). The border of the base should be short of reflections of the cast, since the borders of the completed overdentures, which are of resin rather than of metal, permit adjustments (Fig. 11-24).

The frequent occurrence of undercuts labial to the cuspid abutments precludes extension of the metal base into these areas. An extension 2 or 3

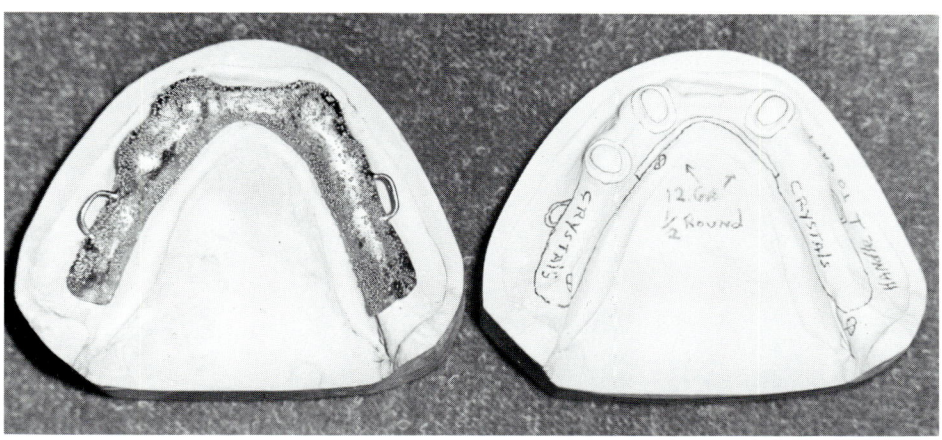

Fig. 11-24. Borders of metal base design are made short of tissue reflections for overdenture borders of resin instead of metal.

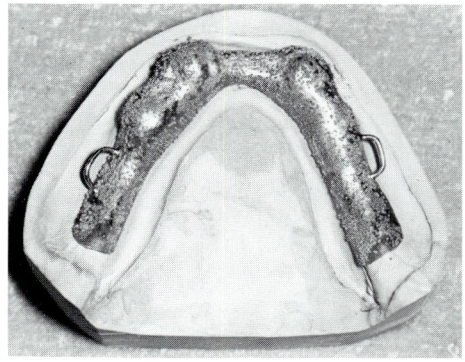

Fig. 11-25. Metal base casting showing handles raised to facilitate handling of base when recording jaw relations. Handles are removed before processing overdenture.

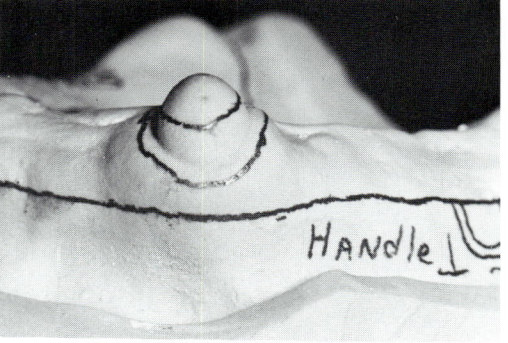

Fig. 11-26. Area of relief around each abutment extending from approximately two thirds of distance up abutment to 1 to 2 mm. beyond coping margin onto gingival tissue. Relief is tapered, being thinnest at incisal extent and thickest over gingival margin.

mm. beyond the gingival margin usually can be obtained without entering undercuts and is facilitated by a slight posterior tilt of the cast during design procedures.

A small loop handle is placed in a raised position on each side of the metal base. The handle should not be in contact with the cast surface (Fig. 11-25). During jaw relation recording procedures, these handles are useful for insertion and removal of the base from the mouth. They are cut off before the final wax-up of the denture.

Relief for copings. Desired relief is indicated on the diagnostic cast. Around each abutment coping the relief area should extend approximately two thirds of the distance up the abutment and taper in thickness from about 0.5 mm. at the gingival margin to 0.0 mm. at the incisal extent of the relief (Fig. 11-26). The relief should extend onto the gingival tissue 1 or 2 mm. beyond the gingival borders of the copings. This design, which minimizes axial contacts, permits a ball and socket contact between the coping and the metal base and reduces lateral stress on the abutment during functional loading of the dentures. The amount of relief should be limited, for too much induces hyperplasia of gingival tissues into the relief space.

Thickness of metal base. The metal base should be thin, particularly over the abutments to avoid interference with the positioning of teeth. Thick bases with needless bulk over the abutment teeth compromise esthetics, but bases should be strong and rigid. The lingual area of mandibular castings can be reinforced by adding a strip of 12-gauge half-round wax to the pattern, extending from the second premolar area to the second premolar on the opposite side (Fig. 11-27). This reinforcement materially increases rigidity with minimal addi-

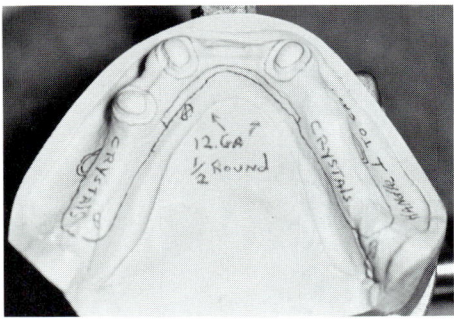

Fig. 11-27. Design for a mandibular metal base with reinforcement indicated. Strip of 12-gauge half-round casting wax extending from premolar area on one side to premolar area on opposite side increases strength and rigidity significantly. Finished castings of this design in chrome cobalt should weigh about 6 to 8 gm.

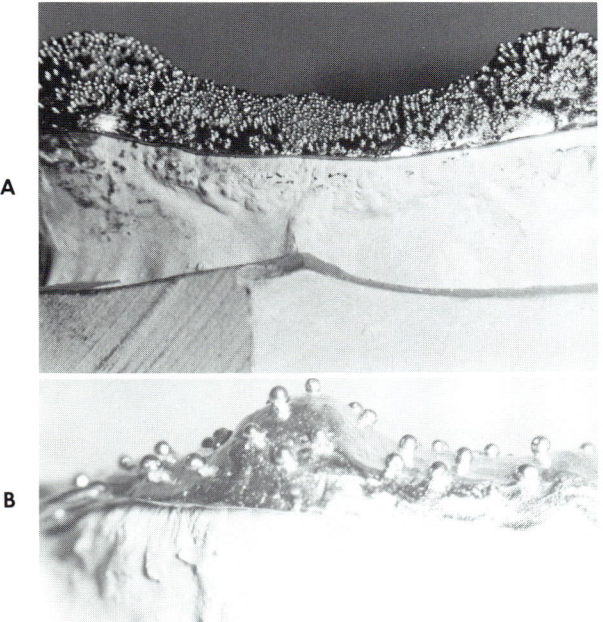

Fig. 11-28. A, Small retentive beads or crystals, which do not interfere with positioning of denture teeth. **B,** Larger retentive beads, which encroach on space available for denture teeth.

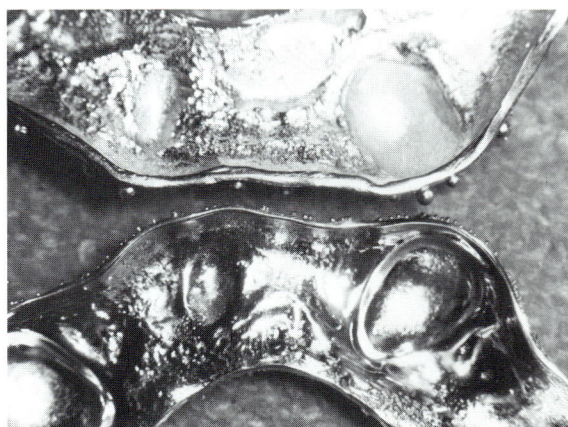

Fig. 11-29. Unnecessarily thick upper casting can make positioning of teeth difficult. Lower casting showing metal base highly polished in areas immediately adjacent to gingival margins around each abutment. Polished casting should be 0.3 to 0.5 mm. thick.

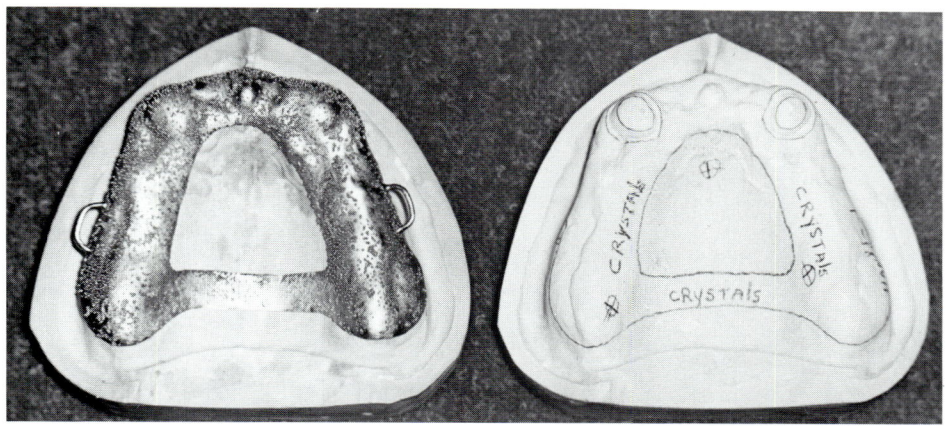

Fig. 11-30. Typical maxillary metal base design showing palatal strap for additional strength and rigidity. Position of handle is similar to that on mandibular bases. Metal base in chrome cobalt is approximately 0.4 mm. thick and weighs about 8 gm.

tional bulk. Chrome-cobalt alloys are ideal for metal base overdentures because the casting can be made light and strong. Type IV gold can be used for metal bases, although cost considerations and weight, especially in the maxillary dentures, are negative factors.

Resin retention. Small beads or crystals are used to retain the denture base resin (Fig. 11-28, *A*). Larger beads should be avoided, for they can interfere with the positioning of denture teeth (Fig. 11-28, *B*).

Finishing and polishing. The metal base is highly polished in the areas immediately adjacent to the gingival tissue around each abutment (Fig. 11-29). A high polish in these critical areas seems to facilitate cleanliness and thereby improve tissue response. The exterior surface of the metal base should be polished to minimize metal display through relatively translucent denture base resins.

Maxillary metal base design considerations

An open palate design is used most frequently for the metal base of a maxillary overdenture (Fig. 11-30). A posterior palatal strap crosses the palate anterior to the posterior palatal seal area. The enclosed ring design provides excellent rigidity with minimal weight. As in the mandibular framework, the casting should be thin. Extensions, retentive beads, handles, and finishing remain essentially the same as for the mandibular denture (Fig. 11-31).

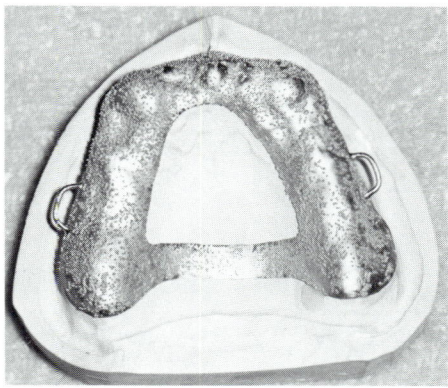

Fig. 11-31. Maxillary metal base with sufficient extension for use as a record base in recording jaw relations. These small castings are incorporated in resin baseplates for recording jaw relations.

Design modifications

Metal base designs can be modified to meet existing requirements. For example, the metal base can be reduced in size so that most of the denture-supporting tissue contact is made through the denture base resin and not through the metal. A small casting joining each abutment permits the denture to be relined and is used when supporting tissues distal to the abutments can be displaced readily (Fig. 11-32). Open mesh frameworks also can be used if relining may be required, particularly in areas of recent surgical procedures (Fig. 11-33). Generally metal-base–supporting tissue con-

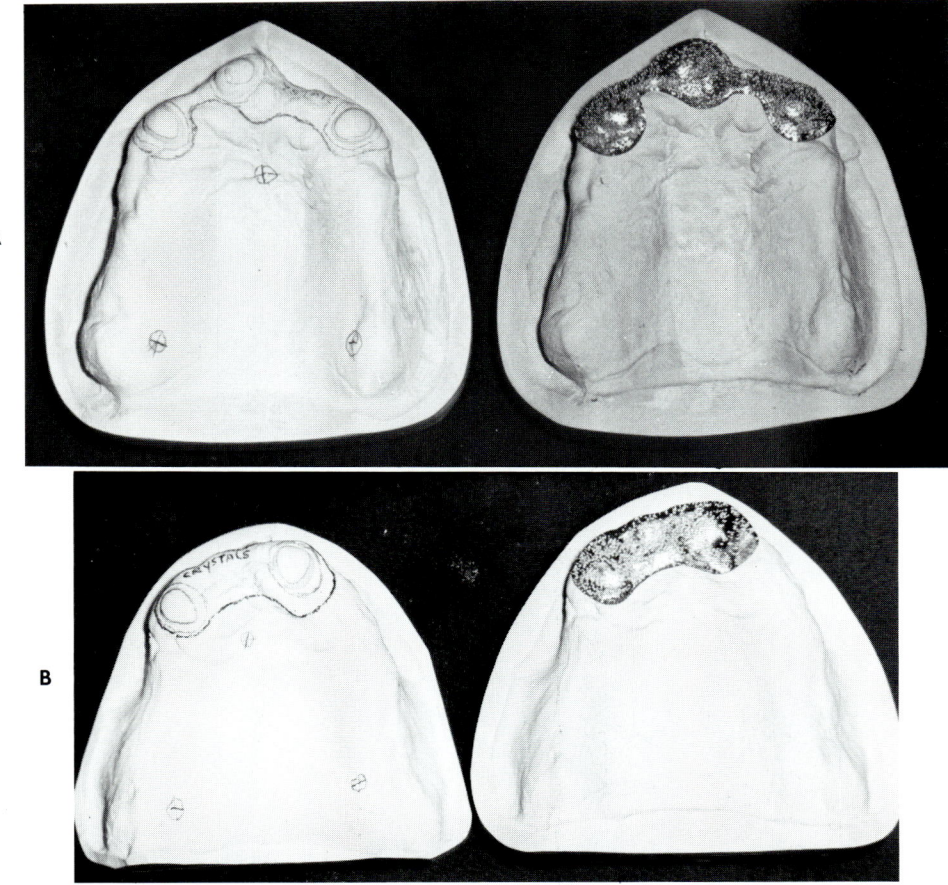

Fig. 11-32. **A,** Small metal overdenture casting covering three abutments. This design retains many advantages of metal bases and makes relining easier. **B,** Another small overdenture casting covering two abutments, a cuspid and a central incisor. Chrome cobalt castings of this design weigh 2 to 3 gm.

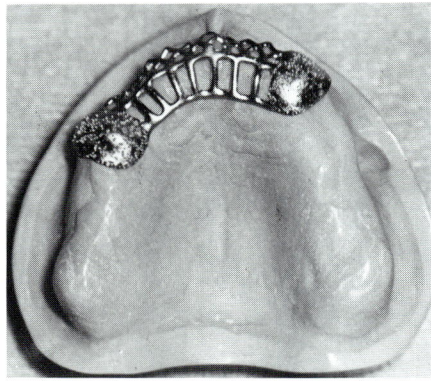

Fig. 11-33. Small maxillary overdenture casting with open mesh between abutments. This design permits "fill-in" applications of autopolymerizing resin to compensate for tissue changes after removal of teeth.

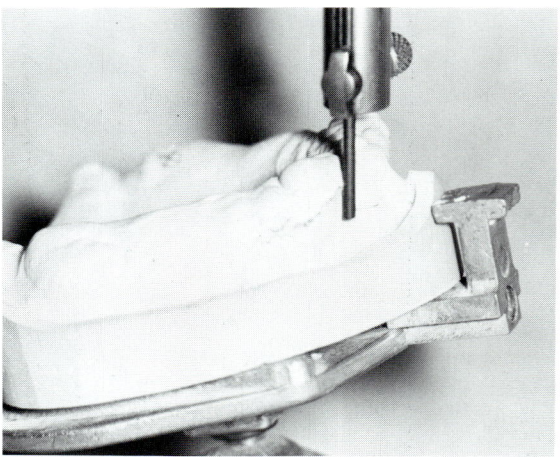

Fig. 11-34. Cast with survey line to indicate undercuts. Posterior tilt was used to lower survey line in anterior area.

tact seems to be preferable to denture-resin–supporting tissue contact.

Procedures for designing diagnostic cast

With the aforementioned considerations as a basis, the design of the metal base is placed to the diagnostic cast in a systematic manner.

1. Place the diagnostic cast on a surveyor, locate the tissue undercuts, and select the tilt. Drawing the survey line on the cast and abutment teeth will indicate the undercuts (Fig. 11-34).

2. Tripod the cast so that the dental laboratory can reestablish the tilt used in completing the design (Fig. 11-35).

3. Draw the extent of the metal base with a brown pencil. Do not extend the metal base into

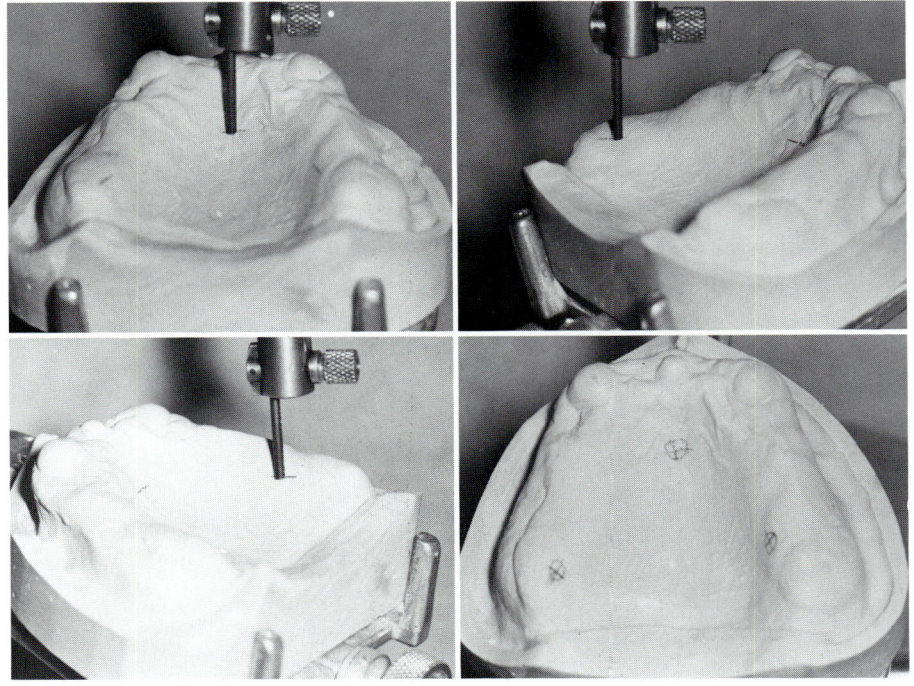

Fig. 11-35. Diagnostic cast tripoded to preserve "tilt" used in designing base. Dental laboratory can use tripod markings to duplicate tilt used in design.

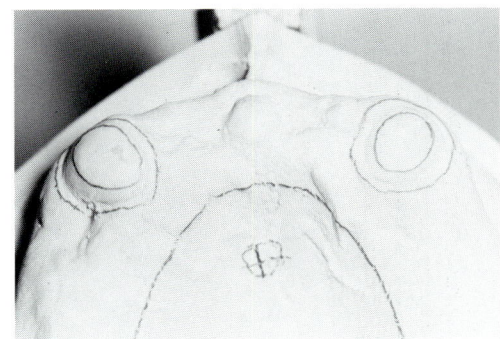

Fig. 11-36. Diagnostic cast with relief indicated. Finished casting should contact abutments only in rounded occlusal or incisal area.

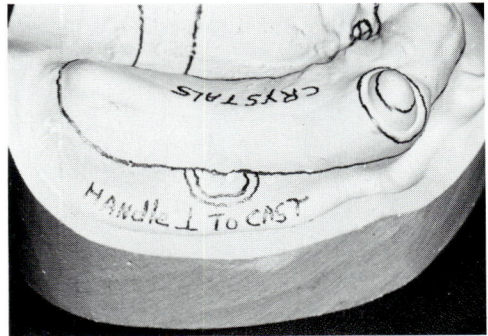

Fig. 11-37. Example of specific directions about handles included in design or instructions. Handles placed in direct contact with tissue by laboratory cannot be used.

the tissue undercuts. Indicate any areas of open mesh.

4. Indicate the desired relief around the abutment teeth with a red pencil (Fig. 11-36).

5. Indicate the type of retention, such as beads or crystals, for the denture base resin.

6. Draw handles in the molar areas, and show that they are to be raised above the cast (Fig. 11-37).

7. Indicate areas of special reinforcement, such as the lingual border of the anterior segment of the mandibular base.

Now the design is complete (Fig. 11-38). The designed cast and the master cast are identified, appropriate work authorizations are prepared, and all are packaged carefully to avoid breakage while enroute to the dental laboratory. The laboratory procedures for fabricating metal bases are presented in Chapter 14.

When the dentist receives the metal base, it should be on the master cast and fit this cast accurately; only a minor adjustment should be necessary. This situation may arise when minute tissue folds or undercuts are not blocked out during fabrication of the metal base.

Metal base try-in

In almost every instance the accuracy of the adaptation is improved by fitting the base to the abutment teeth with Kerr disclosing wax (Fig. 11-39). After the wax is warmed and placed into each abutment indentation, the metal base is seated in the mouth (Fig. 11-40). On removal, the base is examined carefully for any minute bubbles or irregularities that interfere with seating of the base

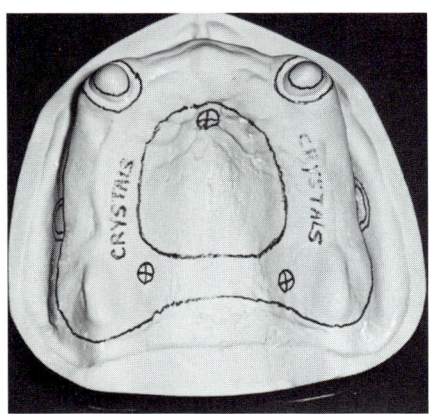

Fig. 11-38. Designed cast for maxillary overdenture.

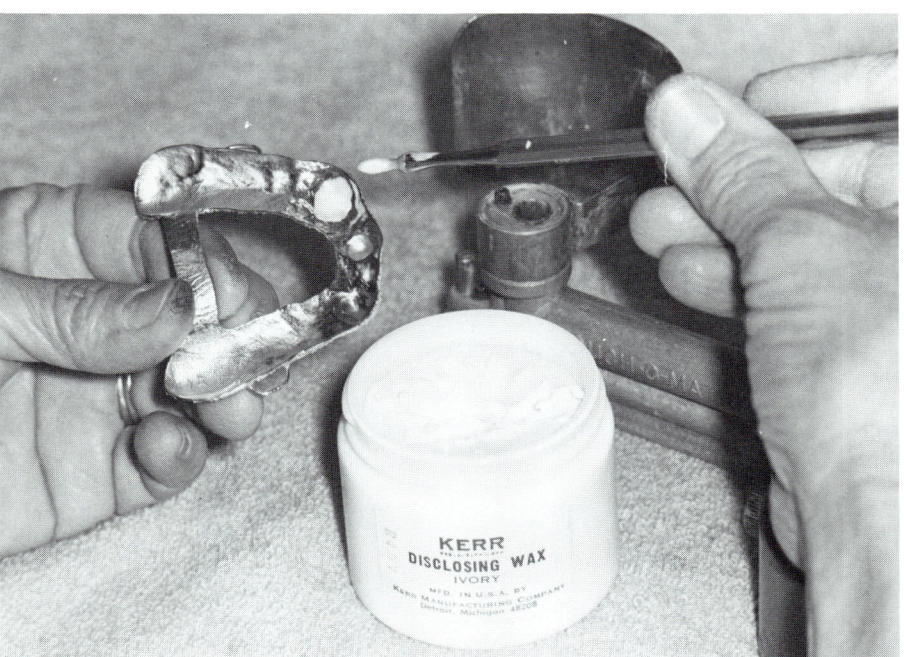

Fig. 11-39. Disclosing wax placed in abutment indentations to verify fit of casting.

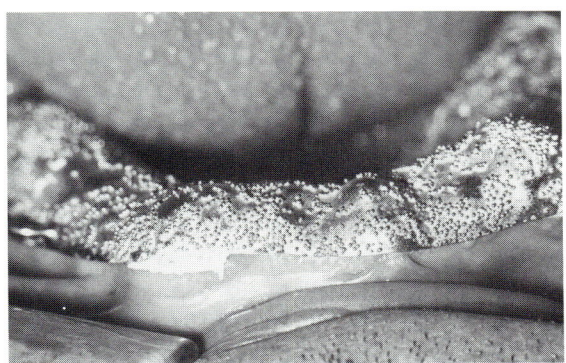

Fig. 11-40. Casting being seated, showing excess wax extruding beneath base.

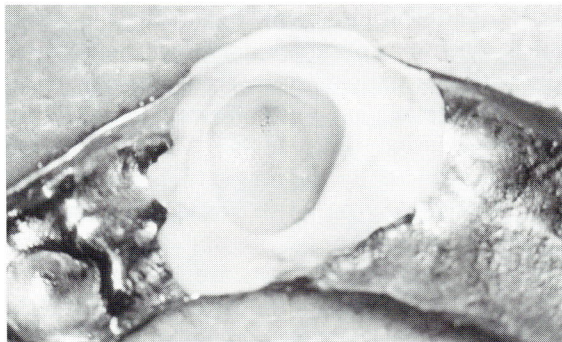

Fig. 11-41. Imperfections that interfere with seating of base, indicated by wax, should be removed with bur and polished.

(Fig. 11-41). These irregularities are removed with a carbide bur in an air rotor. The disclosing wax is removed after each adjustment, and a new coating is applied. Adjustment is continued until an accurate adaptation is confirmed by the disclosing wax. Areas roughened should then be smoothed. Contact between abutments and the base should be indicated in the incisal third of the abutment coping only, with the wax progressively thicker toward the gingival margin. Axial contacts, being undesirable, are removed by grinding the appropriate portion of the metal base.

Jaw relation recording procedures

Jaw relation recording procedures vary according to whether the arch opposing the overdenture is (1) a conventional complete denture, (2) another overdenture, or (3) a natural or restored dentition. Since many methods for recording jaw relations are excellent, our objective is to present only one method that we have found effective for each combination.

Overdenture opposed by complete denture

A frequent treatment situation is a maxillary complete denture to be opposed by a mandibular overdenture. In this combination, an impression of the edentulous arch is obtained by an accepted method and poured in artificial stone. A conventional autopolymerizing resin base with a wax oc-

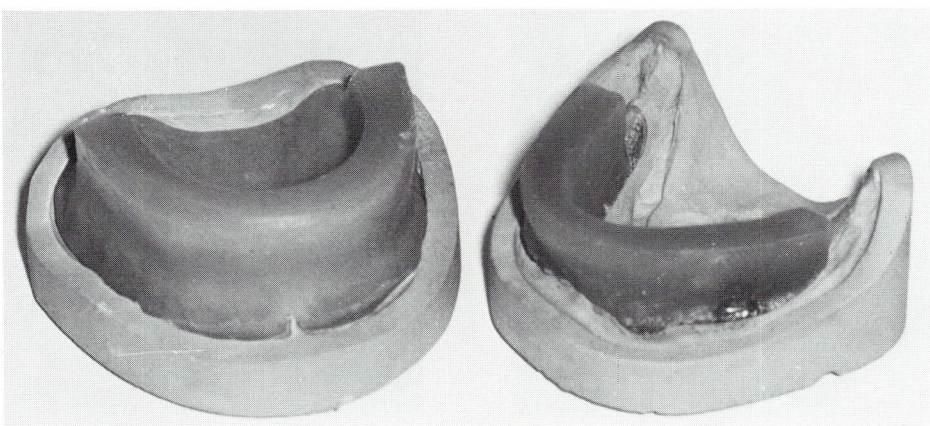

Fig. 11-42. Maxillary baseplate and occlusion rim for conventional complete denture and wax rim on mandibular metal overdenture base.

140 METHODS

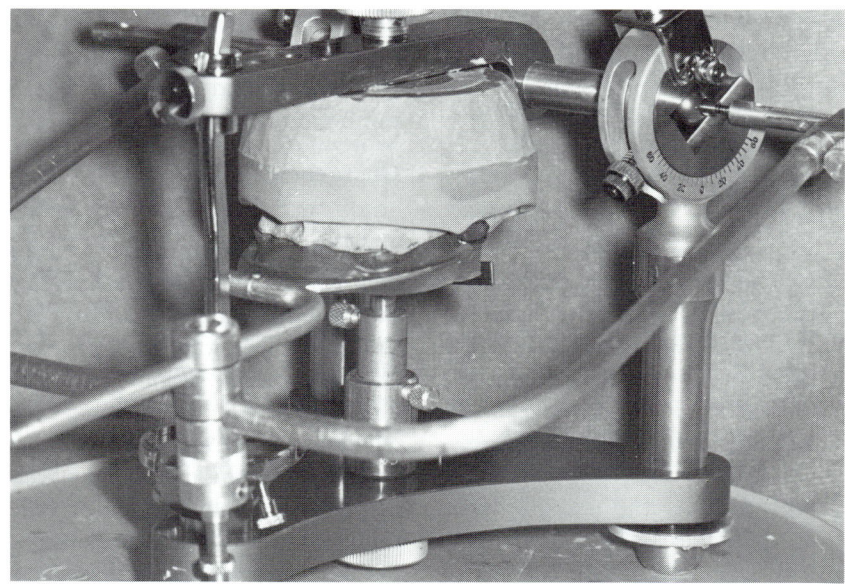

Fig. 11-47. Maxillary cast is mounted in articulator with facebow transfer.

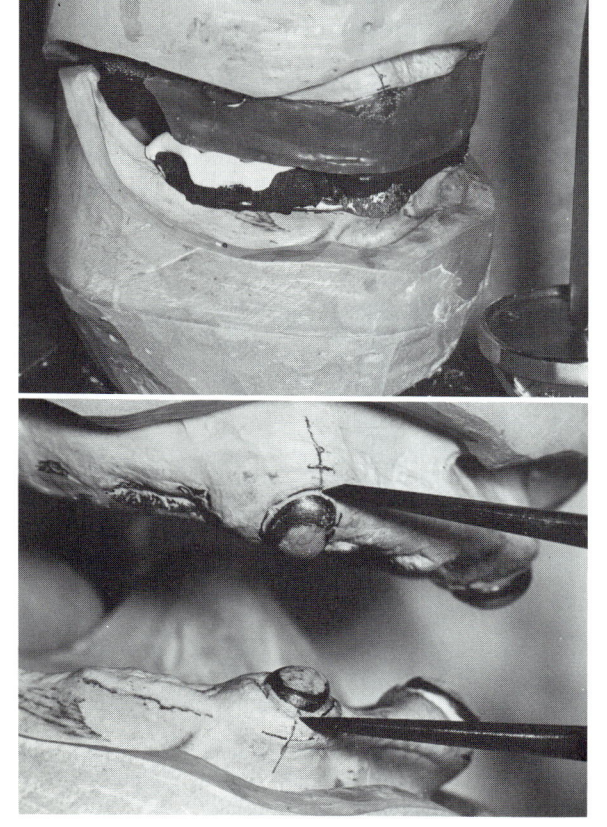

2 or 3 mm., is added to the original measurement. In constructing maxillary and mandibular overdentures, both arches are considered. At this point the maxillary overdenture base does not demonstrate retention; sometimes a thin coating of denture adhesive improves retention during the jaw relation recording procedure. This adhesive must be removed from the metal base before replacing it on the cast.

Jaw relation records. The maxillary wax rim is contoured to provide needed lip support and adjusted to the desired lip line and occlusal plane. The maxillary cast is mounted in the articulator by means of a face-bow transfer (Fig. 11-47). Then the wax rims are adjusted to the desired vertical dimension of occlusion by using the previously discussed pretreatment measurements as a guide. A centric interocclusal record is obtained, and the mandibular cast is mounted in the articulator (Fig. 11-48, *A*). The pretreatment measurement should be confirmed on the mounted casts (Fig. 11-48, *B*). It is essential that the accuracy of the

Fig. 11-48. **A**, Mandibular cast is mounted in articulator by using accurate centric jaw relation record. **B**, Pretreatment measurement between opposing abutment teeth is verified.

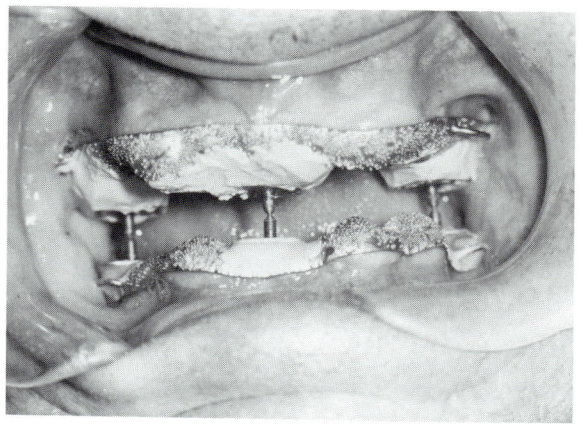

Fig. 11-49. Centric check points are used for verifying jaw relation records. Technique is discussed in Chapter 16.

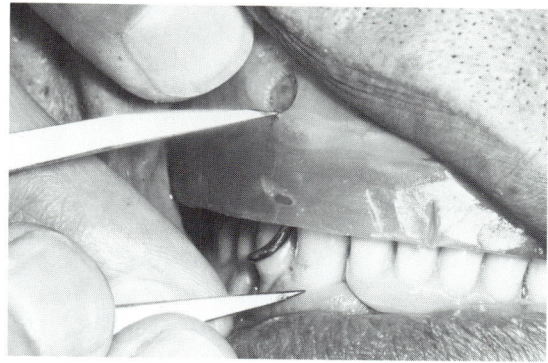

Fig. 11-50. Pretreatment measurements are made between abutment tooth and opposing tooth to help in determining vertical dimension of occlusion. In this instance, hole in maxillary baseplate allows placement of divider point.

cast mounting should be verified by additional interocclusal records or with centric check points (Fig. 11-49).

Overdenture opposed by natural or restored dentition

Jaw relation procedures for overdentures opposed by natural or reconstructed dentitions can be accomplished by the conventional approaches or by the functionally generated path method described by Meyer (1934). The most usual combination is a maxillary overdenture opposed by a natural or a reconstructed dentition in the mandibular arch. Although such cases can be treated successfully by conventional procedures involving mounting the casts in a suitable articulator on which the occlusion is developed, these combinations are compatible with functionally generated path techniques.

Conventional procedure. In a conventional approach the maxillary cast is mounted on the articulator by means of a face-bow transfer. A wax occlusion rim on the maxillary metal base is contoured appropriately and adjusted to the desired vertical dimension of occlusion. The centric jaw relationship is recorded in a suitable medium, and the mandibular cast mounted in the articulator. Protrusive and lateral eccentric positions can be recorded as needed to make the articulator adjustments. Then the occlusion is developed by using the simulated functional movements of the articulator. Centric, protrusive, and lateral interocclusal records and related remounts can be made after completion of the denture to harmonize further the occlusion and the mandibular movements of the patient. If the opposing occlusion is restored with cast restorations, metal occlusal surfaces are recommended.

Functionally generated path technique.[*] Maxillary overdentures opposed by natural or reconstructed mandibular dentition are especially suitable for the functionally generated path technique as described by Meyer (1951, 1959). In these cases the opposing arch is restored first. If teeth are missing in the opposing dentulous arch, fixed or removable partial dentures are used to restore the functional integrity of the arch. Maxillary natural dentitions opposing edentulous mandibular arches are rare; therefore the technique described pertains largely to the construction of a maxillary overdenture opposed by a mandibular natural dentition.

Tentative jaw relation record. To make a tentative jaw relation record, a wax occlusion rim is applied to the maxillary metal base. The maxillary low lip line is determined, and the wax rim is adjusted for esthetics. The midline is scribed on the wax rim. The maxillary metal base and rim is inserted, and the desired vertical dimension of occlusion is established by using such guides as phonetics, interocclusal space adequacy, and esthetics. Pretreatment measurements between abutments

---
[*]This section was contributed by Kenneth D. Rudd.

and selected index teeth in the opposing arch are invaluable when obtaining the vertical dimension of occlusion (Fig. 11-50). Then the maxillary cast is mounted in an articulator with a conventional face-bow transfer. A centric relation record at the desired vertical dimension of occlusion is made by using a suitable recording medium such as zinc oxide impression paste or slurry-activated artificial stone. A rigid recording medium aids in positioning the cusps of the opposing cast into the indentations. The centric relation record is verified. If the record is acceptable, the casts are related with the interocclusal record, and the mandibular cast is mounted on the articulator with accelerated artificial stone (Fig. 11-51). The recorded vertical dimension of occlusion is rechecked on the casts with dividers after they have been mounted in the articulator (Fig. 11-52).

Baseplate fabrication. An autopolymerizing acrylic resin baseplate is made on the maxillary overdenture cast. It is axiomatic that accurately fitting baseplates are a prerequisite for making accurate jaw relation records. Two autopolymerizing resins are used for making baseplates (Burnett, 1968); a soft-setting resin* is placed in the areas of tissue undercuts and abutments, and a conventional hard-setting resin† is used for strength and rigidity.

---

*Coe soft, Coe Laboratories, Chicago.
†Caulk Repair Material, The L. D. Caulk Co., Milford, Del.

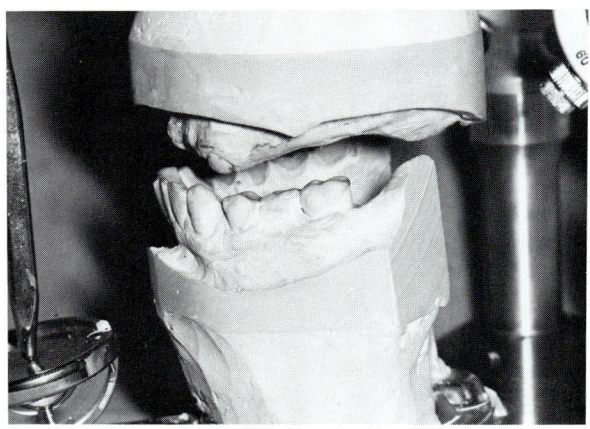

Fig. 11-51. Casts mounted in articulator. Available denture space seems to be adequate.

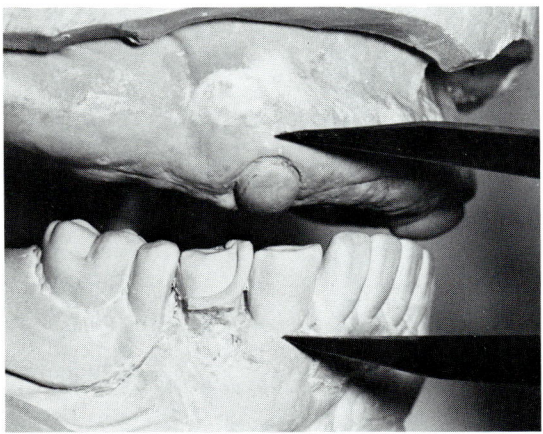

Fig. 11-52. Vertical dimension of occlusion is checked with dividers. Original measurement was from gingival margin to gingival margin. Since metal base covers gingival margin of abutment and usually extends 1 to 2 mm. beyond, the difference is considered.

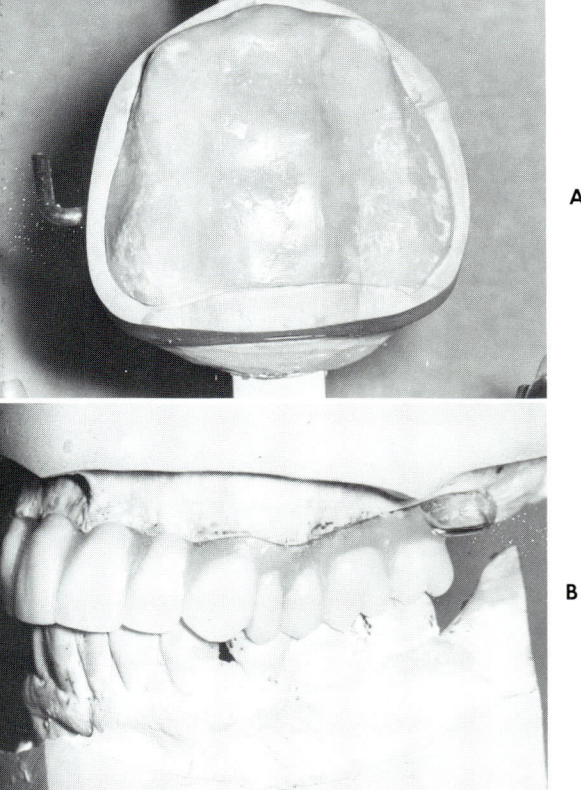

Fig. 11-53. A, Autopolymerizing resin baseplate fabricated on maxillary cast. B, Initial positioning of teeth on articulator.

The master cast is coated with tinfoil substitute. Unless the tissue undercuts are severe, usually it is unnecessary to block them out with wax before adding resin. Soft-curing autopolymerizing resin is mixed with monomer and placed in all undercuts to obturate these areas. More soft resin is sifted around the abutment teeth to reduce the possibility of breakage on separation.

Conventional hard-curing autopolymerizing resin is sifted onto the cast and saturated with monomer to complete the baseplates; then the cast is placed into a pressure container for 30 minutes at a pressure of 30 p.s.i. After setting, the baseplate is removed from the cast, finished, and polished. When constructed in this manner, the baseplate can be removed and replaced on the cast without damage (Fig. 11-53, A). The soft-curing resin also permits extension of the base into moderate undercuts without unnecessary blockout, thereby improving the stability and retention of the baseplate during jaw relation recording procedures.

Positioning teeth. With the previously contoured wax occlusion rim on the metal base as a guide, anterior denture teeth are selected and positioned in the presence of the patient. Then the posterior teeth are positioned on the metal base in the articulator, but no attempt is made to balance the occlusion at this time (Fig. 11-53, B). The metal base with the teeth waxed for try-in is removed from the cast and replaced with the resin baseplate.

Making the compound rim. Black impression compound, heated in a water bath, is used to form an occlusion rim on the resin baseplate. The compound rim is sealed to the baseplate to prevent separation during the "chew in" procedure. The occlusal surfaces of the mandibular cast teeth are lubricated lightly with petrolatum. The occlusal surface of the modeling plastic rim is softened by flaming, and the articulator is closed. The lubricated stone teeth should form distinct indentations on the occlusal surface of the maxillary compound rim (Fig. 11-54). The impression compound rim is cooled and modified by removing the compound on each side of the ridge formed by the central fossa of the mandibular posterior teeth (Fig. 11-55). Enough compound is removed to clear the buccal and lingual cusps, leaving only the compound sulci ridge to maintain the vertical dimension of occlusion (Fig. 11-56). Compound is also removed on the anterior portion of the occlusion rim to clear all anterior teeth by 1 or 2 mm. (Fig. 11-57).

Pretreatment measurements. Before removing the modified compound occlusion rim from the articulator, dividers are used to record the vertical dimension of occlusion. One point of the divider is placed at a selected index point on the lower cast, usually the gingival margin of a tooth opposing an abutment of the overdenture. The other point of the divider extends through a small hole made in the baseplate to the appropriate point on an abutment tooth (Fig. 11-58). This measurement is recorded on the cast (Fig. 11-59). After modifi-

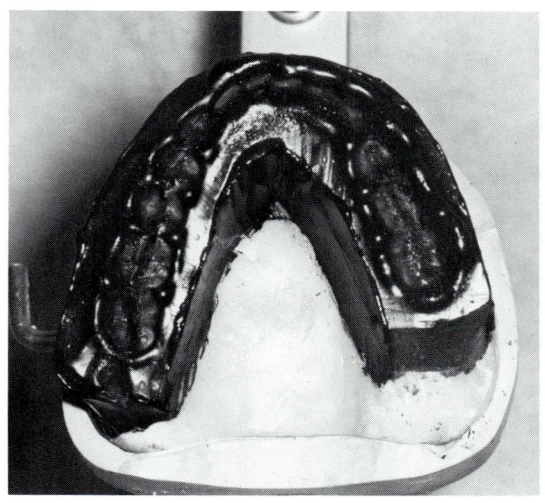

Fig. 11-54. Modeling plastic occlusion rim with indentations formed by opposing mandibular teeth.

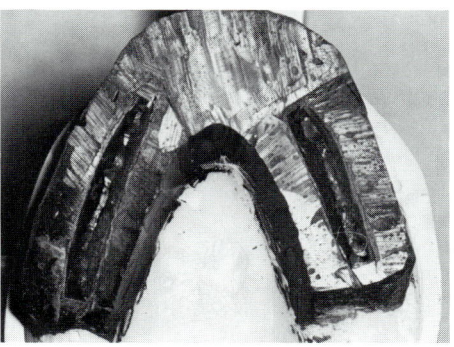

Fig. 11-55. Sulci ridge is formed by removing impression compound on each side of ridge formed by sulci of mandibular teeth. Rim is also reduced so that opposing anterior teeth do not contact rim.

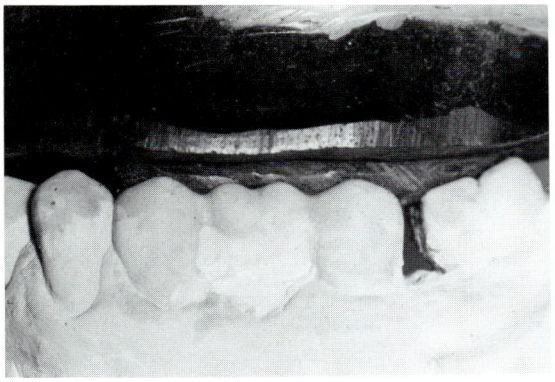

Fig. 11-56. Sulci ridge alone maintains vertical dimension of occlusion.

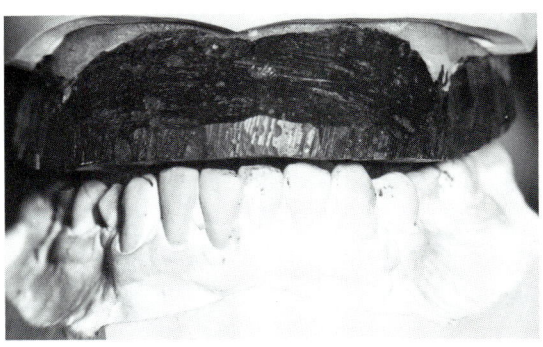

Fig. 11-57. Anterior teeth not contacting the rim.

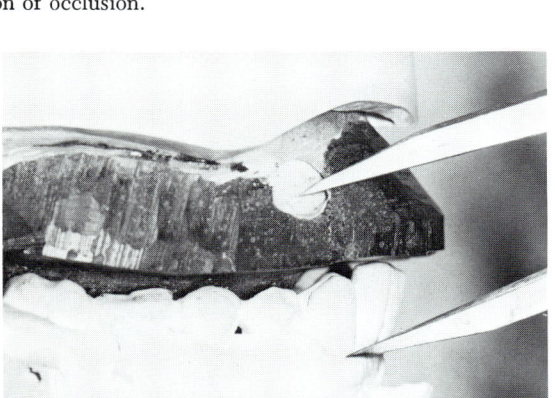

Fig. 11-58. Hole is placed in resin baseplate to expose gingival margin of abutment tooth. Vertical dimension of occlusion is being checked with dividers.

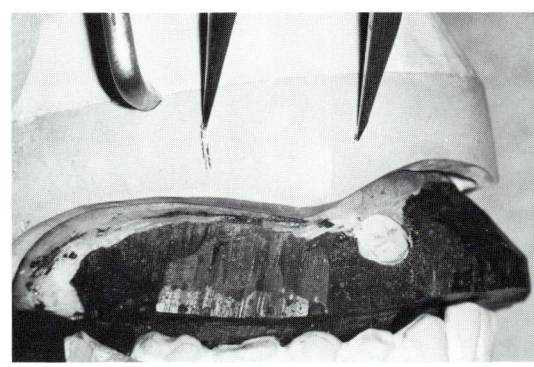

Fig. 11-59. Resultant measurement is recorded on cast for future use.

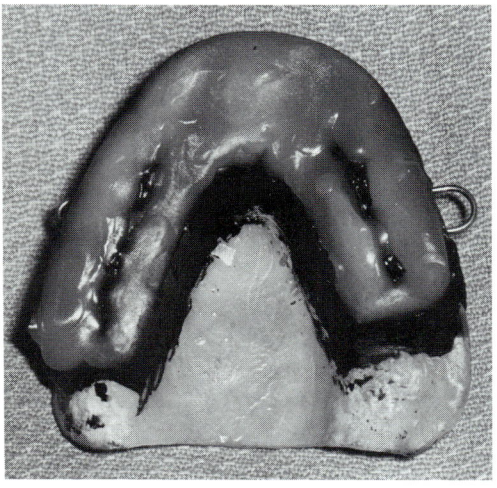

Fig. 11-60. Cuspal path wax placed on modeling plastic occlusion rim. Paper clips embedded in modeling plastic rims to serve as handles when making cuspal path record.

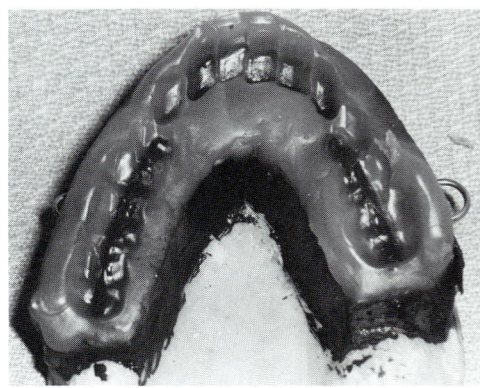

Fig. 11-61. Smooth cuspal path is usually obtained only after several excursions. A thin plastic strip can be attached to occlusion rim to "fence in" or confine wax during "chew in."

cation, the compound occlusion rim is placed in the mouth, and the jaw relation record is verified. The vertical dimension of occlusion is checked to determine the existence of adequate interocclusal distance, and the rim is removed. Errors are corrected by reaccomplishing the jaw relation record.

Wax try-in. The wax-up on the metal base is inserted, and the centric and vertical relation record checked for accuracy. The esthetic result, being of paramount importance, is evaluated critically by the dentist, the patient, and preferably the patient's spouse or close relative. After indicated corrections are made, the wax denture is removed.

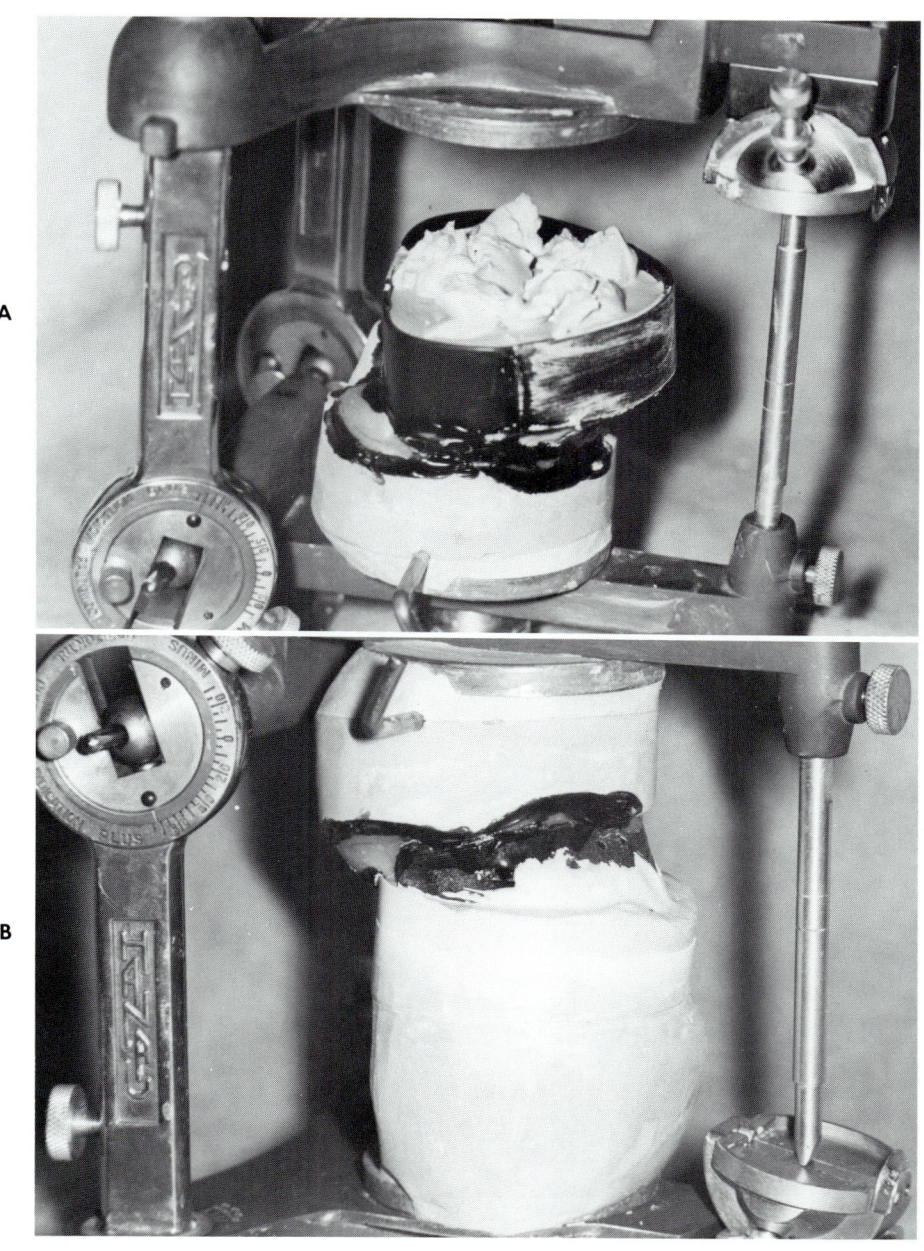

Fig. 11-62. **A**, Cuspal path boxed and poured in vacuum spatulated minimal expansion stone. **B**, Path mounted in articulator. Articulator is used for opening and closing movements only. Condylar slots are set steeply to minimize anteroposterior movement of articulator.

Recording cuspal path. After cuspal path wax* is added to the compound rim, it is inserted in the mouth and the patient is instructed to execute centric closures, as well as protrusive, right, and left lateral movements (Fig. 11-60). The cuspal path wax can be softened by placing it in water at 100° F. for several seconds. Each excursion originates at the most retruded position; on reaching the desired extent it is terminated by opening. Usually a smooth cuspal path is obtained only after several excursions (Fig. 11-61). A completed path exhibits smooth wax contours without tears or separations of wax from the compound rim. Before removing the cuspal path, the vertical dimension is rechecked with dividers.

Pouring the path. On removal from the mouth, the baseplate and the path are rinsed thoroughly in cool water, placed on the cast, sealed with wax, and remounted in the articulator. Then the cuspal path is boxed, poured in vacuum-spatulated minimal expansion stone, and mounted to the lower bow of the articulator (Fig. 11-62). After the stone has set, the wax is removed from the core with clean boiling water (Fig. 11-63).

Adapting denture teeth to core. The waxed denture is replaced on the cast and adapted to the core by using nontoxic water-soluble pigment* (Fig. 11-64) as an indicator. Cast metal occlusals, which are ideal for functionally generated path techniques, can be constructed if desired (Fig. 11-

---

*Korecta-wax (No. 4), Kerr Manufacturing Co., Romulus, Mich.

*Ultramarine blue, nontoxic, Bocour Artist Colors, New York.

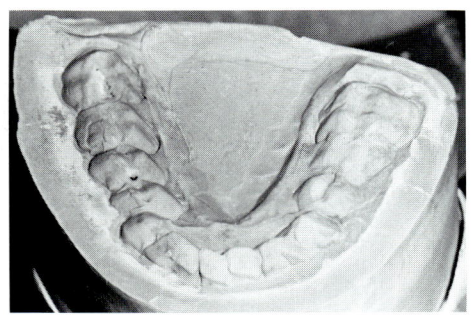

Fig. 11-63. Stone core.

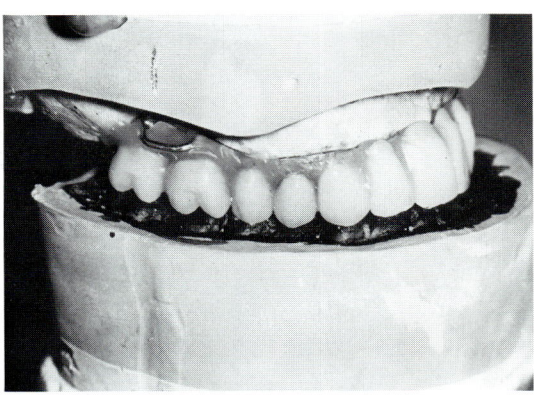

Fig. 11-64. Denture teeth are adapted to core by using nontoxic water-soluble pigment as indicator.

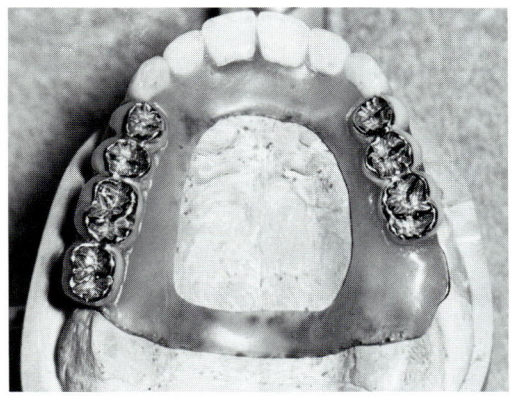

Fig. 11-65. Gold occlusal surfaces have been constructed using functionally generated path concepts.

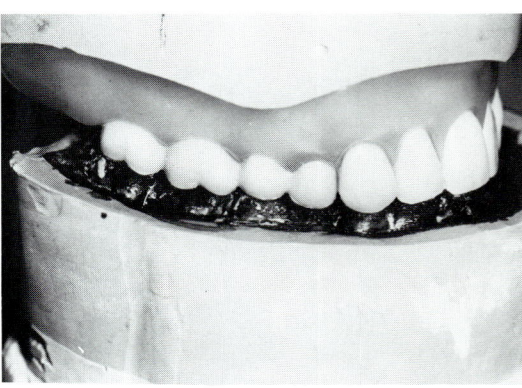

Fig. 11-66. Denture is remounted in articulator after curing. Any change resulting from processing is corrected.

65). A technique for constructing them is described in Chapter 17. The waxed denture is flasked, boiled out, and processed. After curing, the denture is remounted in the articulator and readapted to the stone core as described previously (Fig. 11-66). Then the denture is finished, polished, and thoroughly cleansed with soap and water to remove polishing materials (Fig. 11-67). Overdentures constructed by functionally generated path techniques demonstrate excellent functional harmony with mandibular movements. This procedure is recommended for overdentures opposed by natural or reconstructed dentitions.

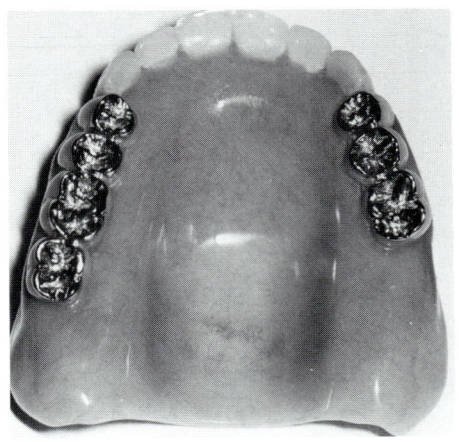

Fig. 11-67. Completed maxillary overdenture with gold occlusal surfaces.

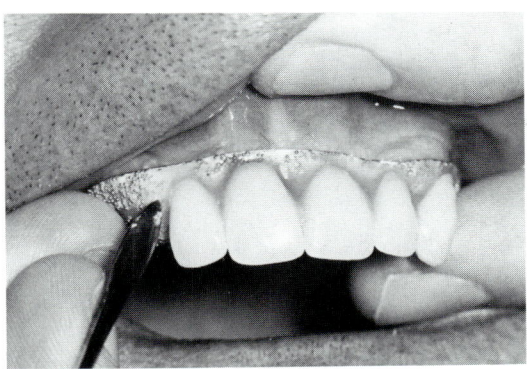

Fig. 11-68. Anterior teeth positioned in patient's mouth. Resin denture teeth are used over abutments; however, porcelain denture teeth can be used elsewhere if desired.

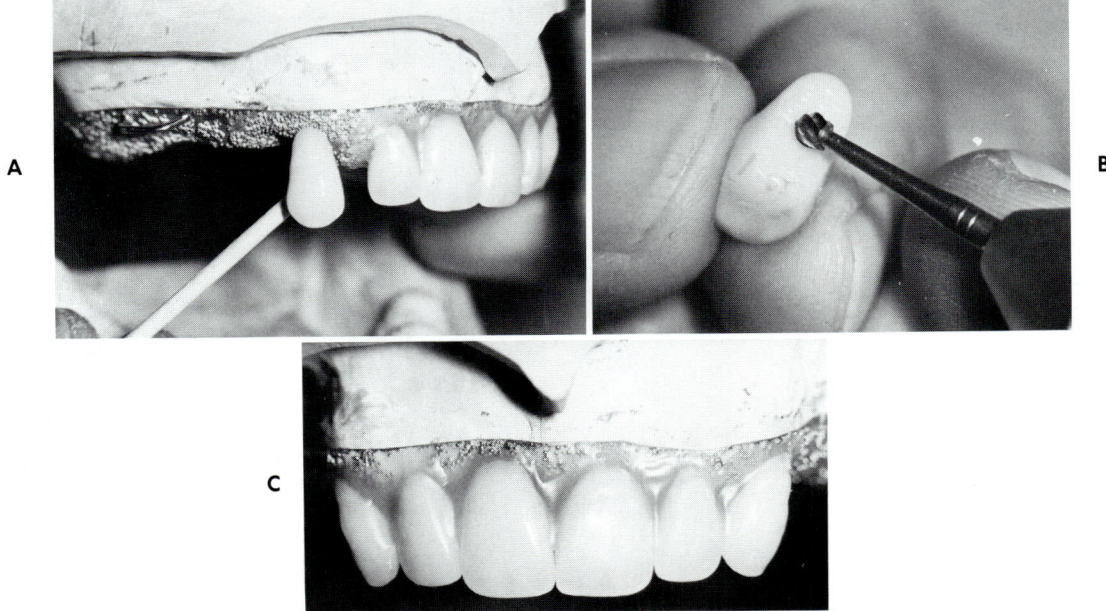

Fig. 11-69. **A,** Resin denture tooth is selected for positioning over abutment. **B,** Denture tooth is hollowed with bur. **C,** Hollowed denture tooth is waxed in place over abutment.

Tooth selection and positioning

Construction procedures for overdentures opposed by a complete denture or another overdenture are more conventional; they are similar to the usual complete denture procedures. Denture teeth of the appropriate mold and shade are selected for positioning on the bases for try-in.

Positioning anterior teeth. Positioning the anterior teeth in the presence of the patient undoubtedly has positive psychologic aspects and further contributes to the overall esthetic result (Fig. 11-68). The presence of abutments assists in the proper placement of denture teeth and, when supplemented with pretreatment casts, removes much of the doubt regarding selection and arrangement of teeth. Porcelain teeth can be used except over abutments, where resin teeth are required.

Positioning abutment teeth. Resin teeth for abutments are selected, hollowed with a bur, and positioned over the abutments on the metal base (Fig. 11-69).

Occlusal scheme. Posterior teeth can be porcelain or resin, anatomic or nonanatomic. When the posterior teeth oppose natural or reconstructed dentitions, metal occlusal surfaces are preferred. Flanges are not added to the metal base for the try-in; they are added to the completed denture (Fig. 11-70). The opinion of the spouse or a close relative is helpful during the wax try-in appointment; frequently the patient is permitted to take the wax-up home for a more leisurely evaluation in familiar surroundings. The patient is cautioned against eating or drinking with the waxed denture. Only after approval of the set-up by both the dentist and the patient is the denture completed.

Flasking and processing the overdenture

After acceptance, the trial denture is waxed for flasking, and the natural contours are simulated for optimal esthetics (Fig. 11-71).

Minimizing processing error. The occlusion is verified with cellophane strips before the casts are removed from the articulator (Fig. 11-72). Flasks that fit together accurately, without rocking, minimize processing error. The flasks are coated lightly with Masque silicone lubricant before the dentures are half-flasked in artificial stone, which preferably is mixed in a mechanical spatulator under reduced atmospheric pressure

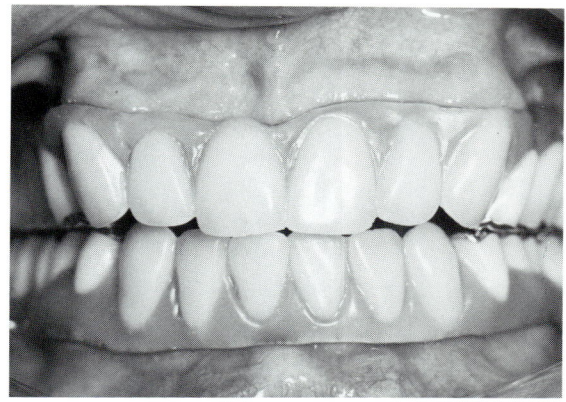

Fig. 11-70. Completed setup is tried in and subjected to usual checks.

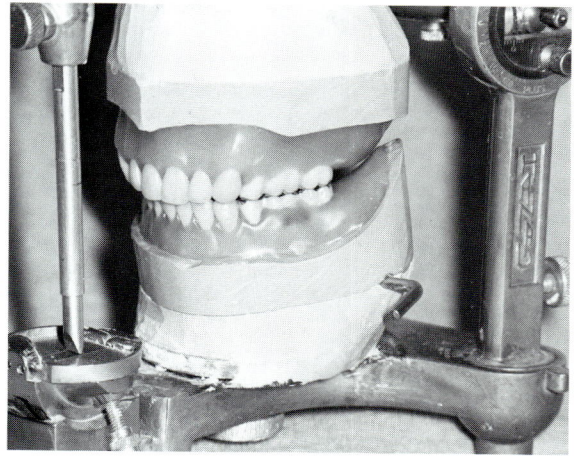

Fig. 11-71. Overdentures are waxed for flasking.

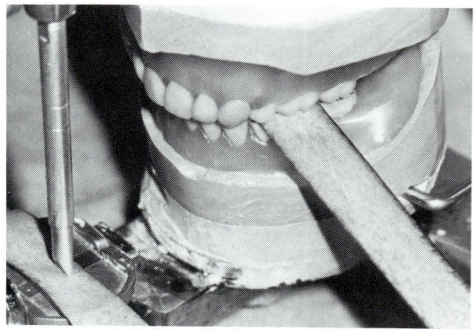

Fig. 11-72. Occlusion of waxed overdenture is checked before removal of casts from articulator.

(Fig. 11-73). After setting, the surface of the stone is coated with a separating medium, and artificial stone is mixed for the second pour. Brushing stone into the interproximal areas of the wax denture minimizes voids and shortens finishing time. Then the flask is filled with the remainder of the second mix with space left for a cap, which is added after setting. The flasked denture should set at least an hour and preferably overnight to allow the stone to achieve increased crushing strength.

Wax elimination. Flasks are placed in clean

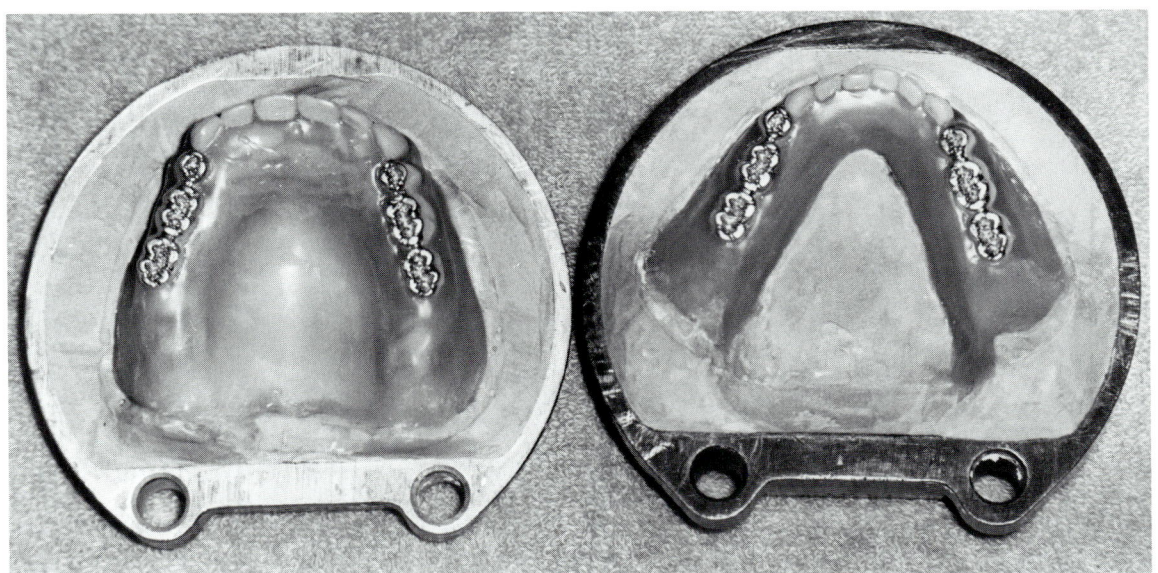

Fig. 11-73. Maxillary and mandibular overdentures have been half flasked.

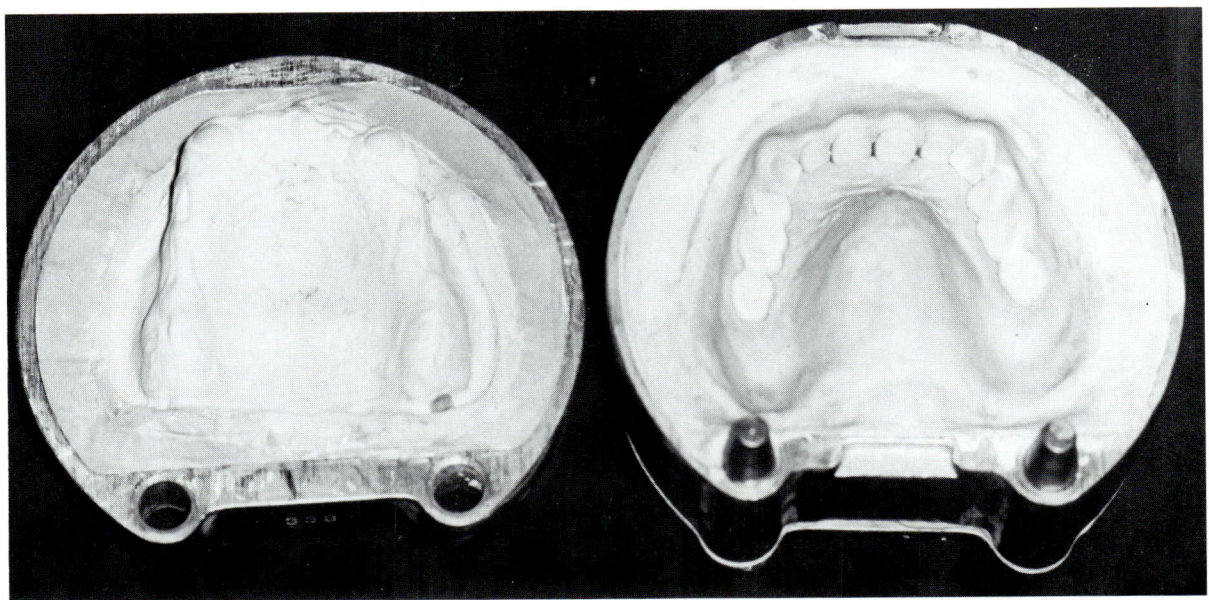

Fig. 11-74. Flasks are flushed with clean boiling water to remove all traces of wax.

boiling water for 4 minutes 15 seconds, and then removed and separated. This period of time allows the wax to soften adequately without liquefying. The metal base is retrieved and placed aside. The open flasks are flushed first with boiling water to which a detergent is added and finally with clean boiling water; then they are placed aside to drain and cool (Fig. 11-74). The metal base is rinsed thoroughly in clean boiling water to remove all traces of wax. After the flasks reach a comfortable handling temperature, the stone of the cope is coated carefully with a tinfoil substitute so as to avoid getting any on the ridge laps of the teeth. This precaution is of special importance for the hollowed-out abutment tooth.

Opaquing the metal base. The metal base is opaqued to prevent undesirable "show-through" under relatively translucent denture base resins (Fig. 11-75). Pink opaquing material* is painted over the part of the base to be covered by denture base resin, and tooth colored opaquing material is applied over the abutments. It is important to allow enough setting time for the opaquing material, for packing the denture too soon displaces the opaquing resin and causes both undesirable streaking and color modification (Fig. 11-76). Then the opaqued metal base is cemented to the cast with a thin mix of zinc oxyphosphate cement (Fig. 11-77). After the cement has set, any excess extruding from under the base is removed. The stone in the drag is coated with a tinfoil substitute, but care is taken to avoid the opaqued metal base.

---

*Justi Opaquer, H. D. Justi & Son, Philadelphia.

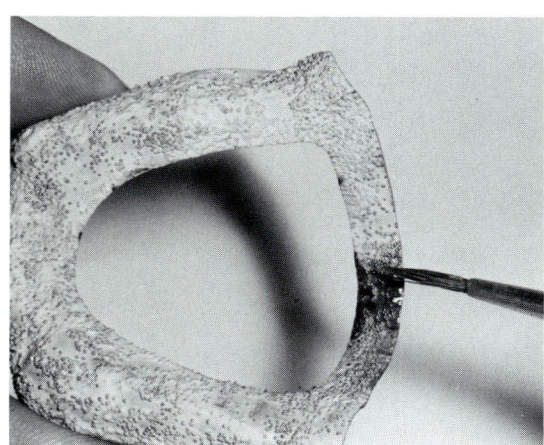

Fig. 11-75. Metal base opaqued to prevent "show through" under denture base resins.

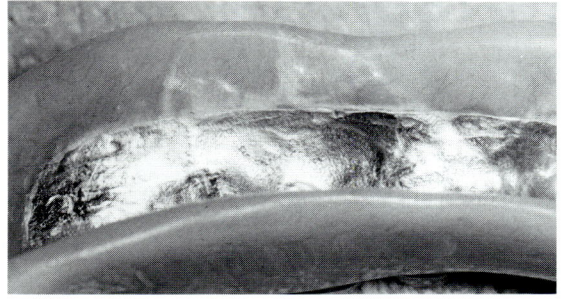

Fig. 11-76. Streaking was caused by packing denture too soon; opaquer had not set.

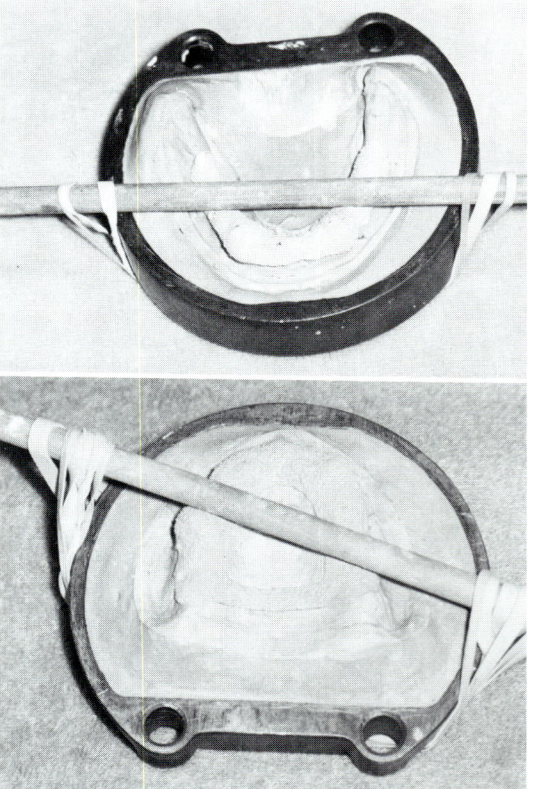

Fig. 11-77. A, Opaqued mandibular metal base being cemented on cast. Dowel rod and rubber bands hold metal base in position. B, Maxillary metal base being cemented on cast.

REMOTE OVERDENTURES **151**

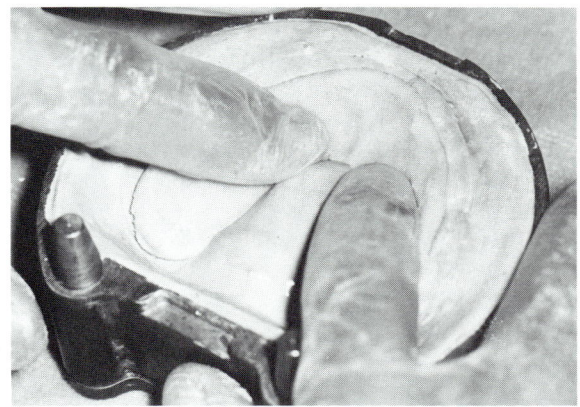

Fig. 11-78. Plastic gloves are used when packing denture base resin.

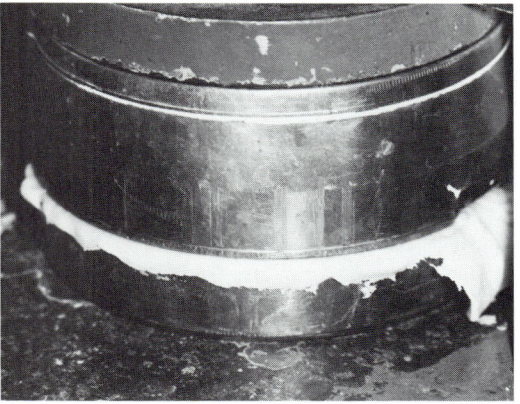

Fig. 11-79. Flask is closed slowly in bench compress. "Single closure" packing procedure is used.

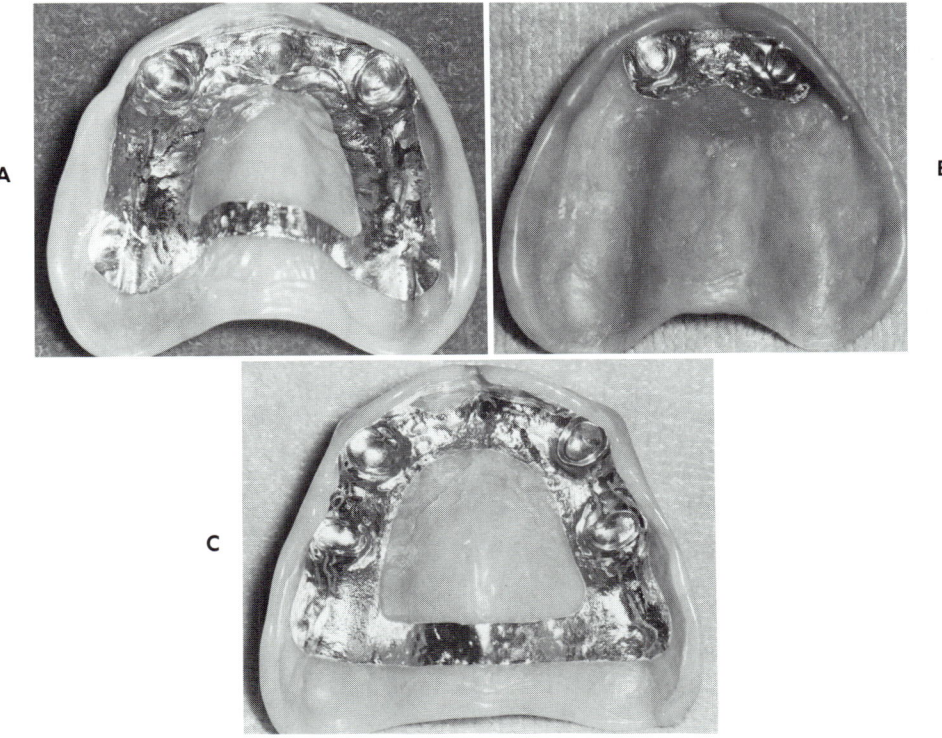

Fig. 11-80. A, Completed maxillary metal base overdenture using cuspid abutments. **B,** Completed maxillary metal base overdenture using smaller metal base. **C,** Maxillary metal base overdenture using four abutments (cuspids and second premolars).

Tooth-colored resin of the appropriate shade is sifted into each abutment indentation in the upper part of the flask and saturated with heat-curing monomer.

Packing the overdenture. The denture base can be tinted at this time if desired. Duraflow,* a denture resin amenable to the single closure packing technique, is mixed according to the manufacturer's recommendations and placed into the flask; plastic gloves are worn to prevent contamination of the resin (Fig. 11-78). The flask is closed slowly in a bench compress until metal-to-metal contact of the flask halves is observed, and the overdentures are subjected to the recommended curing cycle (Fig. 11-79). After curing, the flasks are allowed to bench cool; then the dentures are removed from the flasks and remounted in the articulator. Occlusal discrepancies resulting from processing are corrected before the overdentures are removed from the cast.

Finishing and polishing. The overdentures are removed from the casts and trimmed to the desired border extensions with a lathe-mounted arbor band. A slurry of flour of pumice and water is used with a soft rag wheel to smooth the surface of the resin. Simulated anatomic carvings on polished surfaces of the overdenture can be polished with a handpiece-mounted rubber cup and a slurry of flour of pumice to prevent loss of contour. Flour of pumice is preferred to coarser pumice, for it produces an extremely smooth surface easily polished to a high luster. A stippled surface can be created if desired. Then a high polish can be achieved with a clean fluffy rag wheel and Ti-Gleam No. 341† polishing compound. Porcelain denture teeth, which have been modified by grinding, also should be polished (Morrow and associates, 1973). The overdenture is now completed (Fig. 11-80).

Placing the overdenture

The overdenture should be examined under a good light, preferably under magnification, to locate any bubbles or projections on the tissue surface that need to be removed.

Verifying adaptation. Pressure indicating paste†

---
*Duraflow, Product Research Laboratories, Inc., Cambridge, Mass.
†Ticonium Co., Albany, N. Y.
‡PIP, Mizzy Inc., Clifton Forge, Va.

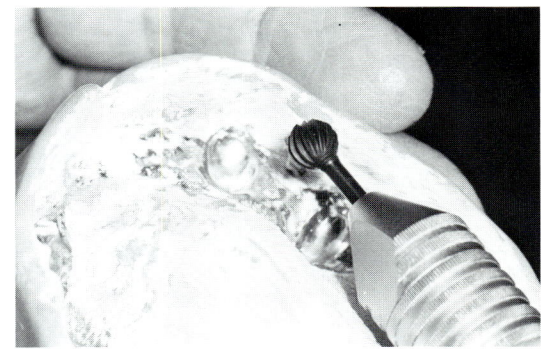

Fig. 11-81. Pressure-indicating paste is brushed on tissue surface of overdenture. Pressure areas identified are adjusted.

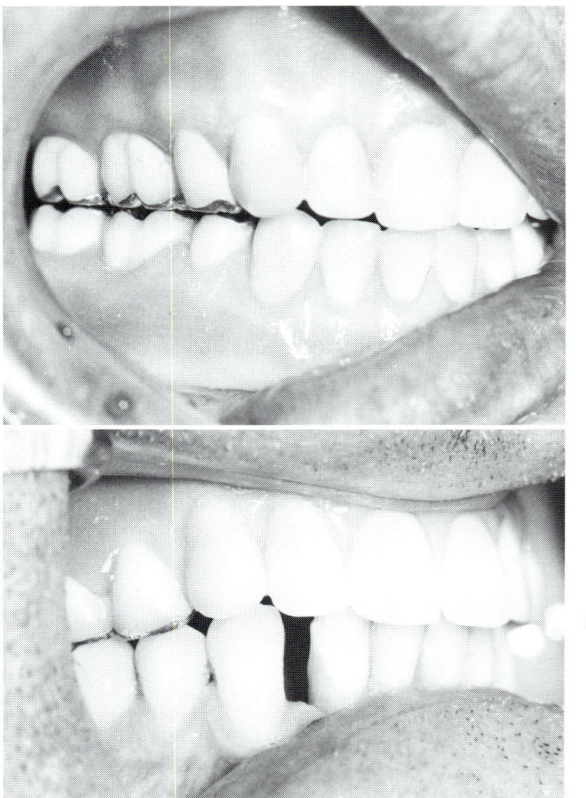

Fig. 11-82. A, Inserted overdentures are checked. In this instance, monoplane occlusion with metal oclusal surfaces is used. B, Maxillary overdenture opposed by natural dentition. Overdenture was constructed by using functionally generated path concept and metal occlusal surfaces.

is brushed on the tissue surface of the overdenture, and pressure areas are identified and adjusted (Fig. 11-81). Border extensions are verified, and the occlusion is examined critically (Fig. 11-82). Disclosing wax is placed in abutment indentations of the overdenture, and the overdenture-abutment contact is evaluated. Abutment contact should exist only in the incisal or occlusal third of the coping.

Postinsertion instructions. An adequate level of oral hygiene is the single most important factor in achieving a reasonable service life from an overdenture.

Overdenture hygiene. Abutments and overdentures must be cleaned regularly and thoroughly to avoid undesirable results. The dentures should be brushed with a soft toothbrush and hand soap. Harsh, abrasive household cleansers and bleaches are to be avoided. Unless contraindicated, the patient is instructed to take out the overdentures at night and place them in a soaking-type denture cleanser compatible with chrome-cobalt alloys. Ultrasonic denture cleansers for home use can also be used to maintain overdenture cleanliness.

Bubble gum massage. Maintenance of the supporting tissues is facilitated by bubble gum massage. Four to six cakes of bubble gum should be chewed at a time for 30 minutes twice a day with the dentures out of the mouth. Initially, it may be necessary to knead the bubble gum in lukewarm water to soften it before chewing. Sugar intake can be restricted by using sugarless gum.

Oral hygiene. Patients should be given detailed oral and written instructions on plaque control procedures for abutment teeth. Disclosing tablets are used to determine the effectiveness of brushing and flossing teeth and to indicate areas in need of special attention. The critical areas are those portions of the tooth adjacent to the gingival margin. Gauze strips approximately ½ by 12 inches can be used in a shoe-shining type of motion to aid in keeping the abutment tooth clean and polished.

Recall appointments. Periodic recall is invaluable to reinforce home care instructions, and overdenture patients derive special benefit from periodic evaluations. The overdenture is a ready-made fluoride application tray, and acidulated phosphate fluoride gel with sequential application of stannous fluoride is used to treat abutment teeth during recall appointments (Fig. 11-83). It must be emphasized continually to the patient that effective home care as well as regular supervision and maintenance by the dentist are significant factors in obtaining a reasonable service life from the overdenture restoration.

Maintenance. Properly constructed metal base overdentures placed on firm, well-healed supporting tissues and stabilized by abutment teeth often do not need relining throughout their service life of 3 to 5 years. If required, the metal base over-

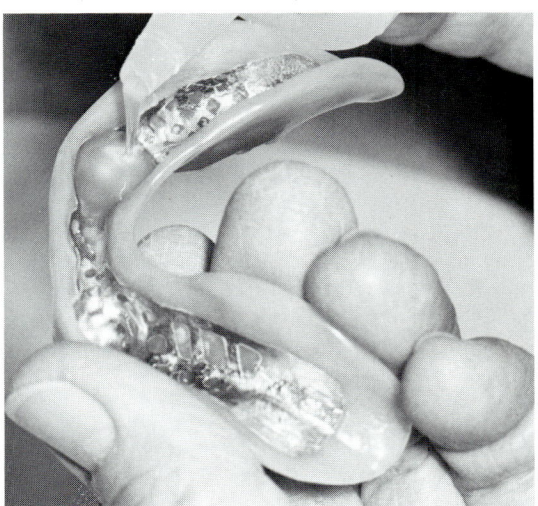

Fig. 11-83. Overdenture being used as fluoride gel tray.

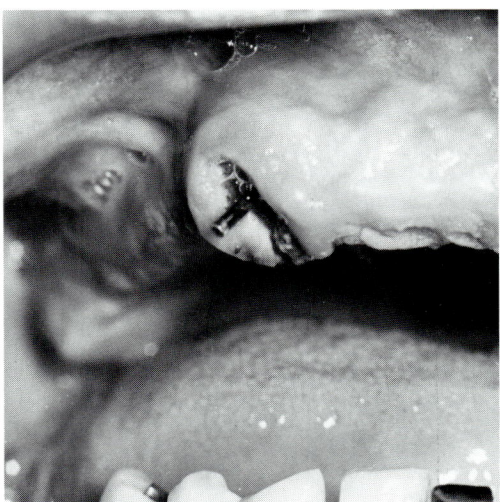

Fig. 11-84. Abutment was lost because of caries.

denture can be relined. The metal base is perforated with a crosscut fissure carbide bur in an air rotor to create areas of retention for the relining resin. After tissue treatment material* is placed in the overdenture, the patient wears the overdenture for 24 hours and functionally molds the impression for the relining. Impression material is removed from the abutment indentations to preserve overdenture-coping relationships. When the impression is deemed acceptable, the occlusion is verified, the overdenture is removed, and a cast is poured. Then the overdenture is mounted in a relining jig, and conventional relining procedures are completed. Resin extruding into the coping indentations is removed with a bur before the relined overdenture is inserted.

A significant advantage of the metal base overdenture is strength. Breakage in service, with the

---

*Coe Comfort, Coe Laboratories, Inc., Chicago, or equivalent.

exception of the occasional fracture of an individual denture tooth is rare. Chipped or broken denture teeth are repaired easily in a conventional manner.

Failures. Failure of an overdenture usually is related to loss of the supporting abutment teeth (Fig. 11-84). Abutment teeth can be lost through caries activity, failure of endodontic treatment, periodontal disease, or trauma. Our experience indicates that loss of abutments from failure of endodontic treatment is exceedingly rare. Abutment teeth with copings are lost from caries activity that is usually gingival to the coping margin. This loss has been reduced significantly by the use of fluoride-containing cements, postinsertion fluoride gel applications, adequate oral hygiene instructions, and good follow-up care.

The majority of abutment tooth losses are due to periodontal disease, almost always in association with inadequate oral hygiene (Fig. 11-85). Abutment loss by periodontal disease can be expected, since most candidates for overdentures have severe periodontal problems from the outset. If, in our enthusiasm to retain teeth, we occasionally select a tooth with a questionable prognosis, it must be remembered also that many severely periodontally involved teeth, after suitable treatment, perform far beyond expectations as overdenture abutments. As long as teeth with an equivocal prognosis are retained to serve as overdenture abutments, an occasional failure must be expected.

REFERENCES

Applegate, O. C.: The partial denture base, J. Prosthet. Dent. **5**:636-645, 1955.

Brewer, A. A.: Prosthodontic research in progress at the School of Aerospace Medicine, J. Prosthet. Dent. **13**:49-69, 1963.

Burnett, J. V.: Accurate trial denture bases, J. Prosthet. Dent. **19**:338-341, 1968.

McCracken, W. L.: A comparison of tooth borne and tooth-tissue borne removable partial dentures, J. Prosthet. Dent. **3**:375-381, 1953.

Meyer, F. S.: A new, simple and accurate technic for obtaining balanced and functional occlusion, J. Am. Dent. Assoc. **21**:195-203, 1934.

Meyer, F. S.: Building full upper or lower artificial dentures to oppose natural teeth, North West Dent. **30**:112-115, 1951.

Meyer, F. S.: The generated path technique in reconstruction dentistry. Part I. Complete dentures, J. Prosthet. Dent. **9**:354-366, 1959.

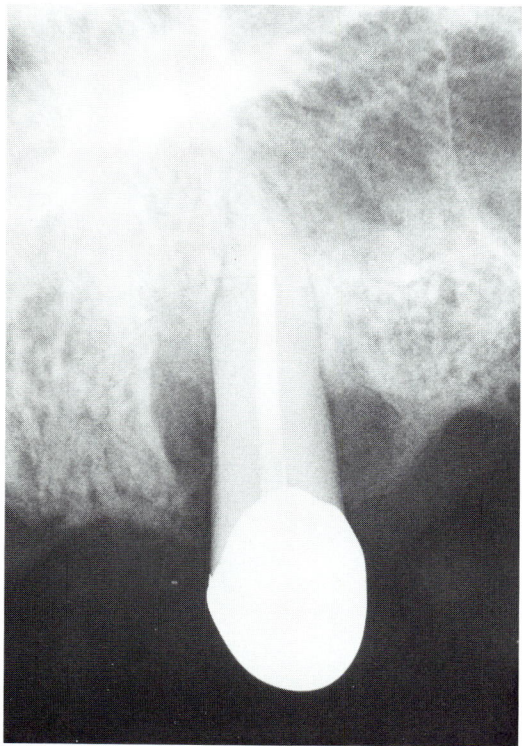

Fig. 11-85. Poor oral hygiene after placement of overdenture resulted in exacerbation of periodontal disease. Abutment prognosis becomes equivocal.

Miller, P.: Complete dentures supported by natural teeth, J. Prosthet. Dent. **8**:924-928, 1958.

Morrow, R. M., Brown, C. E., Larkin, J. D., Bernui, R., and Rudd, K. D.: Evaluation of methods for polishing porcelain denture teeth, J. Prosthet. Dent. **30**:222-226, 1973.

Morrow, R. M., and Rudd, K. D.: A rapid method for accurate cast duplication, J. Prosthet. Dent. **26**:665-668, 1971.

Rantanen, T., Mäkilä, E., Yli-Urpo, A., and Hannu, S.: Investigations of the therapeutic success with dentures retained by precision attachments. I. Root-anchored complete overlay dentures, Suom. Hammaslaak. Toim. **67**: 356-366, 1971.

Rudd, K. D., Morrow, R. M., Brown, C. E., Powell, J. M., and Rahe, A. J.: Comparison of effects of tap water and slurry water on gypsum casts, J. Prosthet. Dent. **24**:563-570, 1970.

12
REMOVABLE PARTIAL OVERDENTURES

ALLEN A. BREWER

A superior removable partial overdenture can be made for many patients by reducing some of the remaining teeth coronally so that the prosthesis can be fabricated over them. This method has several advantages that the more conventional approach lacks.

The crown-root ratio is improved. Teeth that are mobile and have minimal bone support may be retained indefinitely. Endodontic procedures are not always required.

In the presence of a furcation involvement, hemisection and retention of one or two roots is recommended, thereby retaining a hard tissue for vertical support.

Generally the occlusal scheme fabricated with this approach is not only superior to one with crowns and onlays, but it is also less expensive. More pleasing esthetics also can be developed than with alternative methods of treatment.

INITIAL FABRICATION

Frequently a patient needs removable partial overdentures but has some posterior teeth with considerable mobility and little bony support. Sometimes these teeth can be reduced adequately without endodontic therapy. The removable partial overdenture base area covers the soft tissues and the crowns of the teeth that have been reduced. This method makes it possible to avoid resorption of the residual ridge and subsequent settling of the denture base. In addition, the patient

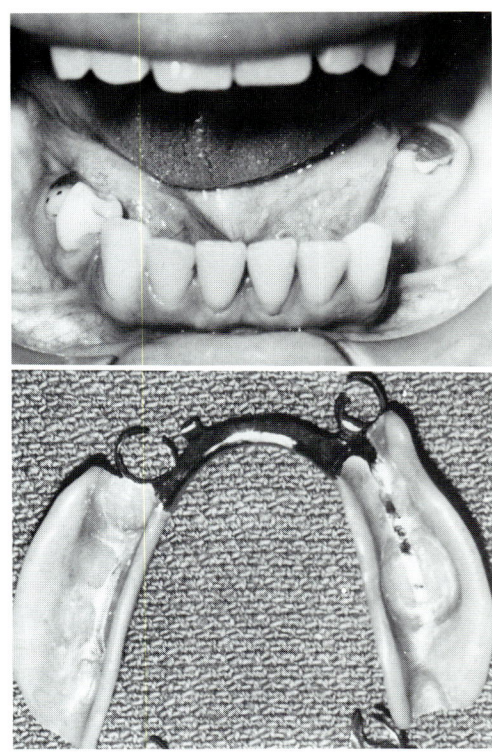

Fig. 12-1. Intraoral view of teeth prepared for removable partial overdenture. Mandibular right second bicuspid and mandibular left first molar have been reduced and restored to support bilateral distal extension bases. (Courtesy Dr. Aaron Fenton, Toronto.)

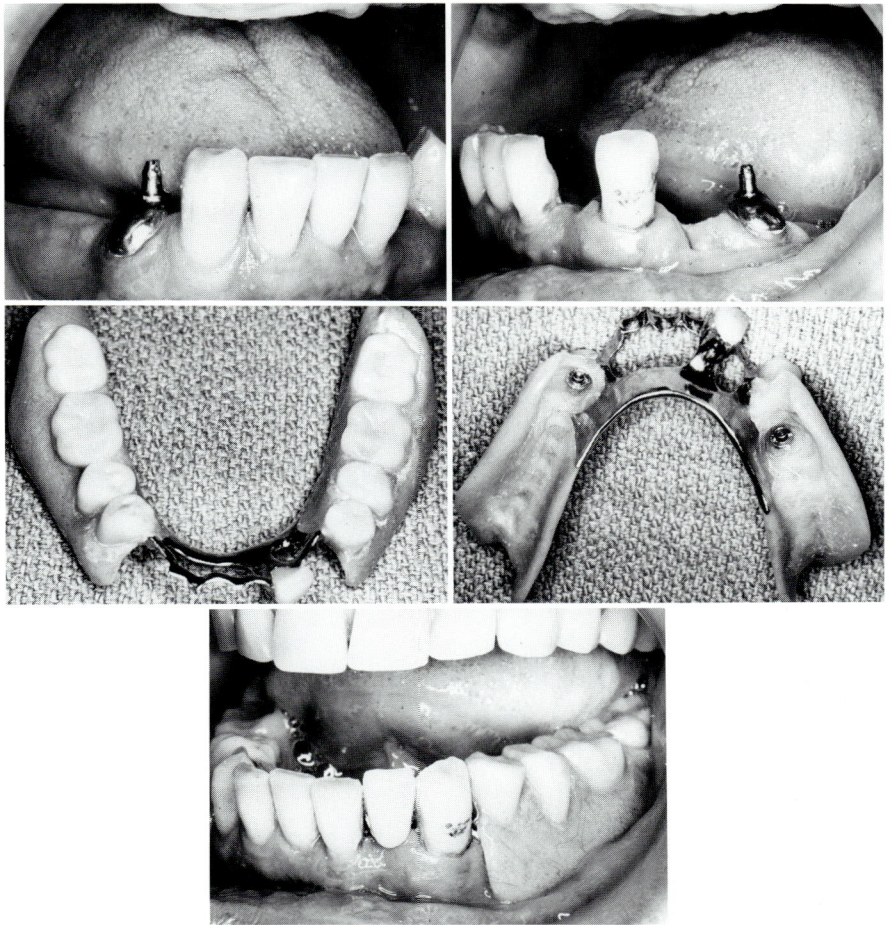

Fig. 12-2. Gerber attachments in place to support and retain bilateral distal extension removable partial overdenture.

enjoys the comfort of biting or masticating on a hard surface (Fig. 12-1).

Attachments such as the Gerber resilient attachment can be used to retain a removable partial overdenture (Fig. 12-2). They eliminate the need for crowns with precision attachments or external clasps. Usually the Gerber resilient attachment is preferred for a distal extension removable partial overdenture.

When anterior teeth are badly eroded or abraded, a removable partial denture may be fabricated over them without preparation or restoration (Fig. 12-3).

Fig. 12-4 illustrates the approach for a patient with only five mandibular anterior teeth remaining. The incisors had little bony support and considerable mobility. The design of the removable partial denture is simplified, since the incisors provide the vertical rest stops necessary and act as indirect retainers.

ALTERATION OF EXISTING REMOVABLE PARTIAL DENTURES

Some teeth are overloaded instead of being supported by a removable partial denture, with the result that frequently extensive bone loss occurs and the teeth become exceedingly mobile. Devitalization and crown reduction improve the crown-root ratio, and the tooth becomes immobile immediately. Teeth treated in this manner may support a removable partial overdenture for many years. An existing partial denture can be altered by using

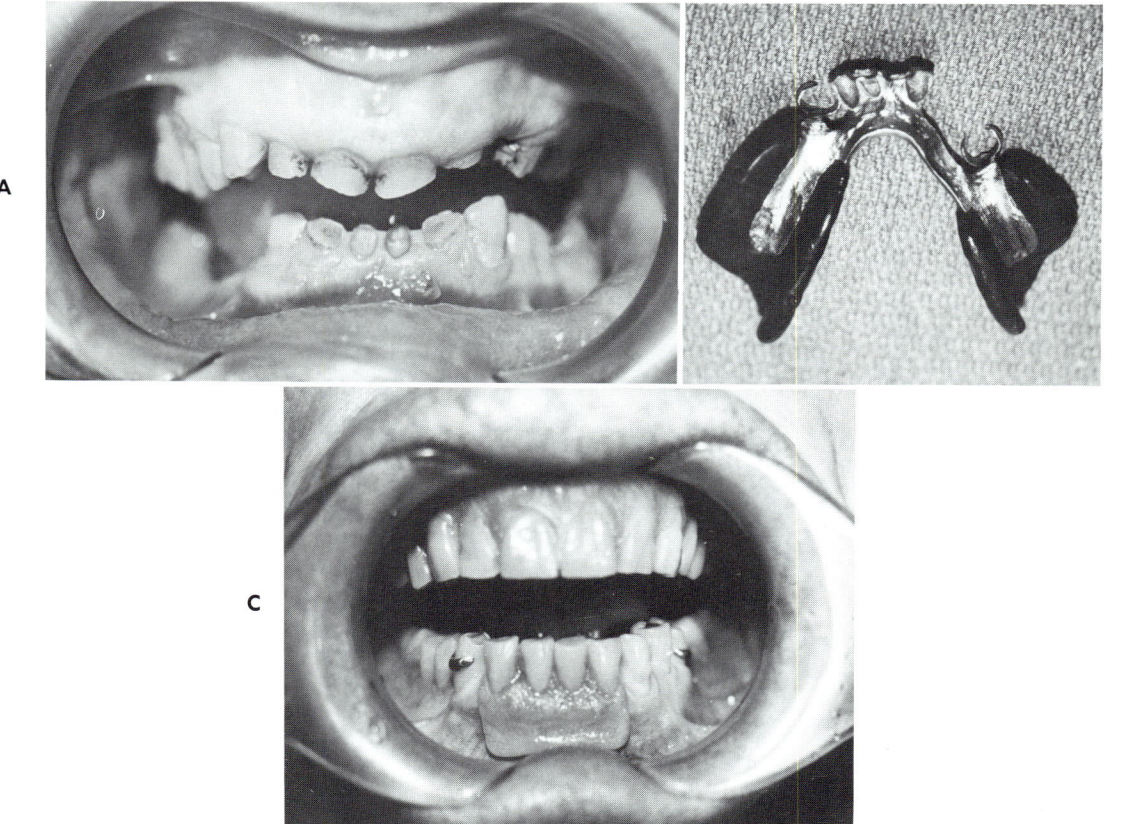

Fig. 12-3. **A,** Eroded and abraded mandibular incisors retained for support of removable partial denture. No restorations are placed in teeth. **B,** Completed casting for removable partial overdenture for patient in **A.** Soft tissue and border extensions in posterior teeth are registered in modeling plastic. **C,** Completed removable partial overdenture after insertion. (Courtesy Dr. Gerald N. Graser, Rochester, N. Y.)

REMOVABLE PARTIAL OVERDENTURES 159

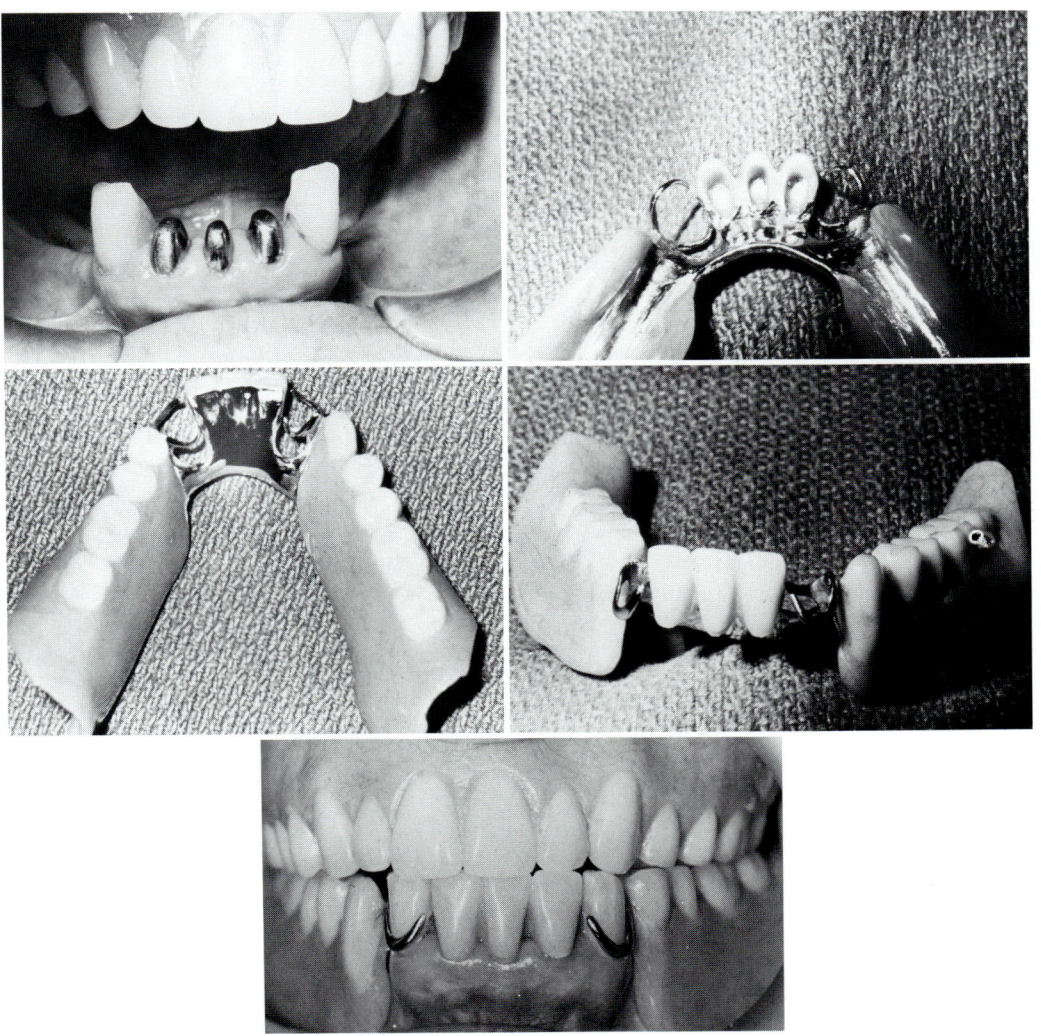

Fig. 12-4. Removable partial overdenture fabricated over three incisor teeth restored with gold copings.

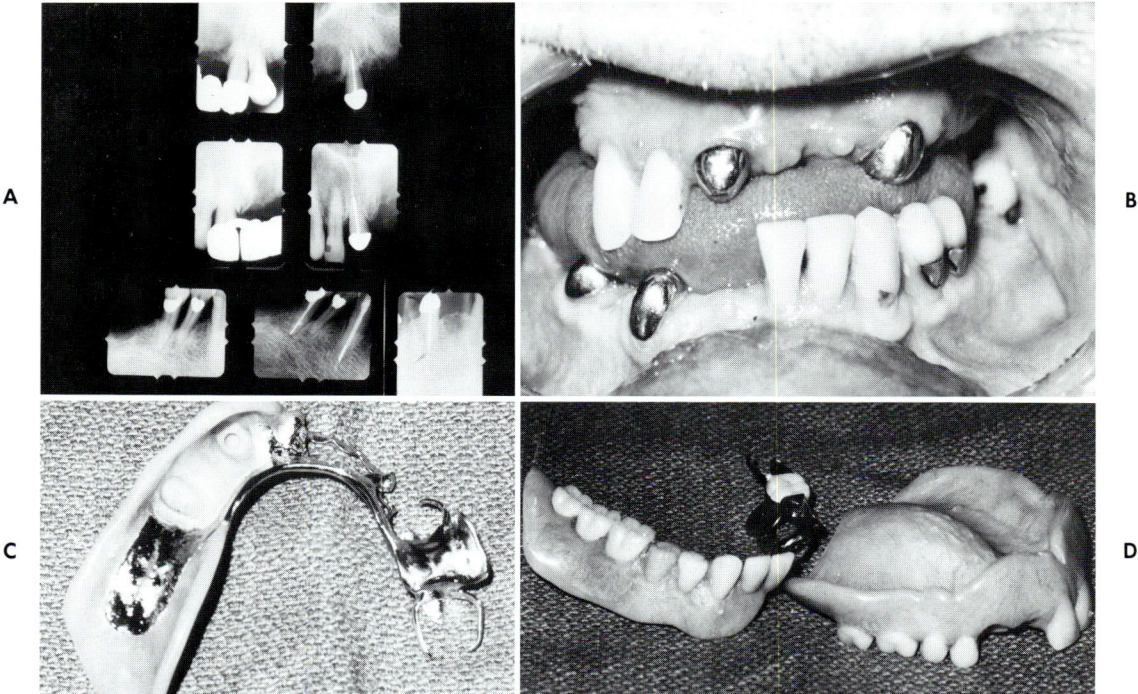

Fig. 12-5. **A,** Radiographs of patient with extensive bone loss and tooth mobility. Mandibular right first bicuspid has been extracted. Devitalization and reduction of other teeth has improved crown-root ratio. **B,** Same patient as in **A.** Teeth have been prepared and restored with gold copings after endodontics. **C,** Existing mandibular partial denture is altered to fit over reduced, restored teeth. **D,** Removable maxillary and mandibular overdentures are fabricated over reduced, restored teeth.

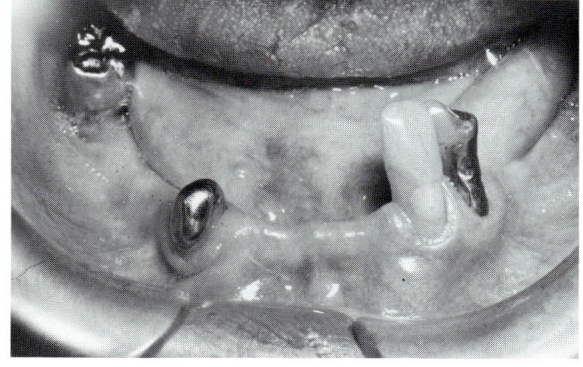

Fig. 12-6. Mandibular right cuspid has been reduced and restored with gold coping after endodontics. Existing removable partial denture is altered to fit over this tooth.

autopolymerizing resin and stock teeth to cover and restore the areas affected. Either the sprinkle method with autopolymerizing resin or flasking and packing with a heat-cure cycle can be used for this purpose (Fig. 12-5).

Although an effort is made to save all teeth that can contribute to a successful prosthesis, situations arise that make it imperative to save "key" teeth. The patient shown in Fig. 12-6 had an almost complete complement of maxillary teeth. Loss of the mandibular teeth would have necessitated extraction of all maxillary teeth to avoid rapid destruction of the mandibular residual ridge. After the right mandibular cuspid became mobile, it was treated endodontically and reduced, and a coping was fabricated. The tooth became firm immediately and was able to support a removable partial overdenture for many years. In addition, this method of treatment delayed resorption of the re-

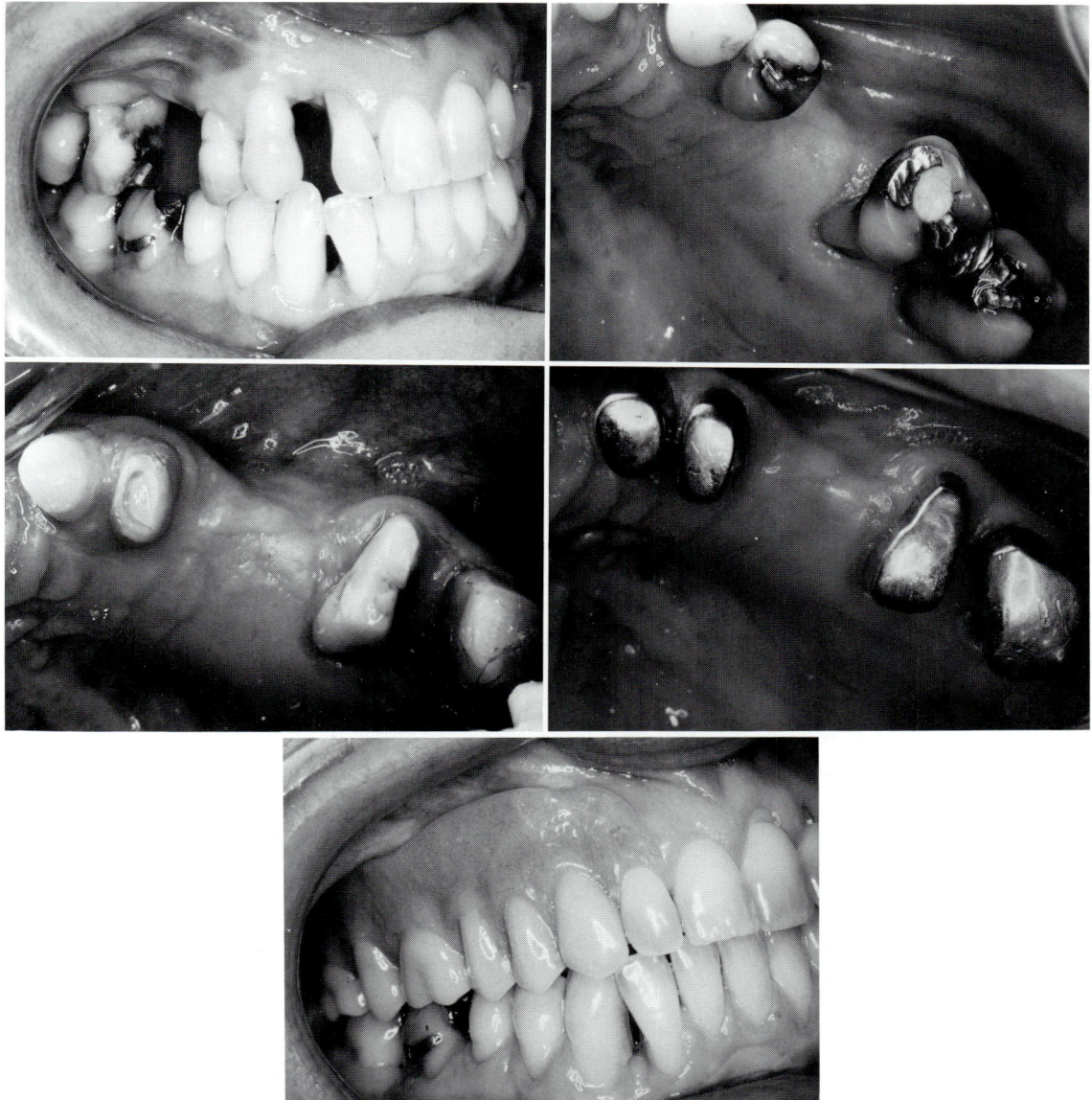

Fig. 12-7. Maxillary right lateral incisor was removed because of extensive bone loss. Remaining teeth on maxillary right side were prepared and restored with gold copings, and unilateral overdenture was provided. (Courtesy Dr. Merrill Mensor, San Mateo, Calif.)

sidual ridge that would have resulted on extraction of the right mandibular cuspid.

UNILATERAL OVERDENTURE

Loss of some teeth in one quadrant of the mouth, when accompanied by extensive bony and soft tissue loss, sometimes makes it extremely difficult to restore function and esthetics adequately. In such situations, use of the unilateral overdenture can be considered (Fig. 12-7).

13

ATTACHMENTS FOR THE OVERDENTURE

MERRILL C. MENSOR, Jr.

The ultimate objective of the prosthetic service is to return the patient to as near a normal function as possible. The basic overdenture concept is to preserve the residual soft and hard tissues. Mechanical stabilization can be improved by incorporating the use of attachments and retentive devices with the basic principles of complete denture prosthetic design.

BASIC PROSTHETIC DESIGN

It is important to realize that the causes of failure inherent in the complete denture prosthesis are not overcome by using attachment fixation. The use of attachments does not authorize the abandonment of basic principles. Failures of the hybrid prosthesis (overdenture with attachment fixation) occur not because of the attachments but because of improper attachment selection and failure of the dentist to develop maximum denture base extension, atmospheric seal and, for mandibular bases, coverage of the retromolar pad.

Improper occlusal records for a hybrid prosthesis can produce the same damaging results to the few remaining teeth as use of improper records for developing an occlusion in conventional removable partial denture treatment. Availability of the proprioceptive elements in the attachment-retained overdenture permits use of gnathologic procedures and, in some instances, anterior disclusion of the posterior teeth as well as the relevant instrumentation if desired.

Use of the attachment introduces another factor in basic prosthetic design, that is, the demand for an exact attachment-prosthesis relationship. For each type of attachment the demand differs, depending on the availability or desirability of resiliency and the overall adaptation of the denture base over the soft and hard tissues of the denture-bearing area. Use of the displacement wash in the final impression minimizes the differential of displaceability with the retained radicular elements and the balance of the soft tissue denture-bearing area.

SUCCESSFUL OVERDENTURES

The paramount consideration in treating the potential overdenture patient is that he is a human being who has potentially emotional as well as frank medicodental problems. No one system of overdentures or attachment fixation of overdentures should be attempted until the patient is evaluated medically and dentally. No elaborate plan of treatment should be presented until the patient realizes the problems of dentures.

The desire and the dental IQ of the patient require consideration when encouraging him to want the overdenture service. Many patients are disturbed emotionally at the suggestion that their remaining teeth be removed. The attachment-retained overdenture affords the patient the idea of a fixed removable bridge instead of dentures, and the patient gains comfort from assurance that natural teeth are used instead of having an important body part removed.

The overdenture procedure in which the patient is programmed to maintain good oral hygiene and plaque control around the teeth copings and the overdenture itself is most successful when the overdenture is made in a step-by-step manner. Then the patient can experience and compare a denture with the attachment-retained overdenture. The patient is given a temporary immediate overdenture for the period of healing after endodontic and surgical procedures. Usually it is accomplished by converting the patient's existing partial denture into a temporary transitional overdenture. The patient is conditioned still more to the "feel" of a denture by not placing retention elements in the attachments until he has had an opportunity to manipulate the new prosthesis. This method of treatment produces the most dramatic results in maintaining the necessary recall control over the patient and appreciation for the service rendered.

MANAGEMENT OF ABUTMENTS

With the exception of the telescope crown overdenture, most systems use endodontically treated teeth to permit maximum reduction of the crown and thereby greatly improve the leverage ratio. When the remaining tooth is not to receive an attachment, 3 to 8 mm. of crown structure is usually left above the residual ridge. This amount depends on the length and form of the root and the portion still surrounded by bone. Multiple abutments also can influence the decision. A cast gold coping can be placed over the exposed surface of an endodontically treated tooth without resorting to a dowel; sometimes pins are used to help retain the coping. An alternative method is to restore the tooth with an alloy or composite resin in the pulp or nerve chamber and then finish it to a polished surface. When an attachment is used, the crown is reduced to the level of the residual ridge, further improving the crown-root ratio. This reduction is necessary to provide room for the attachment and the tooth that covers it in the overdenture.

Periodontal therapy should be completed before final preparation of the tooth. The mechanical advantage of the improved crown-root ratio can be increased and the soft-hard tissue displaceability differential can be reduced by surgical intervention before preparation of the copings. Excessive soft tissue is removed surgically or repositioned over the alveolar ridge, and any bone defects can be filled with a matrix of osseous coagulum to regenerate a buttress of bone for better stabilization (Robinson, 1969). The indication for this type of procedure is found by digital examination of the mucosa for displaceability, periodontal probing for pocket depth, and radiographic review for cratering or angular defects.

Frequently an immediate overdenture is made for a patient with almost a full complement of teeth, most of which are to be lost, and the retained teeth are reduced to accept this overdenture. When the extraction sites are healed, periodontal surgery is accomplished on the retained teeth. After healing, the teeth or roots are prepared for restoration and attachments.

Tooth preparation

Tooth preparation varies with the type of support to be provided. If there is sufficient tooth structure, that is, 3 to 8 mm. of clinical crown for lateral stability of the overdenture, there are several methods of preparation. The teeth can be restored minimally in the pulp chamber or canal with an alloy or composite resin, shaped for retention and release, finished, and polished, or they can be prepared to receive a telescope crown or coping. In using a telescope crown or coping, it is essential to parallel the preparations and provide a definite finish line at the gingiva. When length and parallelism permit, the telescope crown and coping can be more retentive mechanically than the filled and polished clinical crown for the overdenture. The question of whether the tooth should be covered with a telescope crown or coping is determined not only by the mechanical factors desired by the dentist but also by the caries index, oral hygiene, and the patient's ability to pay for this treatment plan.

When the available denture space is insufficient, the roots can be filled with the alloy or composite resin, rounded, and polished, thereby offering vertical support but minimal lateral stability to the overdenture. A coping can be used as a cover for the exposed tooth surface, a minimal preparation made with a definite finish line, and the coping luted with the cement and retained by pins or screws. No dowels are required unless attachment fixation is used; it is a simple procedure to remove

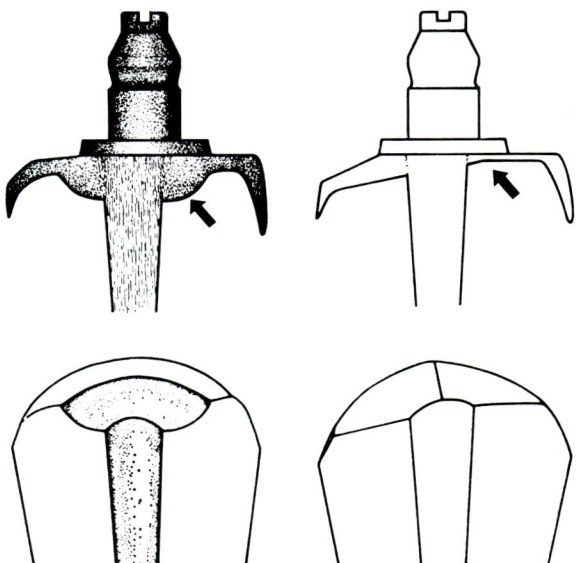

Fig. 13-1. One cause of failure of post coping preparations that carry attachments is the lack of bulk at the attachment-post-coping interphase (right). This causes fracture or opening of the coping. Left drawing illustrates a proper inlay seat that positions coping, prevents rotation, and provides necessary bulk. (Modified from Gerber, A., 1964.)

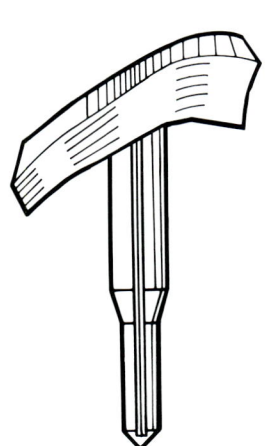

Fig. 13-2. Dowel coping should provide a gradual gingival bulge to protect marginal gingiva. If coping is designed to carry a secondary coping, there should be an occlusogingival bevel to provide a telescopic seal rather than a butt joint.

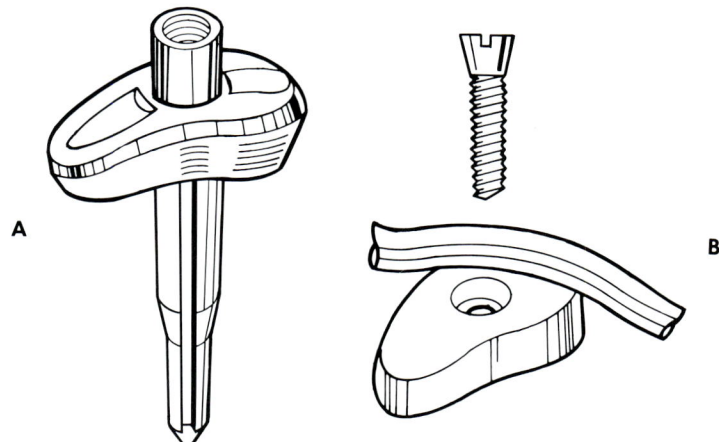

Fig. 13-3. A, If a double crown technique is employed, small locking grooves are cast into root cap to key secondary coping. **B,** Secondary coping can carry a bar attachment and can be secured to the dowel crown by a screw system.

the pin-retained copings or the alloy and composite filling if the tooth is to bear an attachment at a later date. Tooth preparation for a dowel coping is not merely a matter of "flat topping" the root to the alveolar crest. The coping preparation provides retention, stabilization, and a seal for the coping itself (Figs. 13-1 to 13-3) (Gerber, 1964).

Impression technique

The impression technique and materials vary with personal preference. Rubber and silicone elastic materials as well as individual compound impressions allow the dentist to choose silver-plated or stone dies, whereas hydrocolloid impressions permit him to use only stone dies. Incorporation of a dowel in an impression can complicate otherwise routine impression procedures simply because of the divergent paths of entry that can result in tearing or deforming the impression material on removal of the dowel. Therefore it is recommended that several impressions be taken with the dowels in place for transfer, that the dowel copings be fabricated, and that these impressions be related with a secondary master impression. An alternative method is to take an individual or full impression of preparations, join the dowels to the copings with resin, transfer them, solder the dowels to the copings, and prepare the models and dowel copings for subsequent attachment positioning and overdenture fabrication.

Laboratory procedures

The coping is waxed to a low profile and a minimal occlusal thickness of 1 mm., with the exception of the bulk of the inlay seat. It should have marginal bulge to protect the gingival tissue. The occlusal surface of the coping is modified to accept the type of attachment used. The attachments are soldered to the coping after it has been cast and rough finished. The orientation of most stud and bar attachments is established with a parallelometer; exceptions are the Zest anchor, Ginta, and Rothermann attachments, which do not require an exact parallelism. Other exceptions are the plastic pattern type attachments, such as the Quinlivan Snapper and Hader bar joint, which are incorporated directly in the wax-up. Generally the attachment orientation in relation to the coping is dictated by the resin tooth position and the buccolingual and occlusogingival space available.

DOWEL DESIGNS
Customized cast dowels

Waxed dowels require bulk for adaptation of the wax pattern and usually are not long enough to provide resistance against dislodgment. The close tolerance and difficulties in controlling the expansion of the alloys are important to consider when a dowel and coping are waxed together and cast as a unit. The discrepancy is the same as when making an inlay and crown in the same casting. If the expansion for the coping were sufficient, the dowel would be oversized, the coping could not seat, and the dowel could fracture the root during either try-in or cementation because of the wedge effect and the hydrostatic pressure of the cement. This factor can be reduced by preparing a cement release groove down the long axis of the dowel. If the dowel were undersized, the coping would seat properly, but the dowel would be retained by cement only.

Other considerations in using this type of dowel are that it usually has a greater bulk in diameter to achieve the equivalent strength of a prefabricated metal dowel. The length is considerably shorter, and the included angle is generally greater than 5 degrees, so that dowels fabricated in lengths less than 6 mm. and used to carry attachment-bearing copings will contribute to a separation of the coping from the tooth when the attachment functions.

Prefabricated resin patterns

The prefabricated dowel patterns are provided with a matched set of burs for preparing the dowel hole. The technical problems associated with the customized dowel coping are eliminated with the resin dowel because of differences in the coefficient of expansion of the wax pattern to the dowel and, need for only a single casting. The cross-sectional strength of a pattern dowel is considerably less than that of a prefabricated metal dowel of the same size, for the metal dowels are drawn from a high-fusing alloy, different than that used for the copings, and do not have the potential porosity and fracture of a cast dowel. Many patterns are available in the United States and Europe; the systems that use impression pins with copper band impressions give the best results. If the cast dowel is less than 6 mm. long, the taper does not allow the support of an attachment coping, and incomplete seating or fracture of the root may occur during cementation unless a cement release groove is cut in the length of the dowel.

Prefabricated metal dowels

The prefabricated metal dowels have a big advantage over the two previous systems because of the exact fit and high metallurgic strength in the cross-sectional area; they require minimal enlargement of the canal space and strengthen the tooth rather than weaken it. The prefabricated metal dowels have matched sets of burs for exact fit of the preparation. The dowels are machined from high-fusing wrought metal that is specially alloyed for dowel usage. Most of these dowels have cement release grooves, which avoid the possible risk of incomplete seating or root fracture during cementation.

The concept of the tapered root canal dowels can be traced back to Egyptian times and was introduced to provide maximum length to the cross-sectional area. These dowels follow the natural taper of the teeth. As alloys were improved, the cross section and taper were reduced until the included angle was 2 to 5 degrees and the retention was clinically satisfactory.

The parallel-walled dowels, such as the Schenker step pivot, introduced the best mechanical advantage in the dowel coping system other than the threaded dowel. The parallel walls offer complete resistance to dislodgment for the full length of the dowel. Once cemented, the dowel cannot be dislodged because of its adaptation and because the walls of the canal are parallel to each other and the dowel shaft. This type of dowel has been used successfully to retain attachment-bearing copings when the dowel is as short as 4 mm.

The normal dowel coping preparation discussed earlier is ideal for the prefabricated metal dowel. A definite chamfer and an inlay seat are developed occlusally to prevent rotation of the coping and provide bulk for the metallurgical bond of the dowel either from casting to or soldering. Prefabricated metal dowels can be transferred in the initial impression and incorporated in the laboratory wax-up, or they can be joined by luting them with wax or resin to the cast coping on try-in and soldering them after transfer from the mouth. The dowels are notched at the area of the coping to provide a mechanical lock-in both cast to and soldering procedures.

Threaded dowels

Threaded dowels provide mechanical fixation in addition to cementation. The VK and Kurer systems offer excellent retention with the threading. The VK, which is the only system used with a coping, uses a simple, positional method with bar attachments when the teeth are markedly divergent. Another advantage of the threaded dowel is that it aids cementation of the coping by tightening down and gives a positive seal of the coping in the absence of opposing teeth to aid in cementation. A disadvantage with this type of dowel is that the tooth can be fractured during final cementation by using too large a screw for the cross section of the tooth.

Discussion of dowel systems

During the last 18 years the author experienced mechanical retentive failure with the various dowel systems supporting attachments. However, use of the Schenker step pivot as the dowel of choice resulted in no mechanical failures for the last 7 years. Therefore I recommend use of this system for all copings except those that carry bars for divergent teeth; for the latter, the threaded dowel system, known as VK, is recommended.

There are many commercially available dowel systems of European and American* manufacture.

Mooser system (European). The Mooser dowel is produced in three different designs and a variety of lengths and diameters by several manufacturers. It is primarily a taper design with a 5-degree included angle made as a solid dowel, as a screw fixation dowel for the double crown technique, and as a pierced screw post to permit retreatment of the canal. Each type of dowel is manufactured in a special high-fusing precious metal alloy and in stainless steel, with a corresponding series of burs for dowel preparation. The majority of the Mooser dowels have one or more cement release grooves, and the high-fusing alloy can be either cast to or soldered to copings. The Mooser dowel is also available as a plastic dowel kit with related burs under the designation FKG standard plastic pin, without a cement release groove. The Mooser dowel is one of the most popular systems in Europe and, therefore, most readily available.

Stutz pivot (European). The Stutz pivot, developed as a shell dowel system with a 2-degree included angle, consists of a calibrated silver shell 10.5 mm. in length with a shaft diameter of 1.7 mm., and a 14 mm. dowel available in ceramic metal or a high-fusing pivot alloy with a shaft diameter of 1.6 mm. The preparation kit consists of the calibrated burs and a seating tool for the silver shell. For the past decade in the United States the Stutz pivot has enjoyed considerable popularity as a dowel coping system. The concept is to provide a double seal for the canal and a

---

*The American systems and the Kurer screw are available through dental supply houses.

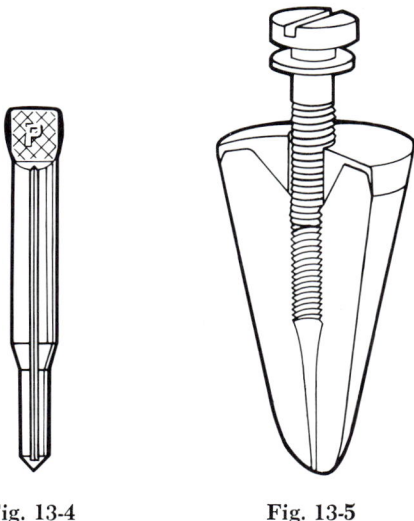
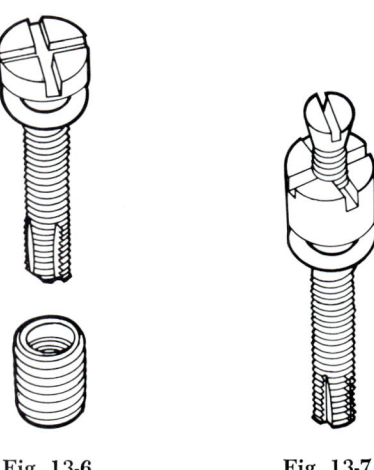

Fig. 13-4. Fig. 13-5. Fig. 13-6. Fig. 13-7.

Fig. 13-4. Schenker step pivot dowel system comes in two configurations, one for small canals and one for large canals. Step compensates for root taper, and parallel walls provide maximum retention in canal.

Fig. 13-5. VK screw cap provides most rigid mechanical fixation of coping. Coping can be cast directly to screw core (Fig. 13-6). Fixation screw is self-tapping.

Fig. 13-6. VK screw consists of a double self-tapping screw and a larger threaded tube to increase diameter for large canals.

Fig. 13-7. VK double screw can be used for fixed removable bridge work and as a base for attachment of superstructures.

metal fit of the post. Unfortunately, the taper must be at least 6 to 8 mm. long to prevent dislodgment and develop an accurate fit. To compensate for the cement elevation in double cementation, which raises the dowel from contact with the silver shell, it is essential that the Stutz dowel be luted to a coping that is cemented to the tooth temporarily and then soldered rather than cast. The Stutz pivot does not have a cement release groove if it is to be used without the silver shell.

Schenker step pivot (European). The Schenker step pivot, introduced in Switzerland 8 years ago, is available in two shaft sizes, 1.4 and 1.9 mm. in diameter, both 15 mm. long (Fig. 13-4). The alloys available are a ceramic metal with the designation "C" on the dowel and a high-fusing pivot alloy with the designation "P." There are two calibrated burs for each size dowel to prepare the two-step dowel hole. The Schenker step pivot dowel has a cement release groove.

Mechanically, parallel-walled dowels are the most retentive. The Schenker step pivot has the ideal design of the dowel systems, for it has not only parallel walls and a cement release groove, but also two steps of different diameters for each post, which afford compensation for the normal root taper. The walls of the canal, being parallel to each other and the dowel, offer maximum resistance to dislodgment. With the exception of the threaded dowel, the Schenker step pivot provides the best coping fixation of any dowel system. The usual technique is to notch the dowel where it joins the coping to produce a mechanical as well as a metallurgical bond by either casting or soldering.

VK screw (European). The threaded dowel of Mooser resembles the canal screw, in principle, but has the weakness of relying on the cement bond of the primary tapered Mooser dowel. The VK (translated from the German for "screw cap") (Fig. 13-5) is unique because of the series of sizes and its adaptability to different size canals through use of the VK canal sleeves. The screws are self-tapping after initial preparation with a Gates No. 5 and a Largo No. 6 reamer. The VK screw system consists of two basic designs for the overdenture: (1) a VK screw for screwing on single primary or secondary root caps (Fig. 13-6) and (2) a double screw as a base to which a superstructure can be attached with the small occlusal screw in the posterior region (Fig. 13-7).

This type of system makes it possible to either

fasten a secondary coping that carries a bar joint or unit or to fasten a bar directly to the primary coping. This system is the method of choice when the abutments are divergent, and it allows flexibility for future planning. When a double coping is used with the VK dowel system, the primary coping is beveled occlusogingivally at a 45-degree angle, and two orientation notches are cut into the occlusal surface of the coping.

Kurer screw (European). The Kurer screw system is identical to the single VK screw. The system has calibrated burs, a dowel threading tool, and the threaded dowel itself. It differs from the VK screw in that its thread is an S shape compared to the Z shape. The thread is pressed into the shaft to eliminate the possible fracture of the screw common to a Z-type design. When used carefully on a nonbrittle, recently treated tooth, it can strengthen the tooth and provide a clinical crown stump. It can serve as a short overdenture post or in combination with a coping.

Whaledent Parapost (American). The Whaledent Parapost consists of a knurled gold dowel with no taper and a cement release groove, a stainless steel dowel of the same design, a temporary aluminum dowel, and a plastic dowel for direct wax-up casting. A bur of the same dimension is used to prepare the dowel space in the canal. The advantage of this system is that it includes a paralleling jig that allows the dentist to prepare secondary pin retentions that can be fabricated with the coping and made parallel to the main dowel.

Parkel CI kit (American). The Parkel CI kit consists of three different burs for preparing the canal, two tapered stainless steel dowels, and two plastic dowels of the same dimension. One is a 12 mm. dowel with a shaft diameter of 1.6 mm. and a 2-degree included angle; the other is a 13 mm. dowel with a shaft diameter of 1.9 mm. and 3-degree included angle. The steel dowel is used to reinforce the tooth or serve in a temporary capacity, whereas the plastic dowel can be used to fabricate a cast dowel coping. The disadvantages of the system are the taper and the lack of a cement release groove.

Kerr Endoposts (American). Kerr Endoposts are a series of calibrated, high-fusing alloy and plastic dowels that exactly fit the endodontic file system, coded on a one-for-one basis from No. 80 to 140. They can be cast or soldered to a coping, or the plastic pattern can be used to fabricate the dowel coping system. The Kerr Endoposts allow the endodontist to prepare an exact dowel space without using additional burs or reamers. The disadvantages are the taper, the lack of a cement release groove, and the length needed for retention because of the small cross-sectional area.

RESEARCH AND EXPERIMENTAL PROCEDURES

Before the work of Körber* at the University of Freiburg in Germany in 1962 and the studies of Fenner, Gerber, and Mühlemann in Zürich, Switzerland, between 1954 and 1956, little more than emperical results were reported on tooth mobility and the effect of attachments on their viability (Fenner and associates, 1956; Gerber, 1964).

Körber showed that a tooth will become dis-

---
*Körber, K. H.: Personal communication, Freiburg/Breisgau, W. Germany, 1964.

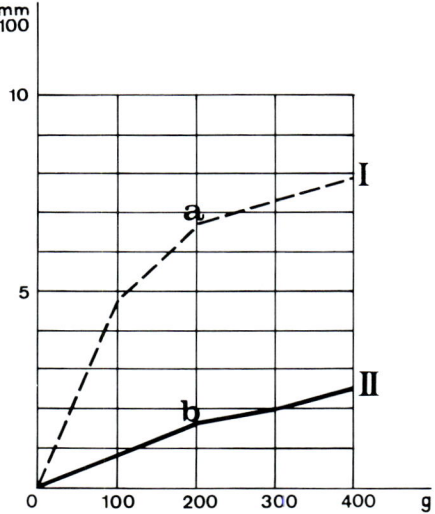

Fig. 13-8. Mobility of teeth was studied and measured in hundredths of a millimeter. A horizontal shearing load of 200 gm. was applied at cementoenamel junction of a central incisor, and displacement was found to be 0.065 mm. (point *a* of curve I). Same load was applied to same tooth by means of a rigid attachment with a reduction of one fourth the value shown at *a*; see point *b*, curve II. Clinical significance is obvious, since a rigid attachment allows hardly any movement of tooth in alveolus. (Modified from Fenner, W., Gerber, A. A., and Mühlemann, H. R.: J. Prosthet. Dent. 6:520-525, 1956.)

torted under loading and produce destructive changes in the periodontium. Fenner's work with Gerber and Mühlemann showed that rigid or cylinder-type attachments allowed hardly any tipping of the tooth, whereas ball-type attachments permitted four times more tipping than that recorded for the cylindrical or rigid type attachments (Fig. 13-8).

Gerber's studies with models (Fig. 13-9) preliminary to the clinical research evaluated both systems under horizontal loads and then with eccentric vertical loads. The results observed were similar mechanically to the clinical results obtained by Fenner from 1954 to 1965. In further studies, Gerber showed that particularly when two attachments are close together or on a mandibular prosthesis, the distal attachment should have a resilient potential as a safety valve to prevent a fulcrum dislodgment of the prosthesis by the bending of the mandible or the flexing of the prosthesis itself.

Dolder (1961), at the University of Zürich, documented more than 20 years' experience with over 800 patients who had successful bar fixation dentures. Dolder's book (1966) on the bar joints and bar units was additional clinical evidence of the success of the concept first introduced in 1898 and popularized by Gilmore 60 years ago.

Bar compared to stud fixation

The splinting of two or more teeth with a bar produces stability similar to the rigid stud type attachment when the overdenture is in place. The question that arises immediately is: if the denture base is so well developed that the bar serves only as a fixation device, what is the difference in the result of splinting obtained in the stud prosthesis and in the bar prosthesis. Theoretically, there is no difference, but the stud type allows independent movement, and, if one tooth is especially weak, the strong tooth can serve as the fulcrum point for movement of the weaker tooth in the prosthesis.

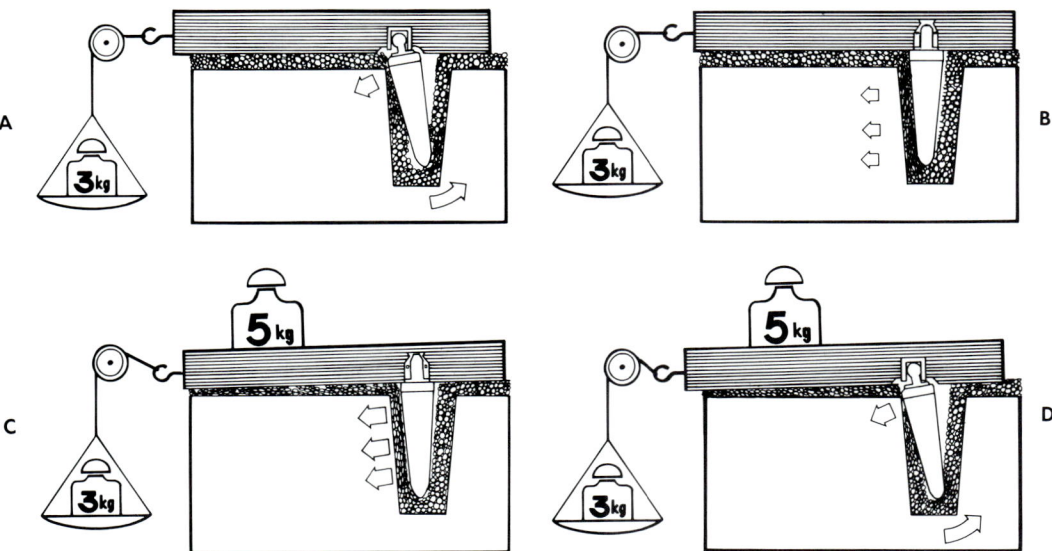

Fig. 13-9. **A,** This analogy represents stretch and compression of periodontal ligament's reaction to forces applied. In this instance, simulated root is connected to denture (beam) by a ball and socket joint, and shearing force of 3 kg. illustrates dynamic load effect and compressional rotation on root. **B,** Experimental model of **A** has a rigid attachment (retention cylinder) substituted for ball and socket. Resultant movement is less than a third of that of **A,** with force (arrows) distributed over entire length of root. **C,** The situation expressed by the models in **B** is simulated for chewing on a free-end saddle by 5 kg. vertical load. There is a slight angular change observed with resultant pressure in alveolus (arrows). **D,** Cylinder has been replaced by ball and socket joint, and experimental loads of **C** again produce results observed in **A**. This push-pull strain exhibits itself as increased mobility in natural tooth and radiographically displays itself as a thickened or widened periodontal ligament.

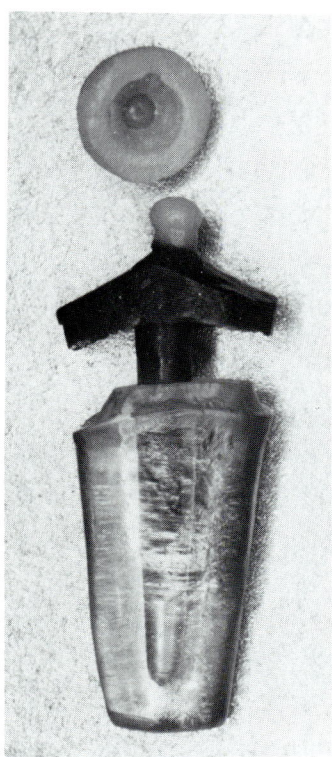

Fig. 13-10. Quinlivan Snapper is a stud attachment that provides simple pattern fabrication. Total height of attachment is 3 mm. Note chamfer preparation on root model.

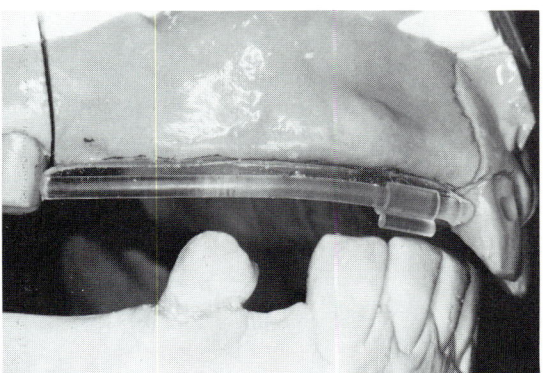

Fig. 13-11. Hader bar joint can be used as a joint or unit. Plastic pattern is a simple and inexpensive method of bar fabrication. Pattern length is sufficient to handle most large span situations.

With the bar units and joints, many times the bar splints in more than one plane. Instead of the prosthesis moving one tooth, all or none move under a functional load. With bar fixation, a stronger and a weaker tooth can be splinted with the result that the stronger tooth strengthens the weaker tooth and the weaker tooth weakens the stronger tooth.

Necessity for simplification

The necessity for simplification in selecting and using attachments for overdenture fixation cannot be overemphasized. There is no need for a highly sophisticated and expensive attachment such as the resilient Gerber, unless the fine resilient movement is desired when the nonresilient Gerber, the Introfix, or the Bona-Cylinder can perform the primary function of positional fixation without additional expense.

As the demand for overdenture service increases concurrently with the need to solve the typical lower denture syndrome of speech problems as well as problems in deglutition and cosmetics, attachments play an important role. The need arises for simple stud systems such as the Quinlivan Snapper* (Fig. 13-10) and the Hader bar joint, which offer easy serviceability and plastic pattern laboratory fabrication (Fig. 13-11). The overall cost is low, for both systems can be cast directly; the coping for the Snapper or the rider in the case of the bar can be made of resin picked up in the mouth or processed in the laboratory. The important consideration is the principle of attachment stabilization of the overdenture, not necessarily which attachment is used.

SELECTION OF ATTACHMENTS

The names of attachment groups, such as the Gerber stud attachment and the Dolder bar joint and bar unit, were developed by the manufacturers or the inventors. The various attachment systems have been organized in a compendium known as the EM attachment selector† (Figs. 13-12 and 13-13), which presents thirty points of information about each attachment (Mensor, 1973). This selector and the EM gauge (Matsuo, 1970) provide a simple color code method of choosing attachments from mounted diagnostic casts. In making the overdenture, only the stud, the bar, and some of

---

*Quinlivan, J.: Personal communication, Buffalo, N. Y., August, 1973.
†Bell International, San Mateo, Calif.

ATTACHMENTS FOR THE OVERDENTURE

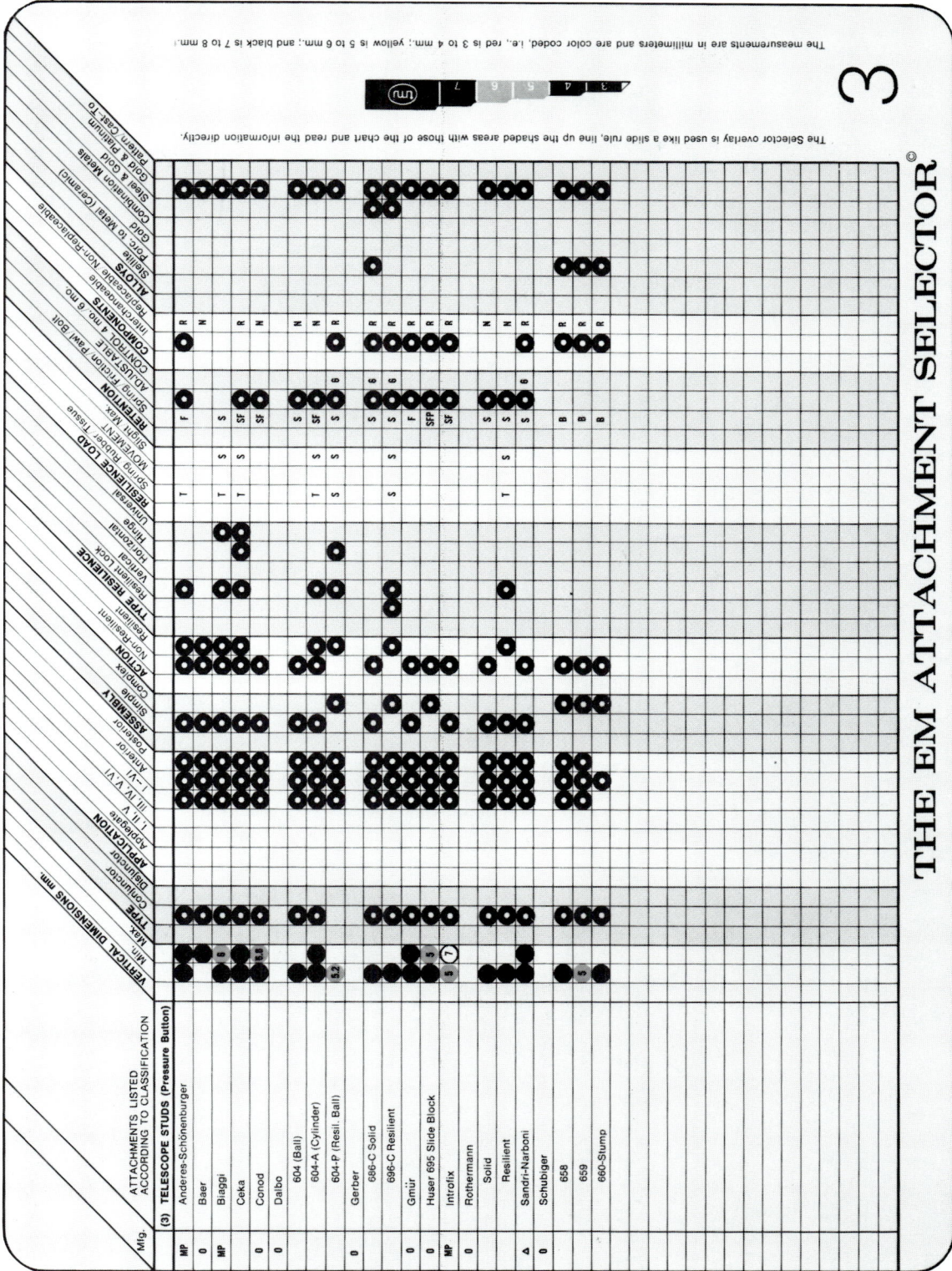

Fig. 13-12. EM attachment selector group 3, card 3, represents almost thirty of the commercially available stud attachments. EM gauge is seen on right side of card. (Courtesy Bell International, Inc., San Mateo, Calif.)

172 METHODS

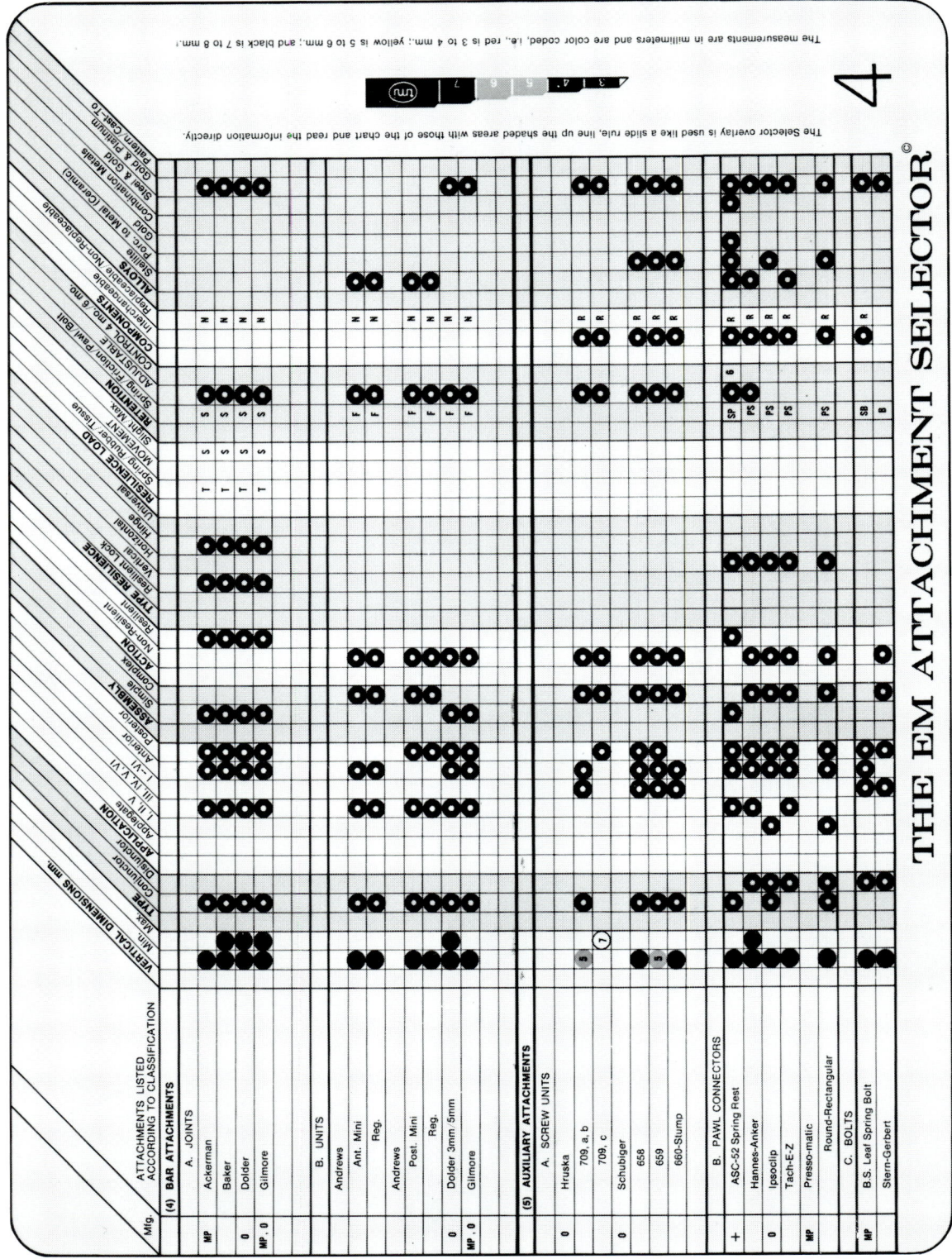

Fig. 13-13. Card 4 of EM attachment selector represents group 4, bar attachments, including joints, units, and some of the auxiliary attachments of group 5. (Courtesy Bell International, Inc, San Mateo, Calif.)

the accessory attachments are of interest. Attachments can be classified according to shape, design, and primary area of use as follows:

Coronal
1. Intracoronal attachments
2. Extracoronal attachments

Radicular
3. Telescope stud attachments (pressure buttons)
4. Bar attachments
   a. Joints
   b. Units

Accessory
5. Auxiliary attachments
   a. Screw units
   b. Pawl connectors
   c. Bolts
   d. Stabilizers/balancers
   e. Interlocks
   f. Pins/screws
   g. Rests

Groups 3 through 5 are primarily related to the overdenture service.

Stud (pressure button) attachments

Most of the stud-type attachments can be considered to be "snap fasteners" and are the simplest in concept, although many, like the resilient Gerber, on initial examination, seem as complicated as a good Swiss watch. Like any device, each system should be studied and the manufacturer's suggestions incorporated. There are no shortcuts to proper fabrication of a hybrid prosthesis; the only shortcut is the attachment itself. Except for the Rothermann series, the simpler the attachment is, the easier it is to use. Some stud attachments, such as the Gerber, are resilient and have a spring return, whereas others, such as the Dalbo cylinder, are tissue-resilient, and still others, such as the Introfix, are nonresilient.

The resilient attachments can be unidirectional or multidirectional and involve both the bar and the telescopic stud attachments. A compensating factor in resilient attachments allows the denture base to be supported entirely by the tissue in function rather than by the tooth.

Resilient studs

Resilient attachment systems are selected to perform a compensatory service and to act as a safety valve for any overload situation. No two resilient attachment systems should oppose each other unless the attachments in the mandibular prosthesis are locked out of function, for the maxillary prosthesis receives additional support from the palatal coverage. This situation arises when two hybrid prostheses oppose each other or a mandibular appliance opposes the maxillary denture. When the mandibular appliance opposes a natural dentition, some provision should be made for movement so that maximal tissue contact of the denture base can be achieved under maximal load. In the well-developed denture base with careful positioning of the attachments, the need for a resilient system becomes questionable. No attempt should be made at equilibrating or establishing permanent records or relining procedures without locking the resilient attachments out of function, because the base would move and produce incorrect markings of the interferences.

The retained root with an attachment offers retention and positional or directional orientation for the appliance. When there is either inadequate technique or inability to develop a well-fitting denture base, the resilient attachment gives some leeway to acceptance of the prosthesis by allowing more base contact and support during function.

Nonresilient studs

The nonresilient stud attachments are used when interocclusal space is limited. They should be used when the teeth are stable or when the dentist does not desire movement or potential movement of the overdenture.

Presentation of stud attachments

The individual attachment systems that are available commercially are discussed with respect to their design, dimensions, indications and contraindications, life expectancy, serviceability, torque to the abutment teeth, advantages, and disadvantages.

The majority of the stud attachments are manufactured in Europe.*

Ancrofix (European). The Ancrofix (Figs. 13-14 and 13-15) is a resilient pressure button system consisting of four parts: a solder base, a replace-

---

*European attachments are available from APM Sterngold, San Mateo, Calif., or from Ultratek, Concord, Calif.

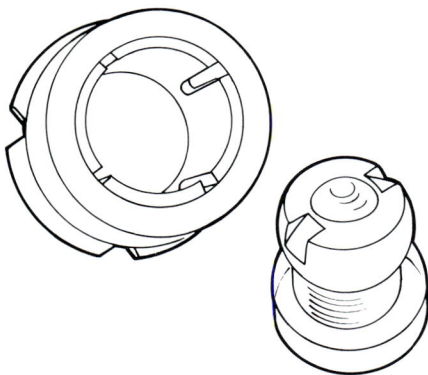

Fig. 13-14. Line drawing of Ancrofix shows threaded stud section and housing with four lamellae surrounded by Teflon ring. Height of this attachment is 3.2 mm.

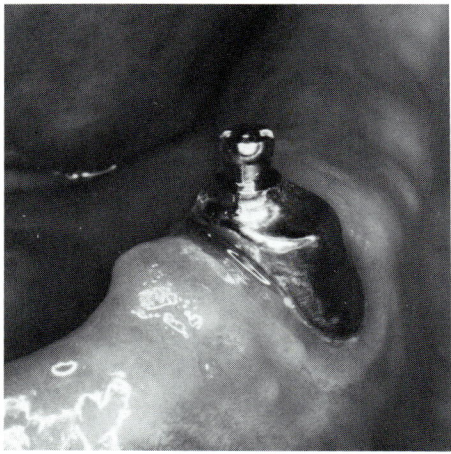

Fig. 13-15. Male portion of Ancrofix is replaceable and has a hemispherical knob that permits rotational movement of attachment. This knob may be reduced to provide rigid stud fixation.

able retention head, a housing with four lamellae that can be activated, and a Teflon ring to allow the lamellae to function in the resin. The overall height is 3.2 mm.

ADVANTAGES

1. The attachment allows rotational movement, which can be deactivated by flattening the knob on the top of the male post. The components can be replaced, and the retention can be adjusted easily, giving the attachment an indefinite life.
2. The solder base is interchangeable with the Introfix attachment, allowing exchange of attachments. The button can be picked up in the mouth with resin or processed in the laboratory.
3. There is no clinically significant torque to the support tooth when the denture base is developed properly.
4. The attachment system is simple and inexpensive.

DISADVANTAGES

1. Use of more than one attachment requires a paralleling mandrel for proper alignment.
2. Improper base development and overtightening of attachments can torque the teeth.
3. Repositioning the attachment during rebasing can damage the Teflon ring.

This attachment is indicated for partial dentures and hybrid prosthesis fixation.

Baer F. G. (European). The Baer F. G. (friction grip) button, which is one of the smallest stud attachments (2.2 mm. high), has an integral post and solder base. The housing has two horizontally opposing lamellae with a PVC (polyvinyl chloride) ring to assure their operation; the lamellae provide adjustable friction grip retention.

ADVANTAGES

1. This attachment can be used when occlusal space is limited.
2. It provides an adjustable friction grip retention.
3. The button can be picked up in the mouth with resin or processed in the laboratory.
4. The system is simple and inexpensive.

DISADVANTAGES

1. The male post cannot be replaced, and it can be subjected to wear from metal-to-metal contact.
2. A mandrel is required for paralleling when two or more attachments are used.
3. The PVC ring can be damaged if the button is repositioned during rebasing procedures.
4. There can be some torque to the teeth if the attachment is too firm and the denture base is not adapted sufficiently.

The attachment is indicated for partial dentures and overdentures when the occlusal space is limited.

Baer snap grip (European). The Baer snap grip is the same as the Baer F. G. except that it is higher (2.6 mm.) and has a stepped cylindrical male post.

ADVANTAGES
1. The snap grip is stronger and more retentive than the F. G.
2. The other advantages are the same as those of the Baer F. G.

DISADVANTAGES
1. The disadvantages and indications are the same as for the Baer F. G.

Biaggi (European). The Biaggi attachment is similar to the Baer series. The male component consists of a solder base with an adjustable split ball. There is a spacing ring for tissue resiliency. The female housing has two adjustable horizontal lamellae (split ring) that thread into the female housing. The movement is vertically tissue borne, and rotational movement is available. The overall height of the attachment is 3.4 mm.

ADVANTAGES
1. Both male and female components provide adjustment for retention.
2. The split ball compensates for metal to metal wear on the male component.
3. The retention lamellae in the female component are replaceable.
4. There is less possibility of torque on the teeth because of the ball-type male component.
5. The button can be picked up in the mouth with resin or processed in the laboratory.
6. The attachment housing is removed easily for rebasing.

DISADVANTAGES
1. A mandrel is required to parallel the attachments if more than one is used.
2. It is essential that rubber be painted over the lamellae to provide space for activation after processing because no PVC ring is provided.
3. The male post is not replaceable.
4. Adjustment is more complex than for other attachments.
5. There is less torque on the tooth, but there is more likelihood of tipping because of the ball configuration.

This attachment is recommended for all overdenture applications when space permits, and it provides rotation, vertical resilience, and fixation.

Bona-Ball anchor (European). The Bona-Ball anchor (Fig. 13-16) consists of a solder base with a sphere, a spacing ring for mounting, and an adjustable housing with four asymmetrical spring

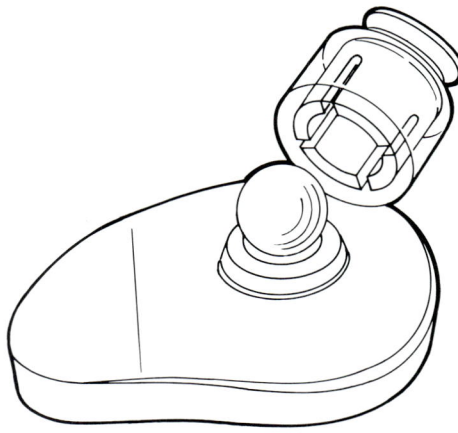

Fig. 13-16. Bona-Ball anchor is an example of a tissue resilient rotational stud attachment.

lamellae that provide the retention. The lamellae are surrounded by a PVC ring to assure their action. The overall height of the attachment is 4 mm.

Accelerated studies* with the Bona-Ball anchor showed that after 50,000 insertions the retention was reduced by about 20%. This diminished retention can be restored by bending the lamellae. Although the sphere is solid to the solder base, this has not been a problem during more than 14 years of service.

ADVANTAGES
1. The attachment provides 0.4 mm. of resilience and rotation if the housing is shimmed during processing.
2. The lamellae are asymmetrical to prevent metal fatigue during insertion and removal.
3. The lamellae provide fine retention adjustment and compensate for wear of the metal ball.
4. The female housing can be picked up in the mouth with resin or processed in the laboratory.
5. The attachment is inexpensive and easy to use.

DISADVANTAGES
1. The male component is not replaceable.
2. A mandrel is required for paralleling two or more attachments.

---

*Dalla-Bona, H.: Personal communication, Biel, Switzerland, June, 1962.

3. There is minimal torque to the tooth, but there is some tipping because of the ball design.
4. The PVC ring can be damaged if the attachment housing is repositioned during rebasing.

The Bona-Ball anchor can be recommended for overdentures when rotation, resilience, and fixation are desired.

Bona-Puffer anchor (European). The Bona-Puffer anchor is of the same design as the Bona-Ball anchor except that the ball is flat on the top, and the female component contains a stainless steel helical coil spring that provides a vertical translation of 0.8 mm. The overall height of the attachment is 5.2 mm.

ADVANTAGES
1. The Bona-Puffer anchor provides rotation and vertical resilience.
2. The spring can be replaced, and the lamellae can be adjusted for retention.
3. The PVC ring provides elasticity for the lamellae to function.
4. The female housing can be picked up in the mouth with resin or processed in the laboratory.
5. The attachment is simple to use and inexpensive.

DISADVANTAGES
1. The attachment provides too much resiliency (0.8 mm.) when the average tissue displaceability is 0.4 mm.
2. The attachment is too bulky in height and diameter.
3. The male component is not replaceable.
4. The PVC ring can be damaged on rebasing or repositioning of the attachment.
5. A mandrel is required for paralleling two or more attachments.

The Bona-Puffer anchor, which has limited use because of its size and function, is *not* recommended for overdentures.

Bona-Cylinder anchor (nonresilient and resilient) (European). The Bona-Cylinder anchor (Fig. 13-17) is similar in design to the Bona-Ball anchor and a miniature telescope crown. The basic design has been used for 14 years, but the number of asymmetrical lamellae has been increased from four to eight to provide a softer but more precise retention. The male post is cylindrical, has a dome-

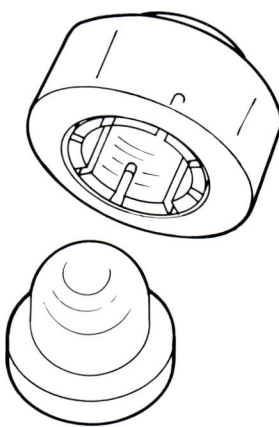

Fig. 13-17. Bona cylinder is, in principle, a miniature telescope crown. The eight asymmetric lamellae provide a softer and more precise retention than earlier model. Overall height is 3.3 mm. (Courtesy MKB Technology, Burlingame, Calif.)

shaped head, and is an integral part of the solder base. A PVC ring surrounds the lamellae. The overall height is 3.3 mm. When a spacer ring is used, the Bona-Cylinder anchor is changed to the resilient form and the height is increased to 3.7 mm.

ADVANTAGES
1. The attachment provides vertical fixation or movement without rotation.
2. The increased lamellae provide softer and more precise retention.
3. If one or two lamellae break, retention in the housing is still adequate.
4. The attachment is small enough for use in areas of limited occlusal space.
5. The PVC ring provides compressibility for the lamellae to function.
6. The attachment can be used as a resilient or a nonresilient anchor.
7. The coping can be picked up in the mouth with resin or processed in the laboratory.
8. The system is one of the least expensive and easiest to use.

DISADVANTAGES
1. The male component is not replaceable.
2. A mandrel is required for paralleling when two or more attachments are used.
3. The PVC ring and the lamellae can be damaged if the housing is repositioned during rebasing.

4. The cylinder configuration can produce some torque on the tooth if the denture base is not adapted accurately.

This attachment is one of the smallest and most popular of the stud attachments in Europe. It is recommended for all overdentures when occlusal space is limited or when only solid fixation or fixation with tissue borne vertical resilience is needed.

Ceka (European). The Ceka attachment is marketed as a so-called universal button/bar attachment.* As a stud attachment, it consists of a solder base with a removable male stud that is conical in shape and has a rounded top with an increased diameter for retention; the male post is quartered vertically into four flexible sections to engage the undersized female housing. Use of a processing spacer enables the Ceka attachment to provide vertical and rotational movement. A newer version of the Ceka stud with a bulkier male post provides relatively rigid fixation. The overall height of the attachment is 4.5 mm.

ADVANTAGES
1. The attachment allows for either solid or resilient fixation.
2. As a resilient attachment, it has vertical and rotational movement.
3. The male lamellae are adjustable, and the male post is replaceable.
4. The taper of the male post reduces the need for absolute parallelism and facilitates insertion and removal.
5. The servicing is easy, and the life expectancy of the attachment exceeds that of the overdenture.
6. The attachment housing can be picked up in the mouth with resin or processed in the laboratory.

DISADVANTAGES
1. The height and excess bulk limit use of the Ceka for the overdenture, because it takes up the space for the replacement tooth.
2. Excessive vertical and rotational movement makes control of occlusion to an exact point impossible.
3. The Ceka requires complex, torque-producing intraoral adjustments.
4. The nonresilient Ceka can produce excessive

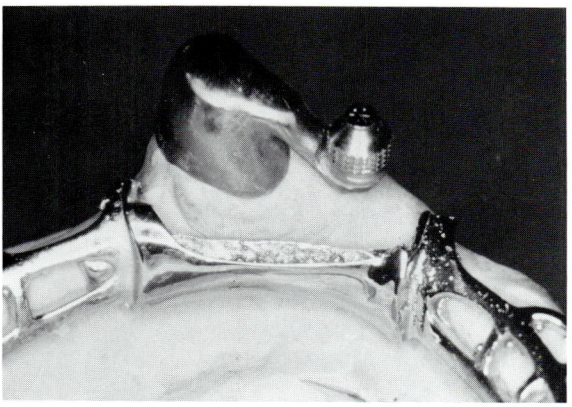

Fig. 13-18. Nonresilient Gerber attachment can be used as an "outrigger" connector and in this particular patient, the only connector for a lower overdenture.

torque on the teeth unless the overdenture base is adapted correctly to the residual ridge.

The Ceka can be used for overdentures when the interocclusal space is sufficient, when vertical and rotational movement is desired, and when the potential leverage is not a consideration, as in the "solid Ceka."

Gerber button (nonresilient and resilient) (European)

Nonresilient Gerber. The Gerber button system is probably the best-known system in the United States.* The nonresilient Gerber button, known also as the Gerber cylinder, consists of five parts: a soldering base, a male post, a retention spring, a retention ring, and a tent-shaped housing (Fig. 13-18). The overall height is 4 mm. The housing is available in 18/8 stainless steel or precious metal, whereas the stud and the solder base are of a special high-fusing alloy. This solder base can be used with the resilient Gerber and the screw block system of Schubiger. This system permits development of a screw bar for maximum splinting and future salvage without rebuilding the entire dowel coping support structure (Fig. 13-19).

ADVANTAGES
1. All component parts are interchangeable and replaceable. The solder base is interchangeable with the other Gerber and the Schu-

---

*Tielman, M.: Personal communication, Chicago, February, 1971.

*Bormes, T.: Personal communication, MKB Technology, San Mateo, Calif., December, 1973.

178 METHODS

biger systems, and the attachment life is indefinite.
2. Retention is internal and replaceable.
3. The housing can be picked up in the mouth with resin or processed in the laboratory.
4. There is solid fixation and minimal torque to the tooth if the denture base is adapted adequately.
5. The special accessory tool kit makes attachment maintenance simple.

DISADVANTAGES
1. The Gerber stud is comparatively expensive in the initial fabrication.
2. The attachment can torque the tooth if the denture base is not adapted adequately.
3. A mandrel is required to parallel the attachments when more than one is used.

Despite some disadvantages, the Gerber stud can be recommended highly for overdenture fixation. The replaceable spring retention and other replaceable parts well outweigh any additional cost or complexity.

Resilient Gerber. The resilient Gerber, also known as the Puffer, is a spring-loaded, vertically resilient attachment, consisting of nine parts and having an overall height of 4.7 mm. It is one of the most sophisticated stud attachments and one of the easiest to use, once the technique is learned. The nine parts are (1) the solder base, interchangeable with the Schubiger and the other Gerber, (2) a different retention post (Figs. 13-20 and 13-21) than used with the solid Gerber, (3) a mounting ring, (4) a threaded bushing, (5) a C-shaped retention ring, (6) a repulsion ring, (7) a return spring, (8) a copper shim 0.4 mm. thick for deactivating the attachment, and (9) a cylindrical housing in 18/8 stainless steel or precious metal. This Gerber button provides mechanical resiliency under a 20 gm. load and requires 2 pounds of force to disengage the locking spring. It is the

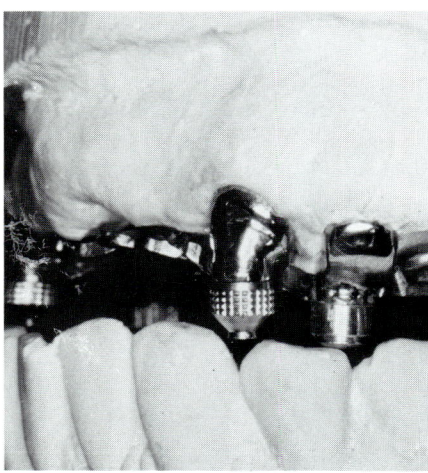

Fig. 13-19. Nonresilient Gerber attachment may be combined with other attachment systems such as Bona cylinder. Note that any reinforcement framework is kept away from attachments, and no soldering is done to join attachments to framework.

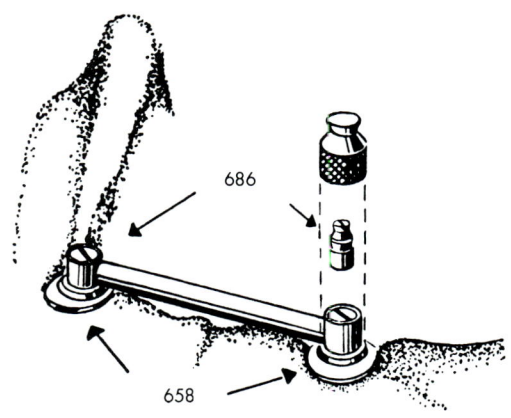

Fig. 13-20. Future plan capability of Gerber/Schubiger system. With same solder base, the prosthesis design can easily be changed from bar to stud support.

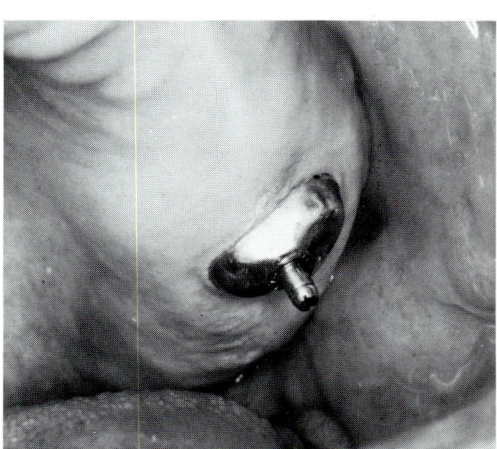

Fig. 13-21. Resilient Gerber attachment may also be used as the only attachment fixation of an overdenture as in this example of upper second molar Gerber stud. Note shape of resilient male stud.

most expensive and most sophisticated of the stud attachments.

ADVANTAGES
1. The soldering base is interchangeable with the solid Gerber and the Schubiger systems to provide design flexibility. All parts are relaceable, making the service life indefinite.
2. The resilient attachment can be made solid by keeping the shim in the housing.
3. Rebasing is simple because of the special processing studs.
4. Assembly and disassembly are relatively easy with the special tool kit. The leverage factors are minimal if the denture base is adapted adequately.
5. The spring-loaded resilience allows the base to adapt under function.
6. The attachment housing can be picked up in the mouth with resin or processed in the laboratory.

DISADVANTAGES
1. The attachment, being bulky, takes up the replacement tooth space.
2. The complexity of the attachment requires more skill on the part of the technician and the dentist.

3. The torque factors should be considered if the denture base is not adapted adequately.
4. The attachment requires control every 4 months for replacement of the resilient spring.
5. A mandrel is required for paralleling more than one attachment, and an expensive tool kit is required for servicing the unit.

The resilient Gerber attachment can be recommended highly when the interocclusal space is adequate. It provides a built-in 4-month recall system for the patient, so that the springs can be changed and the patient's general dental health observed. It is one of the most complex attachments to assemble but the simplest to control.

Introfix (European). The Introfix (Fig. 13-22) is a solid cylinder attachment that can be used for fixed removable bridge work as well as for overdentures. It consists of three parts: (1) a solder base that is common to the Ancrofix anchor, (2) a replaceable and adjustable male friction part, and (3) a female cylindrical housing. The male post is split longitudinally to allow adjustment of retention. The two heights available are 4.7 mm. and 6 mm.

ADVANTAGES
1. The Introfix is simple to use.
2. The components are replaceable, and the interchange with the solder base of the Ancrofix allows for future planning for overdentures.
3. The attachment provides good seating and retention.
4. It can be used in combination with resilient attachments.
5. The service life is indefinite.
6. It is ideal for a rigid overlay denture.

DISADVANTAGES
1. The attachment requires use of a mandrel for paralleling with additional attachments.
2. Usually it is processed in the laboratory.
3. Torque potential is maximum if the denture base is not adapted adequately.

This attachment is recommended for rigid fixation and for future planning of overdentures because of the Ancrofix interchange.

Rothermann system (European). The Rothermann system has enjoyed a tremendous popularity in its original form because of its low height and simple assembly. The new design introduced in

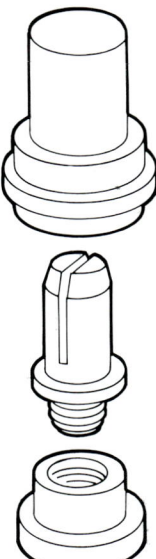

Fig. 13-22. The Introfix consists of three main parts: the solder base, the retention cylinder, and the housing. The solder base is interchangeable with the Ancrofix.

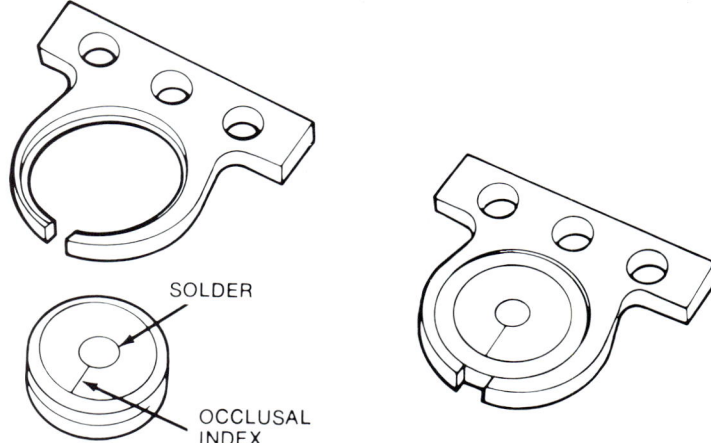

Fig. 13-23. New Rothermann attachment has an integral C clip and retention bar fabricated in a highly elastic alloy. Stud has a solder core built in for freehand soldering. Usual orientation is retention bar lingual to tooth. The only alignment required is that notch on stud face opening of C ring. (Courtesy MKB Technology, Burlingame, Calif.)

1972 (Fig. 13-23) prevents the frequent breakage of the ring that was typical of the older unit.

Rothermann nonresilient. The Rothermann nonresilient attachment consists of two parts: a male stud with a solder core for freehand soldering to a coping and a female clip, consisting of a perforated retention beam with a split C ring extension. The attachments do not require mandrels for alignment and are inexpensive. The overall height is 1.1 mm. Torque is of an absolute minimum.

ADVANTAGES
1. The attachment is low in height; it is the shortest attachment available.
2. Minimal retention can be obtained by spreading the retention ring.
3. No parallelometer is required, and the attachment can be aligned on teeth divergent as much as 10 degrees more or less from the long axis.
4. Freehand soldering reduces laboratory time and cost.

DISADVANTAGES
1. There is no provision for C ring activation; it is necessary to paint on rubber during processing to provide space for this function.
2. Laboratory processing is the method of choice for initial fabrication or relining.
3. Rebasing is difficult despite a rebasing stud.
4. There is lingual bulk in the orientation of the attachment.

The Rothermann attachment is recommended for overdenture fixation when space is limited, teeth are divergent, and light fixation is essential.

Rothermann resilient. The Rothermann resilient attachment consists of the same type of stud and retention loop as the Rothermann nonresilient attachment, but the overall height of the male stud is 1.7 mm. (Figs. 13-24 and 13-25). There are two spacers for assembling, so that the attachment can allow some tissue-borne vertical and rotational movement. All the features, advantages, and disadvantages of the Rothermann nonresilient attachment apply here. The Rothermann resilient attachment is recommended for overdentures when space is limited, the teeth are divergent, and vertical as well as rotational movement is desired in addition to fixation. There is no torque to the teeth because of the movement.

Schubiger screw block (European). The Schubiger screw block system consists of a short screw

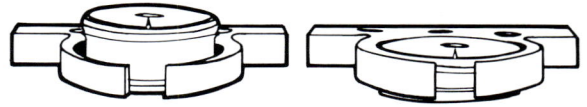

Fig. 13-24. Difference in resilient and nonresilient Rothermann is in height of male portion. Resilient system (left) is 1.7 mm. high compared to nonresilient system (right) at 1.1 mm. (Courtesy MKB Technology, Burlingame, Calif.)

ATTACHMENTS FOR THE OVERDENTURE 181

block for bar fixation, a larger one for fixed removable bridge work, and an individual cap core system. The basic Schubiger (Fig. 13-26), which is used for overdentures, consists of three parts: the solder base common to the Gerber system, a sleeve in ceramic metal, and a cap nut. The overall height is 2.8 mm.; the system is used to connect bar joints and bar units to the anchor teeth and to serve as a connector for bars when the teeth are markedly divergent (Fig. 13-27).

ADVANTAGES
1. The Schubiger system allows complete flexibility in future planning with the Gerber system without necessity for dowel coping support replacement.
2. It provides for bar fixation.
3. It permits conversion from bar to individual stud fixation (Gerber).

DISADVANTAGES
1. A mandrel is required for paralleling, and a special screwdriver is required for setting the attachment.
2. Assembling is complex and expensive.

The Schubiger attachment is recommended for bar fixation on divergent teeth and for future planning with weak abutments that require conversion to Gerber stud fixation of the overdenture.

Ginta (American).* The Ginta attachment is

---
*Whaledent, Inc., New York.

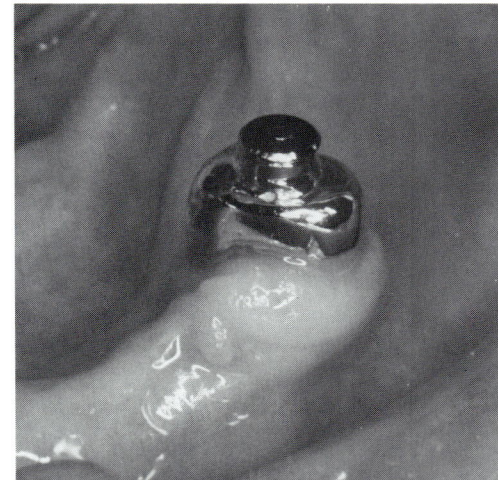
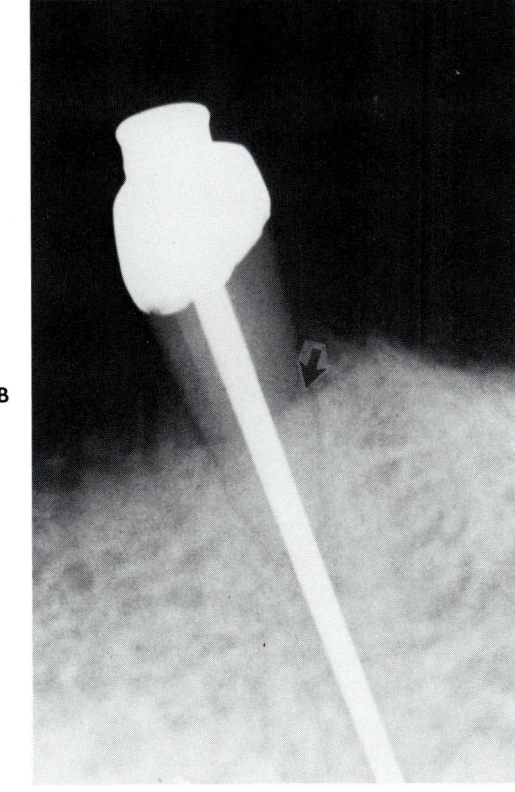

Fig. 13-25. **A,** Rothermann attachment can be used on a single tooth or in combination with other attachments. In this application, it is being used in conjunction with an endosseous implant. **B,** Radiographic view shows Rothermann, coping, and endosseous implant. Initial mobility of this tooth preoperatively was 3+, yet in this combination it can support an attachment and overdenture.

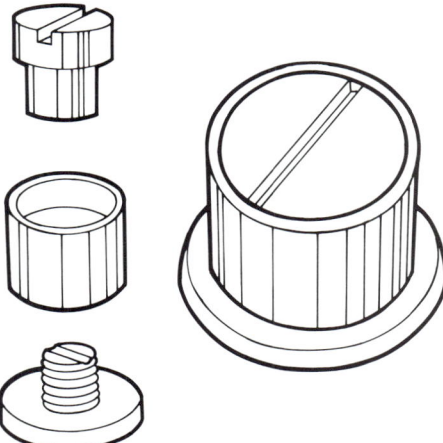

Fig. 13-26. This basic Schubiger consists of three parts: solder base, a ceramic metal sleeve, and a cap nut that looks like a screw.

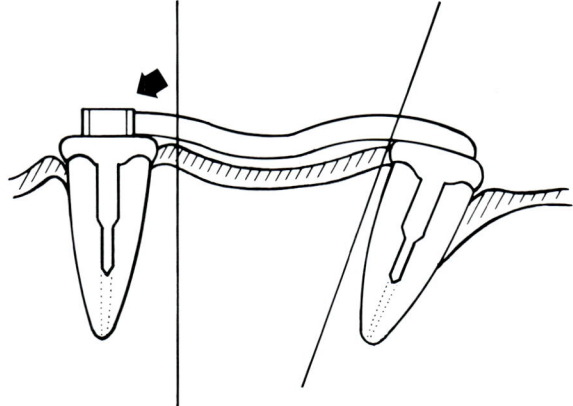

Fig. 13-27. When two teeth are markedly nonparallel, they may have bar fixation using a Schubiger attachment. Bar is soldered on one coping, and attachment is placed on strongest of the two teeth for future salvage or conversion to stud fixation.

similar to the Zest anchor system in that a metal sleeve is cemented into an endodontically treated root either with or without a cast coping. The sleeve receives a longitudinal double spring with a retention bend. This spring is engaged in the resin of the prosthesis and spring-slips the denture to the root. There is slight horizontal and vertical mobility with the Ginta, and the system is easy to use. There is no torque or leverage on the root. The overall length for the dowel space is 7 mm., but the sleeve can be reduced to as little as 5 mm.; the retention knob is 2 mm.

ADVANTAGES
1. Serviceability is easy, for the spring can be bent to increase retention or replaced easily by a resin pick-up in the mouth.
2. Parallelism is not essential with the Ginta.
3. It can be used in as short a dowel space as 5 mm.
4. There is no torque of the tooth.

DISADVANTAGES
1. Assembling is complex.
2. The patient can find insertion difficult and can puncture the gingiva or gingival sulcus.
3. Plaque control of the internal socket is difficult for the older patient.
4. There is too much mobility, instead of fixation of the overdenture.

The Ginta attachment, like the Zest anchor, can be recommended as an overdenture connector, but the design is too new to have a successful clinical history.

*Quinlivan Snapper (American).** The Quinlivan Snapper is a ball-shaped resin casting pattern for the male component and a prefabricated resin cap with an O ring that fits the male ball-shaped stud. The male pattern is incorporated in the coping wax-up and cast directly with the coping and dowel. The plastic cap is picked up in the mouth with resin by the completed denture base. The O ring provides the retention and can be replaced easily. The design allows rotational movement but no torque to the tooth. The overall height is 3 mm. This attachment is inexpensive, provides good retention, and is easy to use.

ADVANTAGES
1. The Quinlivan Snapper can be used on divergent abutments.
2. It requires no mandrels or special tools.
3. The attachment is short enough to be used in limited space areas.
4. It provides fixation with rotational movement.
5. It is picked up easily in the mouth with resin or replaced by a resin pick-up.
6. The O ring can be changed easily.
7. The assembly procedure is simple and uncomplicated.

DISADVANTAGES
1. The male component, which is cast, could have porosity in the stem.
2. It is necessary to cut out the resin cap for repositioning.
3. Infrequent wear of the male component has been observed.

The Quinlivan Snapper can be recommended for all overdenture procedures in which vertical resiliency or rigid fixation is not required.

Zest anchor (American).† The Zest anchor consists of a sleeve similar to the Ginta attachment and a nylon male post with a "ball head" that resembles a "reverse Gerber." The original concept was developed by Carl Axel Gross‡ in Sweden in 1954 and then introduced in the United States by

---
*Quinlivan, J.: Personal communication, Buffalo, N. Y., Aug., 1973.
†American Precision Metals, Burlingame, Calif.
‡Goraneson, P.: Personal communication, Göteborg, Sweden, Nov., 1972.

Max Zuest.* The system is designed to be used with or without a coping. As a noncoping attachment, a dowel space is tapped and the sleeve is cemented to the reduced clinical root. The male post can be processed in the laboratory, but usually it is a chairside procedure in which the nylon post is placed in the sleeve and is picked up in the denture resin. The leverage and the torque on the tooth can be considered zero. The overall sleeve length is 6 mm., and it can be reduced to 3 mm. The total length of the nylon post with the pick-up base is 5 mm., making it 2 mm. higher than the root surface for the resin pick-up.

ADVANTAGES

1. This attachment serves well as a temporary fixation for a transitional denture.
2. There are no leverage or torque factors.
3. The attachment can be used without a dowel or coping.
4. Pick-up in the denture with resin is easy.
5. It does not require paralleling.
6. It can be used on divergent teeth.
7. It provides slight vertical and rotational movement.
8. It is simple to use and inexpensive.

DISADVANTAGES

1. There is no coping, with the result that the root face is exposed in a caries-susceptible mouth.
2. The sleeve requires meticulous hygiene for plaque control.
3. The nylon studs have a water absorption problem that causes them to bend, break, or prevent entry of the attachment.
4. Studs can require replacement as frequently as every 2 to 4 months.
5. Stud bending prevents proper seating when many are used in the same mouth.

The Zest anchor can be used successfully as an overdenture connector. The system lends itself ideally to a nonlaboratory technique. Care is required because of the short life of the nylon studs.

Zest Mini. The Zest anchor female component is also available in a so-called Mini configuration† in which the diameter has been reduced to 3.5 mm. and the length has been reduced to 3.25 mm. This reduction in size solves the problem of parallelism in divergent root application and makes the Zest usable on lower anteriors and upper lateral incisors. This configuration has retention grooves that permit direct casting to the female component when a coping is desired. The same centering sleeves and male posts are used as for the standard Zest anchor. The same statements relevant to the standard Zest anchor are applicable to the Mini. The ball can be removed on the male post to provide a rest rather than a retention when multiple Zest attachments are used. Two retentive male posts are usually sufficient for anchorage to stabilize an overdenture when one is used on each side of the arch.

BAR ATTACHMENTS

Bar attachments are divided into two groups: bar units and bar joints. They give fixation for the overdenture and spinting for the remaining teeth. Bar units, as the name implies, provide rigid fixation for the overdenture, whereas bar joints permit some degree of rotational or resilient movement or both.

Bar units

Bar units are selected on the basis of the space available, the shape and curvature of the ridge, and the type of defect to be replaced. Bar units are ideal for gross tissue defect replacement as well as for support of an overdenture. A bar joint can be converted to the function of a bar unit by bending it into a shape other than that supplied by the manufacturer. The primary functions of bar units are splinting and carrying the appliance positionally. Most laboratory-fabricated bars, such as the Gaerny or Steiger-Boitel bars, are considered to be bar units (Gaerny, 1972; Steiger and Boitel, 1959). The height available, the type of occlusal surface, and the type of denture tooth are the only factors that limit their size, position, and design.

The usual bar attachment splints two or more teeth together (Fig. 13-28). Most prefabricated bars are made of a high-strength alloy, so that size plays no part in the selection of short-span cases. If splinting alone is considered, theoretically a long reach, for instance, between a molar and cuspid, requires a larger cross-section of bar than a cuspid-to-cuspid splint. This usage produces a rule

---

*Zuest, M.: Personal communication, San Diego, Calif., June, 1973.
†Zuest, M.: Personal communication, San Diego, Calif., March, 1974.

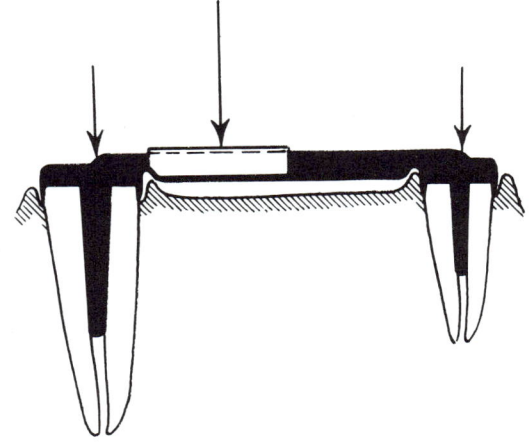

Fig. 13-28. Bar joints and bar units serve to splint two or more teeth together. In example from Dolder, arrows show dowel copings, bar, and rider clip.

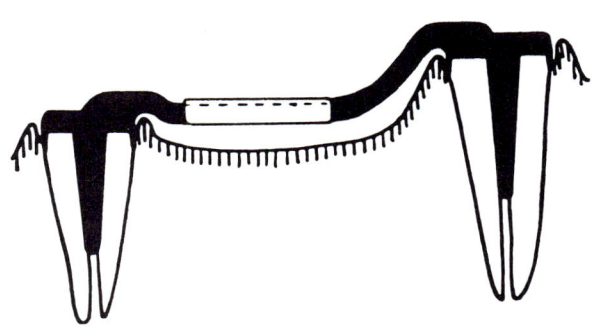

Fig. 13-29. Prof. Dolder emphasizes that Dolder bar can and should be bent to conform to ridge and that rider should be segmented to fit straight sections.

of direct proportion of the cross-section to the length of span; it is considered more important in the laboratory-fabricated bar because of the type of alloy used in contrast to the commercially available prefabricated units.

The major determinant in selecting the proper size of bar is the space available in the specific case to ensure rigidity of the splint. It is always desirable to select the largest possible size for the space without affecting the vertical relationship, occlusion, or contour of the prosthesis.

The splinting effect and strength of the restoration also are controlled by the number of abutments and their location as well as by the dimension of the bar. Properly designed bar cases have the retention, retention adjustment, and wear in the female portion of the attachment, eliminating the bar wear and the necessity for a bar of large diameter. The only compelling reason for using a large-diameter bar is the necessity to span a long edentulous area, so that the bar is subjected to heavy forces.

The Dolder bar has been used most in discussions of the bar system. Preiskel (1968, 1973) has given part of both the first and the second editions of his book to a discussion of the Dolder bar joints and units. An in-depth review of Dolder's writing (1959, 1961, 1966) reveals that the Dolder bar system can be bent and shaped to approach any ridge configuration (Fig. 13-29). Both the inventor, Dolder,* and the manufacturers recommend its use in this broad application. Technically, any bending, cutting, or soldering of bar attachments requires annealing, followed by a heat treatment to restore the crystalline structure alignment and the original strength to the alloy. Cutting, bending, and soldering produce a weaker bar than bending alone because of the different crystal structure of the solder joint.

Except for the Baker clip and the Andrews bar, the bar attachments described are of European design and manufacture.

Andrews bar (American). The Andrews bar consists of a series of curved austinetic friction bars of different radii with corresponding retentive riders.

ADVANTAGE

1. None.

DISADVANTAGES

1. It requires complicated mechanical joining and soldering of a nonprecious metal bar to a coping.
2. It has excessive bulk.

The Andrews bar is not recommended for overdentures.

Ceka bar unit (European). The Ceka bar unit is of the same height as the Ceka bar joint, that is, 4.5 mm., and consists of one or more basic Ceka

---

*Dolder, E. J.: Personal communication, Zürich, Switzerland, 1963.

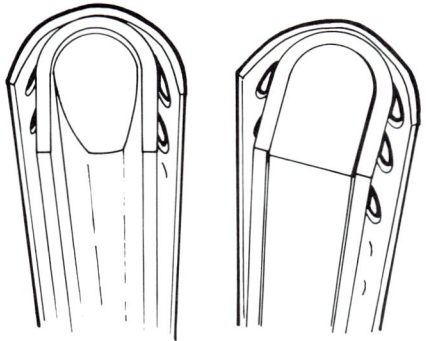

Fig. 13-30. Dolder bar has two basic shapes. Bar joint (left) is "egg"-shaped to allow movement, and bar unit (right) is a "church window" configuration and is rigid. Note improved mechanical retention on both riders.

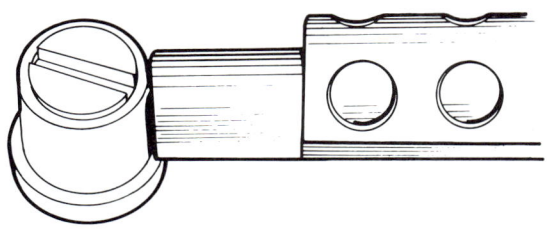

Fig. 13-31. Dolder bar may be joined to sleeve of Schubiger stud and be used as a fixed removable bar unit. Note retention available for resin on rider channel.

studs incorporated in a rectangular bar. The Ceka bar uses an exact-fitting Ceka stud, which is a tapered split flange with a ball tip. The stud can be separated from the base, which is incorporated in the denture.

ADVANTAGES
1. The male stud is replaceable and interchangeable with the Ceka bar joint stud.
2. The stud retention unit is adjustable and can be picked up in the mouth with resin.
3. Insertion in the mouth is easy.

DISADVANTAGES
1. The system is expensive and requires exceptional skill.
2. There is too much bulk.

The Ceka bar is used for overdentures, but it is not recommended because of the bulk and complexity.

C. M. bar (European). The C. M. bar is a prefabricated bar 100 mm. by 10 mm. by 1.8 mm., which is provided with a copper template for the milling technique. The bar section can be used to splint several roots, and, with the aid of the template, it can be made to fit the ridge. The rider can be cast to fit the bar, or a square Gilmore rider designed to fit a 1.8 mm. bar section may be used.

ADVANTAGES
1. Time is saved in fabrication, rather than milling.
2. The wrought metal is stronger.
3. The rider can be picked up in the mouth with resin.

DISADVANTAGES
1. It is extremely bulky.
2. It is too expensive when the advantages of other systems are considered.

Generally it is not recommended for the overdenture.

Dolder bar unit (European). The Dolder bar unit (Fig. 13-30) has a "church window" profile in contrast to the "egg" shape of the joint. It consists of the bar and the same rider, but it has retention mesh for the joint. The unit is rigid and is available in a standard size, 4.65 mm. in height, and a micro-size, 3.6 mm. in height. This bar can be jointed to divergent teeth by use of the Schubiger system (Fig. 13-31), illustrated earlier.

ADVANTAGES
1. Rider sections can be segmented and adjusted for retention.
2. The bar and rider are available in two sizes.
3. The rider makes a good frictional fit.

DISADVANTAGES
1. It is too bulky in all dimensions.
2. Retention in the denture complicates rebasing or repositioning procedures.
3. It is too expensive.
4. The bulk has a negative effect on the esthetic results.

The Dolder bar unit is used for overdentures, but it is not recommended highly because of the bulk, cost, and esthetic problems.

M. P. channels (European). The M. P. channels consist of a series of four rectangular bars and channels provided in 2 or 20 cm. lengths. All of the bars are 1.1 mm. wide, three are 6 mm. high, and one is 3 mm. high (Fig. 13-32). The channels or riders are supplied in three heights: 3.5, 6.5, and 6.35 mm. They allow splinting and adaptation of a milled bar without the usual expense. It is neces-

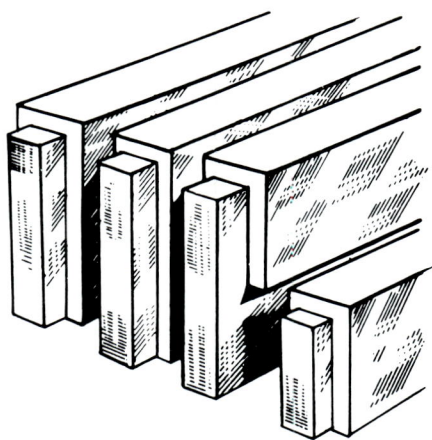

Fig. 13-32. These are the four configurations of M. P. channels and consist of a bar with its appropriate rider channel. These units save many hours of laboratory time and are more rigid metallurgically than any cast system of same dimension.

sary to cut retention into the channels for the resin fixation in the denture.

ADVANTAGES
1. They are less expensive than milled bars.
2. There are four different sizes.
3. They are stronger than cast bars.

DISADVANTAGES
1. They are expensive.
2. They offer no advantage over other systems for the overdenture.

Generally the M. P. channels are not recommended for the overdenture, although, in combination with the pawl connectors, they can provide good fixation at an increased cost.

Discussion

It is essential to realize that there are single-sleeve and multiple-sleeve configurations of the riders. Multiple-sleeve riders, such as the Ackermann, the C. M., and the Baker, which are short segments, allow maximum contouring of the bar to follow the ridge shape and permit the dentist to increase retention by the number of riders used rather than by the tension of a single rider sleeve. The single sleeve, such as the Dolder bar rider, is used generally in straight segments, but it can be sectioned to serve as a multiple-sleeve system when desired. It should be understood also that a wrought bar has better physical characteristics than a cast bar, and it requires far less expenditure of time and material than the fabrication of a cast and precision milled bar.

Bar joints

Ackermann (European). The Ackermann system is a bar and rider attachment. The riders are clips that have retention wings in a linguofacial orientation and measure 3.6 mm. in length. The clip is used on three types of bars: a round bar 1.8 mm., an oval bar 1.5 by 2.5 mm., and an egg-shaped bar 1.65 by 2.5 mm. The bar is available in a variety of lengths, the most common being 5 mm., 10 mm., and 15 mm. The round bar is the most popular of the Ackermann series, for it can be bent most easily and adapted to the irregularities of the ridge. The riders have brass spacers for processing. This system is popular for bar joint fixation and often is incorporated with a screw block fixation on the copings.

ADVANTAGES
1. The bar can be bent easily to follow the ridge contour.
2. The clips are in short segments, so that many curved sections can be developed.
3. The clips are adjustable for all degrees of retention.
4. The copper shim provides vertical and rotational movement after fabrication.
5. The bar does not present great bulk.
6. Three different bar configurations are available.

DISADVANTAGE
1. The retention wings run in the wrong direction for resin pick-up in the mouth.

Generally this bar is recommended for the overdenture because of its size and adaptability.

Baker clip (American). The Baker clip is a small joint connector available in two sizes, one to fit a 12-gauge bar and one to fit a 14-gauge bar. Both sections are 6 mm. in length, and there are no retention wings. The retention is obtained by soldering a loop, bending the ends, or notching the surface. The length of the clip permits division into two units. It is readily available in the United States.

ADVANTAGES
1. The Baker clip is adjustable for retention and provides rotational movement.
2. It is readily available.

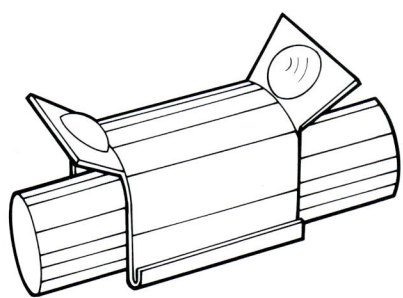

Fig. 13-33. C. M. clip is a rider system 2.7 mm. high with resin retention wings. It comes in two configurations, one with short blades, one with long blades. Short form is most popular and can be used to replace Hader rider.

3. It can be divided into two units.

DISADVANTAGES

1. Retention for the clip is not provided.
2. Soldering retentive loops decreases the elasticity of the clip.
3. It provides joint movement only.

The Baker clip is used for overdentures, but it is not recommended because of the availability of more versatile clips with built-in retention.

C. M. clip (European). The C. M. clip is similar to the Ackermann in design. The retention wings are at both ends on the top side of the rider. It is supplied in two configurations, one with short flanges (Fig. 13-33) and one with long flanges; the shorter one is more popular. It has a shim of 0.5 mm. for the postfabrication vertical movement and a rider bar with a diameter of 1.9 mm. The rider is 2.7 mm. high and 2.6 mm. long.

ADVANTAGES

1. The clip is provided with retention in the best orientation for laboratory processing or resin pick-up in the mouth.
2. The shim provides resilience and rotation, or rotation alone if the shim is not used.

DISADVANTAGE

1. The bars can be only 1.8 mm. to 1.9 mm. in diameter.

The C. M. clip is ideal for the overdenture and particularly for resin pick-up in the mouth because of the retention wing orientation.

Ceka bar joint (European). The Ceka bar consists of a series of one or more Ceka retention elements in a rectangular bar configuration. The Ceka retention unit consists of the replaceable split-flange male stud that is tapered longitudinally with a ball-shaped head. The stud is adjustable for a clip-type retention and is replaceable in the metal solder base that is incorporated in the denture. The overall height is 4.5 mm. added to the bulk of the bar faciolingually. Systems identical to the Ceka are the Regulex 51 bar (C. M.), the Wolf attachment (Heraeus), the Universal-Anker (Degussa), and the KC (König).

ADVANTAGES

1. The retention elements provide fixation with tissue-borne universal movement.
2. The retention elements are replaceable.
3. The retention elements can be picked up in the mouth with resin.

DISADVANTAGES

1. The cost is high.
2. It has too much bulk.

This attachment is used for overdentures, but is not recommended because of the bulk.

Dolder bar joint (European). The Dolder bar joint consists of egg-shaped bars of any length (Fig. 13-30), a brass spacer to provide resilience, and a rider channel with an integral retention flange. The joint consists of two configurations, a standard size 4.65 mm. overall height and a Micro-Dolder bar with an overall height of 3.6 mm. The rider channels can be used as supplied or sectioned into smaller clips. The retention mesh affords the best retention of all clips in the resin base.

ADVANTAGES

1. Two heights are available.
2. The rider and the bar are available in any length.
3. Retention mesh is the best of all found in attachment riders in the denture base.
4. A shim allows vertical and rotational movement.

DISADVANTAGES

1. There is too much bulk even in the micro-size faciolingually.
2. Retention mesh allows too much retention of the rider in the denture for repositioning or rebasing.
3. It is expensive and requires exceptional skill for its use.

The Dolder Micro unit is recommended for overdentures, but the cosmetic effect of the bulk must be considered in any application.

Hader bar joint (European). The Hader bar joint

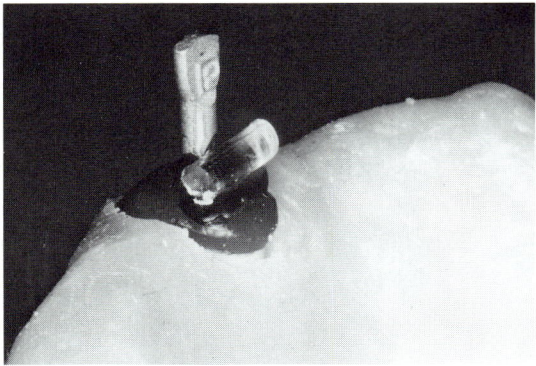

Fig. 13-34. Hader bar joint, which is 1.8 mm. in diameter, may be incorporated on individual crowns for studlike fixation. Here plastic rider has been reduced in length and height and made a part of direct casting with coping wax-up and Schenker step pivot.

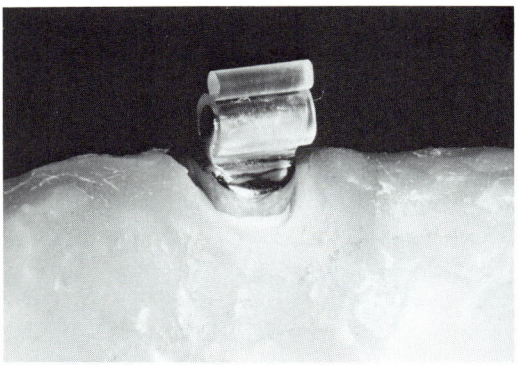

Fig. 13-35. This is replaceable plastic rider on completed casting referred to in Fig. 13-34. Note that bar position is to lingual aspect of crown to reduce bulk and provide space for teeth. Bar attachment, such as Hader bar joint, may be employed in similar fashion to stud attachments or it may join several copings in function of a connector and splint.

(Fig. 13-34) consists of prefabricated plastic forms: 5 mm. plastic bar sections, keyhole in shape, with the greatest bulk being the 1.9 mm. round bar section, processing clips, a series of resilient plastic rider clips 5 mm. long by 4 mm. high, and rider seater tool. The unique features of this system are that the bars can be cast in any restorative alloy or nonprecious alloy, and the patients can service the riders themselves (Fig. 13-35). It is the least expensive of the bar joint systems, and there is no torque to the teeth.

ADVANTAGES
1. Preformed plastic bars allow fabrication in any alloy.
2. The retention is replaceable by the patient or dentist.
3. A metal rider can be picked up with resin and substituted for the plastic rider if more retention is needed.
4. It has the capability to follow anteroposterior gingival contours.
5. The assembly technique is simple.

DISADVANTAGES
1. The rider is too bulky occlusogingivally in contrast to a metal clip.
2. The rider retention is decreased too rapidly.
3. There is no tension adjustment; increased retention must be obtained by adding metal riders.

The Hader bar joint can be recommended for overdentures because of the resin bar pattern feature as well as the riders themselves. The rider clips allow minimum retention and serve as good intermediate "training clips" until metal riders can be substituted.

AUXILIARY ATTACHMENTS

Auxiliary attachments for overdentures consist of the various sizes of screws that can be used to retain bars or a secondary coping carrying bars, and the pawl connectors, which are used to provide or increase the retention of bar units.

Screws

Screws have the advantage of providing removable bar fixation splinting by the use of secondary copings on the roots or as a method of bar placement on divergent teeth.

Pawl connectors

Presso-matic (European). The Presso-matic is a pawl connector available in two lengths (2.2 mm. and 3 mm.) and with two configurations (flanged taper or smooth taper). The diameter of the Presso-matic is 2.6 mm. The Presso-matic consists of a housing, a plunger, a nylon cushion, and a recessed locking screw. These connectors can be either soldered in or cast to the bar or rider.

ADVANTAGES
1. These connectors provide a positive seat and

ATTACHMENTS FOR THE OVERDENTURE   189

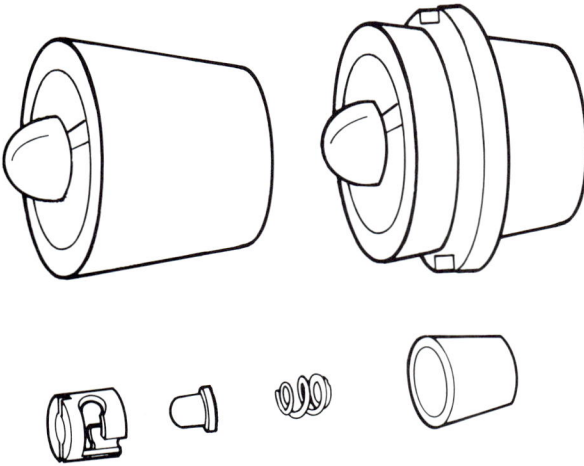

Fig. 13-36. Ipso-Clip is representative of all plunger type pawl connectors. The two assembled units are serviceable from plunger side. Ring configuration is for direct "cast to" or porcelain bonded to metal technique, whereas "smooth" surface is for soldering into bar or rider. Notice bayonet type closure for Ipso-Clip in disassembled unit. Presso-matic series is closed by a screw plug. Both systems are available in regular and high-fusing metal and come with service plugs either on back or plunger side.

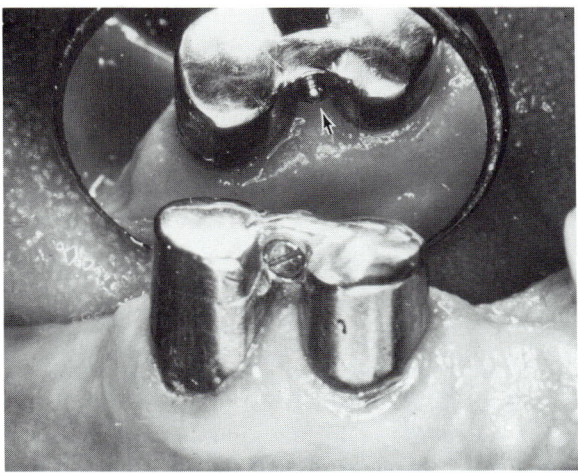

Fig. 13-37. Ipso-Clips are soldered or cast into bars to provide "click" retention. Mini-Presso-matics are smallest pawl connectors providing excellent retention for short bar units. Facial view shows access screw; mirror image shows pawl plunger (arrow).

retention for the riders that is verified by the "click" sound when they are seated.
2. They also give the bar system an indefinite service life because the retention elements are replaceable.

DISADVANTAGES
1. There is an increased bulk buccolingually with the attachment.
2. Skilled technical assistance is required for assembly.

Mini-Presso-matic (European). The Mini-Presso-matic is a pawl connector that is used to increase the retention of a bar unit. It is only 1.75 mm. long and has a 3.2 mm. diameter, and it consists of an alloy shell, a stud plunger, a stainless steel spring, and a recessed screw.

ADVANTAGES
1. This unit is less bulky than the Presso-matic, although it provides the same "click" retention.
2. It is also designed to be cast to the rider.
3. The plunger and spring, being replaceable, provide indefinite service life to the connector.

DISADVANTAGE
1. The extra-small size requires meticulous care in assembly and service, for any damage to the thread housing cannot be rectified.

Ipso-Clip (European). This attachment is a pawl connector that is used to increase or provide retention for bar units or their riders. It consists of two different designs, depending on whether the plunger is to be serviced from the back side or the plunger side (Figs. 13-36 and 13-37). It consists of a taper housing, a stud plunger, a stainless steel spring, and a screw plate. The Ipso-Clip is provided in both cast and soldering alloys. The dimensions are 2.5 mm. by a tapered 2.4 to 2.9 mm. in diameter.

ADVANTAGES
1. This attachment provides positive "click" fixation of the bar rider unit and has an indefinite service life because of the replaceable plunger and spring.
2. Its length is between that of the Presso-matic and the Mini-Presso-matic.
3. The male closure is a bayonet lock instead of a threaded lock, as in the Presso-matic, and is less subject to damage from mishandling.

DISADVANTAGES
1. The increased bulk limits its use.

2. The exceptional skill needed for the laboratory procedures increases the cost of the assembly.

PROCEDURES TO AVOID

It is essential to realize that not all patients can be treated with attachment-retained overdentures.

Patient selection mistakes

1. Teeth that are too mobile to carry attachments should not be used.
2. Patients with crippling arthritis or poor dexterity should be evaluated thoroughly, for they are poor candidates for manipulating the prosthesis or maintaining the gingival and coping hygiene.
3. Some patients have a history of rampant decay and high acidity because of personal hygiene habits or systemic problems. These problems have caused and will continue to cause failure of the coping.

Preinsertion technical mistakes

1. The copings and wax-up of the overdenture are not tried in before processing.
2. In an attempt to over-improve the cosmetics, improper jaw relation records can be registered by over-opening.
3. In trying to obtain an extra millimeter of dowel length, the root is perforated laterally. Unless a dentist performs the endodontics himself, it is desirable to have the endodontist prepare the dowel space.
4. The normal denture border extension and seal are not developed. Improper extension and seal overload an attachment and torque the abutment teeth, with subsequent accelerated loss of support. There is no shortcut to proved full-denture techniques with the attachment-retained overdenture.

Postinsertion technical mistakes

1. The patient is asked to remove the prosthesis without receiving personal instruction. The attachments are so retentive that they usually release in one direction and can extract a weak abutment tooth if the patient attempts to remove the overdenture forcibly.
2. The patient does not receive instructions as to what he can expect from the mechanics of the attachments and the overdenture as well as the frequency of spring and retention control service requirements.

SUMMARY

There are many attachment systems of the bar or stud type that increases the stability of an overdenture. In selecting an attachment, it is always essential to consider the skill of the dentist-laboratory team as well as the dexterity of the patient and to strive for the most easily used system that improves stabilization.

The leverage factors on the teeth also are important and are related directly to the fit on the denture base. If there is a clinically perfect adaptation and atmospheric seal as well as a well-developed occlusion, leverage plays no role. Other aspects to consider are the amount of osseous support and mobility of the individual tooth units. Some splinting is gained from the prosthesis for individual abutment support, but splinting is increased by using bar fixation. In effect, splinting weakens the stronger tooth while it strengthens the weaker tooth. As a rule, simplicity in design, ease of maintenance, and minimum leverage should be paramount in selection. Use of guides such as the EM gauge and attachment selector* significantly reduces the confusion in selecting attachments and increases the working armamentarium for overdenture stabilization (Mensor, 1973).

---

*Bell International, San Mateo, Calif.

REFERENCES

Dolder, E. J.: Die Steg-Gelenk-Prothese im Unterkiefer, DDZ **14**:1-2, 11-15, 1959.
Dolder, E. J.: The bar joint mandibular denture, J. Prosthet. Dent. **11**:689-707, 1961.
Dolder, E. J.: Steg-Prothetik, Heidelberg, 1966, Dr. Alfred Hüthig Verlag GMBH.
Fenner, W., Gerber, A. A., and Mühlemann, H. R.: Tooth mobility changes during treatment with partial denture prosthesis, J. Prosthet. Dent. **6**:520-525, 1956.
Gaerny, A.: Removable closure of the interdental space (C.I.S.), Chicago, Die Quintessenz.
Gerber, A. A.: Retentions Zylinder Retentions Puffer, Biel, Switzerland, 1964, Cendres & Metaux, S. A.
Matsuo, E.: ASC-52, 1970, Kanawaga, Japan.
Mensor, M. C., Jr.: Classification and selection of attachments, J. Prosthet. Dent. **20**:494-497, 1973.
Preiskel, H. W.: Precision attachments in dentistry, ed. 2, London, 1973, Henry Kimpton, Publishers.
Robinson, R. E.: Osseous coagulum for bone induction, J. Periodontol. **40**:503-510, 1969.
Steiger, A. A., and Boitel, R. H.: Precision work for partial dentures, Zürich, 1959, Berichtahaus.

14

LABORATORY PROCEDURES FOR METAL BASES

PETER R. REINER

The materials and laboratory procedures used in fabricating a metal base are the same as those used for chrome cobalt removable partial denture frameworks. In the techniques to be described, Ticonium* metal, investment, and duplicating materials are used. However, it must be emphasized that most of the acceptable chrome series of alloys commonly used in commercial laboratories can be substituted by modifying the technical procedures. The constant is a balanced system, that is, the use of a metal, duplicating material, and investment series that has been developed to produce a predictable end product on a regular basis. The chrome alloys lend themselves well to the fabrication of an overdenture metal base, and their cost, strength, and the inherent lightness are distinct advantages.

As mentioned in Chapter 11, Type IV gold alloys can be used after suitable modification of the technique and materials. The increased weight of the gold prosthesis can be helpful on some mandibular dentures. The disadvantages of weight on maxillary dentures can be overcome by using smaller unit castings. Gold alloys have another advantage when laboratory facilities do not include chrome cobalt casting equipment. However, the rapidly escalating cost of gold alloys has severely restricted their use in most instances and allowed the chrome series of alloys to predominate.

The objective of this chapter is to describe a technique that produces a light, reasonably rigid, well-fitting, economical chrome-cobalt metal base that is clinically acceptable.

SURVEY AND DESIGN: GENERAL CONSIDERATIONS

Like a removable partial denture framework, a metal base should be designed by a clinician. This design is drawn carefully on a reasonably accurate diagnostic cast with soft crayon pencils, and this cast is tripoded to indicate the desired tilt. The prescription form must state clearly all instructions pertinent to fabrication of the metal base. A carefully conceived, well-designed, and annotated diagnostic cast is probably the most valuable tool that a clinician can have for relating his information to the laboratory technician. Survey and design procedures are discussed in Chapter 11.

In most instances the basic design of the metal base will be in one of the following five general categories (Fig. 14-1):

1. A unit casting using the anterior abutments cross arch bilaterally and including the tissues of the edentulous area between the abutments. Castings of this design are small and light in weight, can be unobtrusive when placed in the overdenture base, increase cross-arch strength, minimize

---

*Premium 100 alloy, Ticonium Division, CMP Industries, Albany, N. Y.

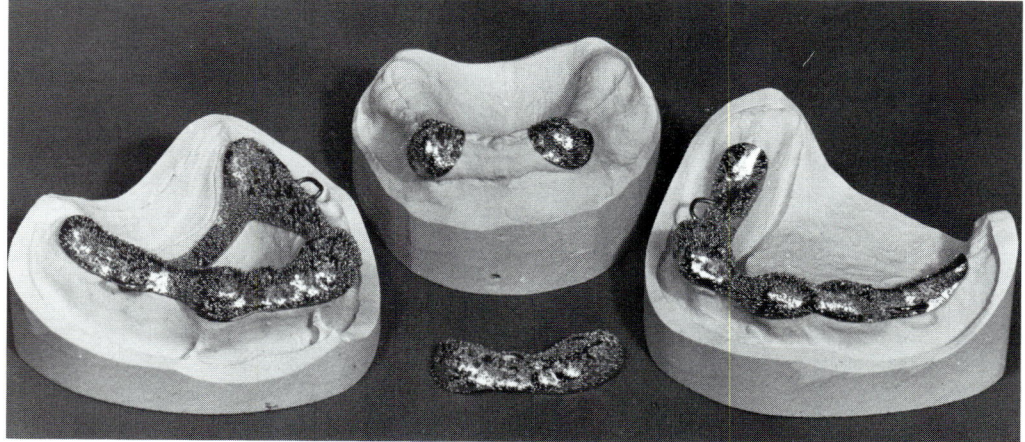

Fig. 14-1. Typical overdenture metal bases. From left to right on cast, a circular bar, individual bases, and conventional full-arch mandibular casting. Small unit casting (minibase) in foreground.

midline fractures, and simplify stabilization of abutments. This relatively simple design facilitates fabrication by the laboratory and allows for possible relining of the overdenture. Sometimes the small casting is referred to as a "minibase."

2. A unit casting using the anterior abutments cross arch bilaterally and including distal extensions to posterior abutments or residual ridges or both. This design permits use of the metal casting as the record base during jaw relation recording procedures.

3. The maxillary circular bar design, similar to the preceding design, but including a posterior palatal strap that is placed anterior to the posterior palatal seal area.

4. Individual abutment unit castings. Although they also can be placed unobtrusively in the overdenture base, they do not provide the strength obtained with other designs.

5. Designs using partial denture-overdenture combinations, as discussed in Chapter 12.

The first three designs can be modified by incorporating open retention for denture base resin in any area in which subsequent corrective procedures such as relining may be required. However, modifications of this type may encroach on available denture space as a result of the relief wax used in the areas modified.

Modifications of designs to meet specific requirements are based on both the ingenuity of the clinician-technician team and the technical feasibility. Simplicity of design is a virtue in most instances. It must be emphasized that designs including cross-arch involvement of the anterior ridge area with the metal base have the advantage of giving the definitive prosthesis greater strength.

Inasmuch as cuspid or cuspid-premolar abutments are involved anteriorly in the majority of overdentures, the midline area between these abutments is subjected to considerable force. The retention of teeth for abutments and the resultant maintenance of bone structure reduce the space that the denture can occupy. Minimal denture space necessitates thinner denture resin and generally makes a weaker overdenture. Use of high-impact resins partially solves the problem of denture breakage in this area; however, inclusion of a metal denture base between these anterior abutments eliminates the problem.

EXAMINING CASTS

First of all, the technician must examine the designed diagnostic cast and the master cast carefully and thoroughly. He or she also takes note of any instructions on the prescription form. It is essential to make certain that all traces of tinfoil substitute used in previous laboratory procedures are removed from the master cast to prevent rough areas on the investment cast.

Then the master cast is placed securely on a suitable surveying table and given the proper tilt, as indicated by the diagnostic cast. Care must be exercised in securing the master cast to the surveying table. Considerable time and effort have been expended by the clinician in producing the master cast. Border areas and anterior frenum areas have been determined carefully during impression procedures. The thickness of the base of the master cast is somewhat critical to its placement on the surveying table. Unless care is exercised, the anterior gripping jaw of the table, when tightened firmly, can crush or chip the anterior border of the cast as well as the frenum attachment (Fig. 14-2). Ideally, the cast is thick enough to permit gripping by the table in a more rigid area of the base. If this placement is impossible, usually the cast can be reversed on the table and held firmly without damage to the cast. Once mounted, the undesirable undercuts on the cast are indicated clearly with a carbon marker. They include the abutments and all tissue undercuts at or near the proposed border areas of the base of the cast. All other undesirable tissue undercuts are marked in the same manner as for a removable partial denture.

GENERAL BLOCKOUT PROCEDURES

A blockout wax that is heat stable at the storage temperature of the duplicating hydrocolloid is used. The wax must be of a color that contrasts markedly with that of the cast material to assure complete removal of tags of excess wax during blockout. All blockout instruments must have smooth, rounded edges to prevent scraping or abrasion of the cast surface (Fig. 14-3).

Abutment blockout

All axial surfaces of the individual abutments are blocked out by using a smooth tapered block-

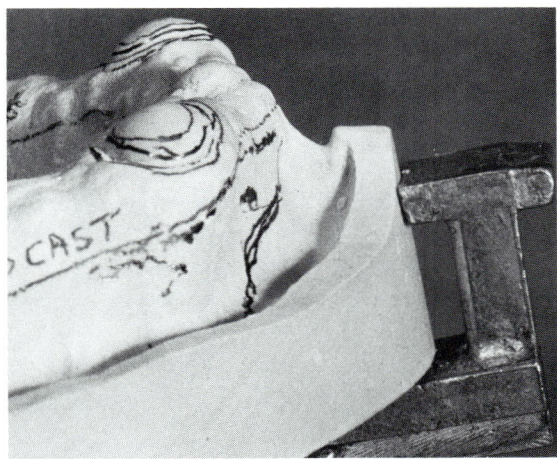

Fig. 14-2. Gripping jaw of cast holder, which, if tightened firmly, can fracture cast.

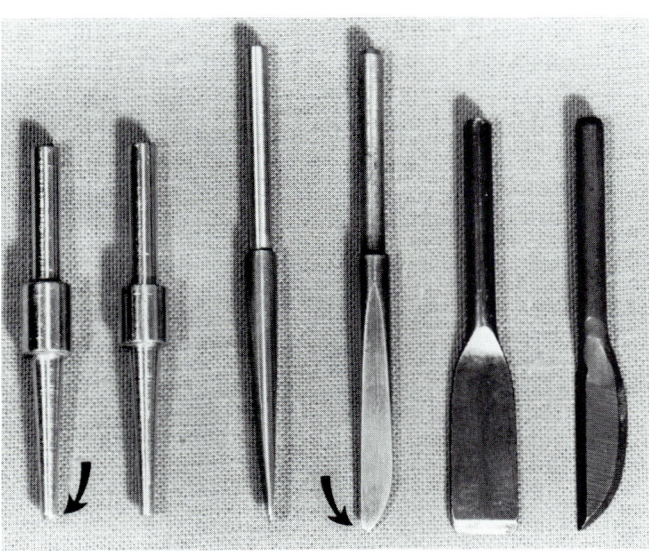

Fig. 14-3. Blockout tools, which must be modified by smoothing sharp edges (arrows) to prevent scraping cast during use. Two tools on right require modification before use.

out tool and a surveyor. A round-tip blade cutting tool that has a taper of 2 or 3 degrees is used for the procedure to permit the degree of freedom required in the finished casting. A surveyor is essential in abutment blockout, for "eyeballing" is risky unless the abutments are excedingly short. The position of the abutment in relation to a path of insertion can be extremely deceptive at times, even to the trained eye. Inadequate blockout can result in a tight abutment casting that requires excessive finishing, which may even result in a hole in a thin casting. Overblocking can cause undesirable tissue hyperplasia around the abutments and make the casting bulkier than necessary, thereby reducing the effective denture or artificial tooth space available at the time of set up.

A very thin layer of blockout wax is applied to the tissues immediately adjacent to and surrounding each abutment. It softens the texture of the metal casting in this area and makes subsequent finishing and polishing easier. The wax layer must be thin to avoid overblocking.

In most instances, no wax is applied to the incisal portion of the abutment (Fig. 14-4), for it is the definitive bearing area of the finished casting. The only exception to this procedure arises when it is necessary to fill in voids or other minimal distortions that occur when making the impression and pouring the cast. Voids and distortions are minimal on an acceptable master cast.

A careful flaming of the wax on and around the abutment is permissible and desirable for a smooth duplication and a smooth casting. Extreme care must be taken during this procedure, and best results are obtained with an alcohol torch.

Tissue blockout

Facial undercuts from the gingival survey line toward the mucobuccal fold also are blocked out with a surveyor. Generally this blocking out is necessary only from the premolar area on one side of the cast to the premolar area on the other side, but it applies to both maxillary and mandibular casts. Lingual tissue undercuts on mandibular casts are treated similarly (Fig. 14-5).

Small amounts of wax are added to other tissue areas within the borders of the design to minimize tissue defects and soften sharp contours. The areas include those in and around the incisive papilla on the maxillary cast, as well as the surgical scars and deep tissue creases, which are subdued by additions of wax (Fig. 14-6). Generally the aim of the procedure is to create a smooth cast surface and a smooth, passively fitting casting. All areas on which wax is placed are flamed gently to assure a smooth surface. Any gross border undercuts that remain are blocked out with modeling clay or baseplate wax.

The total blockout includes the creation of a smooth cast that can be removed passively, without strain, from the duplicating material when the refractory cast is to be poured. This requirement is important, for forcefully retrieving a cast from the duplicating material can produce serious distortions in the duplicate cast, and the result is an ill-fitting casting.

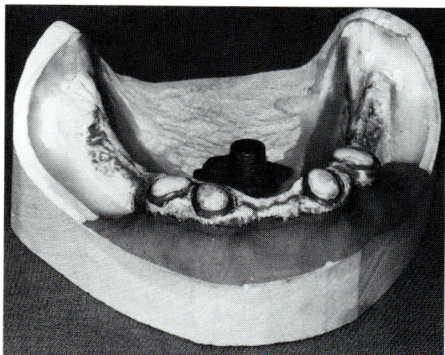

Fig. 14-4. Bearing surface of abutment on which no wax is placed except to correct minute defects on cast.

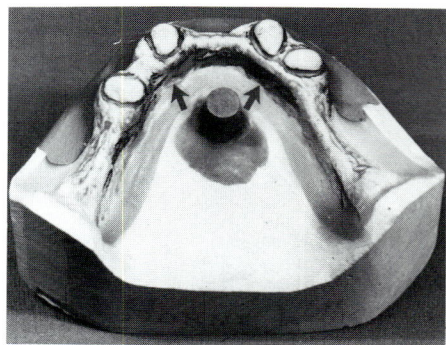

Fig. 14-5. Mandibular cast with lingual tissue undercuts, which must be blocked out.

Cast preparation for spruing

Through-the-cast spruing is used in this technique. On maxillary casts using a circular bar design, the sprue cone is affixed to the center of the palate of the master cast. In the majority of other designs the sprue cone is placed on the anterior slope of the palatal vault. Sprue cones on mandibular casts are centered in the tongue space between the ridges and approximately 20 mm. lingual to the anterior ridge area (Fig. 14-5).

On maxillary casts, wax is flowed onto the rugae area between the sprue cone and the palatal border (Fig. 14-6) of the proposed design to permit a more passive removal of the cast from the duplicating material and a smooth, nonturbulent flow of metal from the sprue to the case at the time of casting. This procedure can be important in obtaining thin castings.

Mandibular cases are treated similarly. The lingual border area of the cast between the sprue and the proposed lingual portion of design is filled in with wax (Fig. 14-5) to permit a smooth, straight-line flow of metal into the case.

A cast sealer is not used on the surface of the master cast before the addition of blockout wax. Experience has shown that this sealer often peels in some areas during the wetting stage of the duplicating process, especially on master casts poured into rubber base impression materials. Peeling also occurs on master casts that are not thoroughly dry before the addition of the sealer, and the result is a rough refractory cast if the sealer peels during duplication. This situation is most apparent at the tips of the abutments, which are critical areas. The design is not drawn on the master cast with crayon pencils, for they penetrate the cast surface, are difficult to remove from the cast, and can stain the acrylic resin. If it is deemed necessary to draw the design on the master cast, a pink or red crayon pencil is recommended, for these colors blend well with the acrylic resin in the event of contamination. Similarly, a red or pink blockout wax is recommended. Now the master cast is ready for duplication (Fig. 14-7).

PREPARATION FOR DUPLICATION

The master cast is placed with the base up in clear slurry water* and preferably soaked overnight to allow for adequate surface wetting and air displacement from the cast. Use of clear slurry water

---

*Solution made by soaking stone debris or particles in a container of water for 48 hours. The resultant supernatant solution is used for soaking casts, for it does not dissolve them.

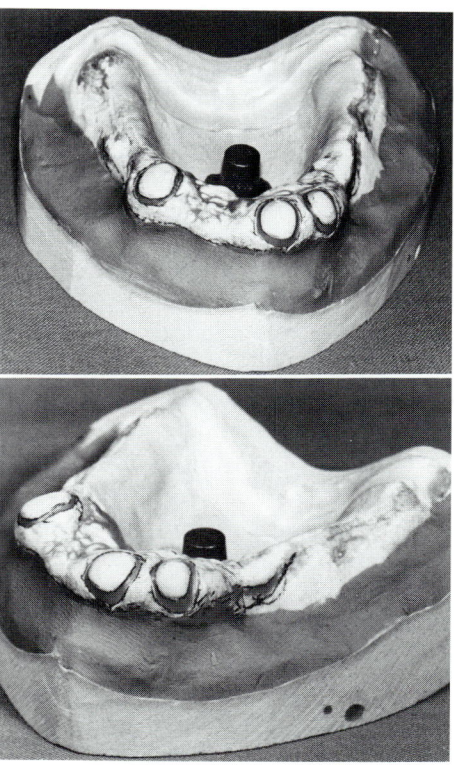

Fig. 14-7. Master cast ready for duplication. Deep tissue undercuts in mucobuccal fold blocked out with modeling clay.

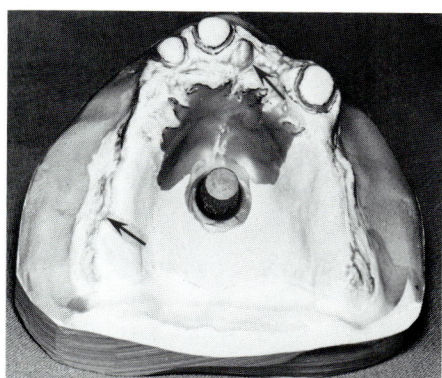

Fig. 14-6. Wax has been flowed into tissue creases and around incisive papilla. Wax has been flowed onto rugae area between sprue cone and palatal border.

196 METHODS

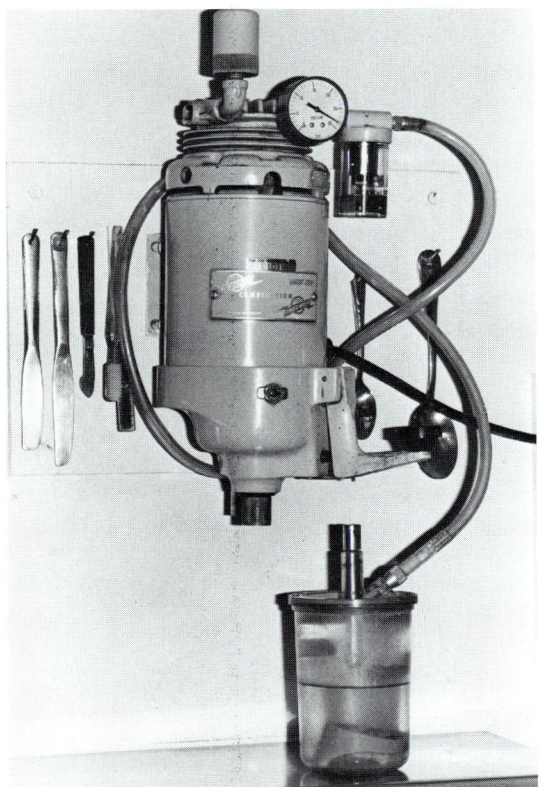

Fig. 14-8. Cast immersed in clear slurry water at reduced atmospheric pressure to shorten soaking time.

prevents damage to the surface of the cast during soaking. A quicker method is to place the master cast in clear slurry water with the base up for an hour, then fully immerse it in the same position in clear slurry water and vacuum it at reduced atmospheric pressure for 3 to 5 minutes* (Fig. 14-8). This method adequately wets the cast and removes air from the internal portions. Adequate wetting of the surface of the cast and air displacement before duplication are essential. Failure to wet the surface of the cast causes the hydrocolloid to stick to the cast, and it can distort the surface when removed. If all of the air in the cast is not displaced before duplication, the heat of the duplicating hydrocolloid causes this air to rise to the surface of the cast and produces many nodules. Proper preparation of the refractory cast gives it a smooth surface with a resultant smooth casting.

---

*Combination Vac-U-Vestor and power mixer, Whip-Mix Corp., Louisville, Ky.

After the cast is adequately wet and air-free, all surface water is removed with a gentle blast of compressed air; however, excessive surface drying must be avoided. Free water on the surface of the cast dilutes the hydrocolloid immediately adjacent to the cast surface and can result in distortion.

DUPLICATING CASTS

The master cast is centered in a suitable duplicating flask and held in position by small amounts of modeling clay. To be suitable, the flask is one that permits the hydrocolloid to cool toward the base of the flask and down onto the cast. The flask also must be large enough for a reasonable amount of hydrocolloid to surround the cast. The duplicating hydrocolloid must be compatible with the refractory material to satisfy the requirement for a balanced system. The fit of the casting is less than ideal if the setting and hygroscopic expansion of the refractory material are not correct.

The flask is filled with a gentle stream of hydrocolloid and placed in a suitable cooling tray. The water temperature and the cooling time must be compatible with the manufacturer's recommendations, and rapid or excessive cooling must be avoided.

Pouring refractory cast

The refractory material selected must be weighed carefully, and the water or liquid portion must be measured accurately according to the manufacturer's specifications. The water-powder ratio is determined carefully and adjusted as needed to achieve the relative fit of the casting. Generally large castings require more expansion than smaller ones. All refractory material is vacuum mixed to make the surface of the cast dense and free of voids.

Removal of master cast from duplicating material

Accuracy dictates a strain-free, passive removal of the master cast from the duplicating material, and blockout procedures facilitate this action. Before removal of the cast from the duplicating material, a substantial wedge of the hydrocolloid is cut away, leaving enough of the base of the cast exposed to permit a firm finger grasp on the master cast. Removal of this wedge of hydrocolloid reduces the drag force on the material and makes

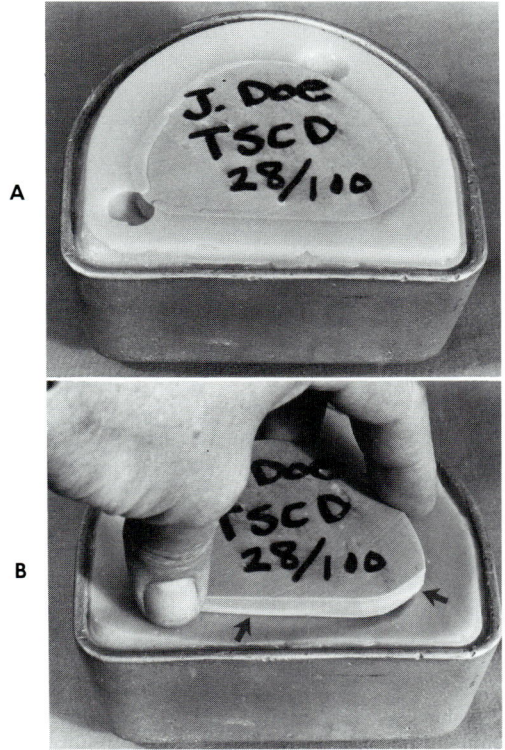

Fig. 14-9. **A**, Duplicating flask with master cast after removal of base of flask. **B**, Wedge of hydrocolloid removed to permit firm finger grasp on cast.

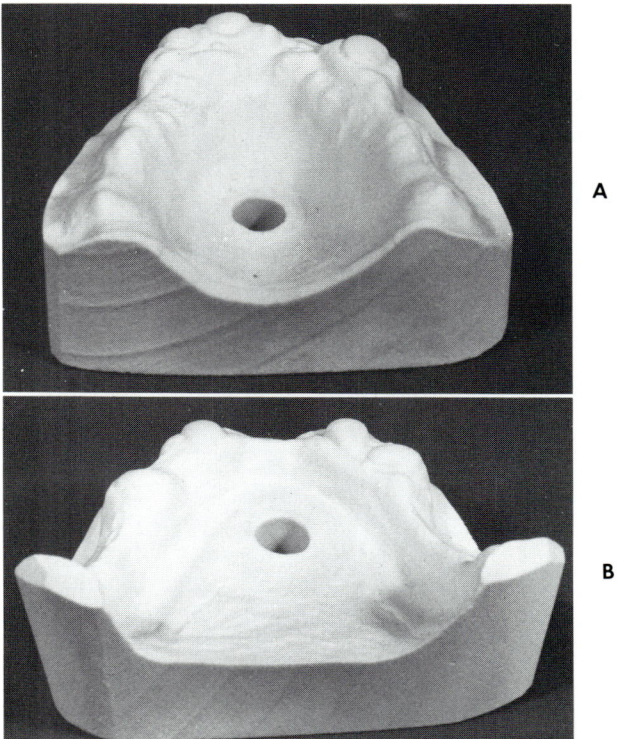

Fig. 14-10. **A**, Maxillary refractory cast with smooth surface. **B**, Mandibular refractory cast.

passive removal easier (Fig. 14-9), which is important. The cast is removed quickly with a vertical pull; torsion is to be avoided.

The stainless steel sprue former is placed in the impression in the hydrocolloid formed by the cone attached to the master cast. Then the vacuum-mixed refractory material is vibrated gently into the mold until it reaches the top of the previously cut out portion of the hydrocolloid. The flask is placed in a vibration-free area to set for the period recommended by the manufacturer, but not for less than an hour. A timer is used for accuracy; rushing the setting time results in inadequate expansion or surface inaccuracy or both. When the setting time has expired, the refractory cast is retrieved carefully from the hydrocolloid and set aside for additional maturation of the surface. Often it is desirable to reduplicate the master cast while it is still wet. A second or duplicate refractory cast can save considerable time in the event that the original is a miscast. Since overdenture castings must be thin, miscasts result occasionally.

Trimming refractory cast

The refractory cast is wet thoroughly in clear slurry water, placed on a wet cast trimmer, and trimmed to the desired size. The fingers must not touch any area included in the design during this procedure, for the cast is soft, and abrasion of the cast surface will occur. After trimming, the cast is rinsed thoroughly in clear slurry water to remove all traces of the grinding, and free water is removed from the cast by an air blast. Improper cleaning of the refractory cast can result in a rough casting. Under high illumination the duplicate refractory cast is compared closely with the master cast for accuracy. Surface defects and nodules are removed, and the sprue hole is smoothed and leveled with the cast surface. Few surface defects should be noted if all procedures are carried out properly (Fig. 14-10).

Inasmuch as further maturation of the cast surface occurs, it is preferable to wait until the next day to dry the refractory cast and dip it in wax. This delay allows the surface to become harder and more durable. The manufacturer's recommendations are followed exactly during the drying and dipping.

WAX-UP
General considerations

The wax-up, being a crucial stage in the fabrication of the metal base, must be accomplished neatly and carefully under high illumination. Unlike removable partial denture frameworks, thinning of the general bulk of the overdenture casting by grinding is difficult. Therefore it is essential to control the thickness of the casting during the wax-up, so that it is uniformly thin. Gauged, adhesive wax* is used in most of the wax-up (Fig. 14-11), for it is reasonably tough, it adapts and flames well, and it stays where it was put.

The only problem with the wax is its natural color, which makes high illumination essential for the technician to find surface defects. However, since crayon pencil design outlines can be seen through the wax, the border can be placed accurately, which is a distinct advantage. The adhesive wax sheets are available in a variety of gauges; 22- and 24-gauge sheets are adequate in most instances. They are superior to the resin pattern sheets used for partial denture wax-ups, for they remain adherent to the cast surface and do not rebound or "pull up" from depressed cast surfaces. The application of tacky liquid and retention crystal placement is accomplished more easily than with the resin pattern material. Adhesive wax can be adapted over abutments readily and sealed easily. Adhesive wax is not merely an asset but an essential item in waxing metal bases of uniform thickness for overdentures.

Technical considerations

The outline of the proposed design is transferred accurately from the diagnostic cast to the refractory cast with a soft crayon pencil; the pencil marks do not abrade the surfaces of the cast, and they burn out clean. A small amount of soft blue pattern wax is flowed around the gingival area of each abutment (Fig. 14-12). This wax is flamed with a torch to assure a smooth blend with the surface of the cast. The tissue-bearing portions of the wax-up are done in sections with pieces of adhesive wax of the desired gauge. The aim is to produce a light, thin, rigid casting; however it is equally important to have the casting complete, and the gauge of wax selected determines both.

---
*Casting wax, pressure-sensitive adhesive coated, The Kindt-Collins Co., Cleveland; Stalite, pressure-sensitive adhesive coated wax, Stalite, Inc., Hialeah, Fla.

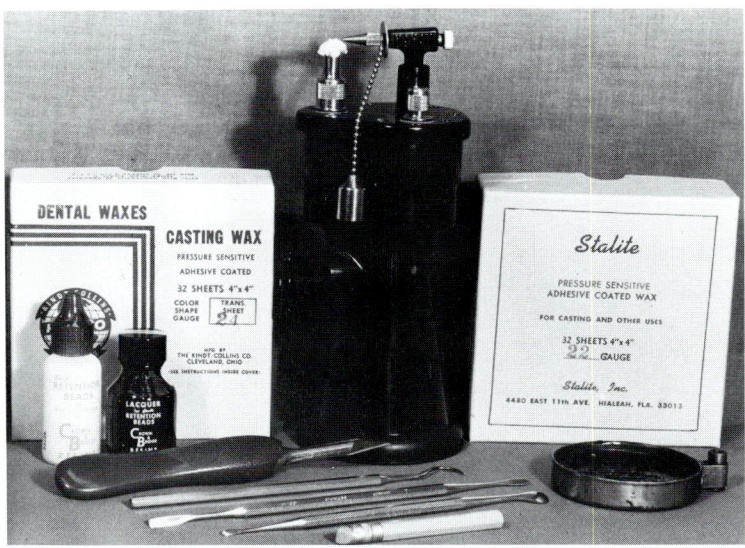

Fig. 14-11. Armamentarium for waxing overdenture metal base.

On larger metal bases 22-gauge adhesive wax is used for most of the wax-up; 24-gauge wax can be used over abutments and in areas that need to be especially thin, and 24- or 26-gauge wax can be used for smaller castings. Gauged wax sheets that are thinner than 24-gauge are difficult to handle. In most instances, the skill of the technician dictates the choice of gauge.

As mentioned previously, the wax-up is completed in sections. Application of the wax in this manner makes adaptation to the convexities of the cast easier and minimizes tearing and overthinning. Large, relatively flat surfaces can be covered with one piece of wax (Fig. 14-12). The abutments and the surrounding tissue are waxed last, for they are more difficult to do than other areas. Wax has a "memory," and in colder climates or in cool laboratories it becomes slightly sluggish in sheet form and tears more easily when adapted over convex surfaces. For best results each adhesive wax section is warmed slightly under a light bulb prior to placement on the cast, so that it will adapt better and tear less easily. Generally adhesive wax is tough wax and handles well. It is adapted slowly to the cast with finger pressure and worked down from one side to the other. It must not be stretched over valleys but worked into them as they are approached, especially in the rugae area; likewise it must be worked over sharply convex tissue surfaces. Once a section is adapted reasonably well, firm finger pressure can be applied to adapt it further. Some thinning will occur. A blunt, smooth, wedge-shaped pencil eraser further aids adaptation in depressed areas of the cast.

A technician soon learns how large a section to place at one time. The wax-up is completed piecemeal until the abutments are approached, and each section is joined to the other with soft blue pattern wax. It is desirable to overwax the borders of the case by extending the borders several millimeters to seal them with pattern wax. The thickness of the sealed area varies from that of the finished casting; however, the metal can be cut to a uniform thickness at the border outline during finishing. All sections and borders must be adapted closely and sealed down to the surface of the cast to prevent the refractory material from running under during the investing.

As was mentioned earlier, abutment waxing is the most critical portion of the wax-up. Inasmuch as uniformity of thickness is essential, undue thinning of the wax during adaptation must be avoided. Wax is trimmed away from the abutment until there is a 5 mm. space around the abutment. A dulled No. 23 scalpel blade is used, and care is taken to avoid cutting into the cast.

In most instances a single piece of wax can be used for the abutment and surrounding tissues. A piece larger than the area to be covered is warmed and placed distal to the abutment in approximation to the last adjacent section (Fig. 14-13). The wax is adapted slowly and carefully up to and over the abutment. The distal or lingual surface can be adapted first. If the distal surface is done

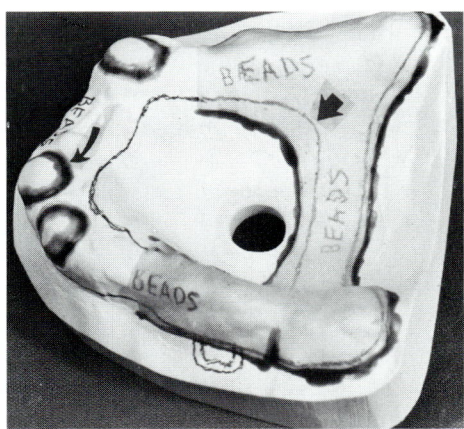

Fig. 14-12. Soft pattern wax flowed around gingival area of abutments. Large, relatively flat tissue areas can frequently be covered with one piece of adhesive wax. Note border outline visible through translucent wax (large arrow).

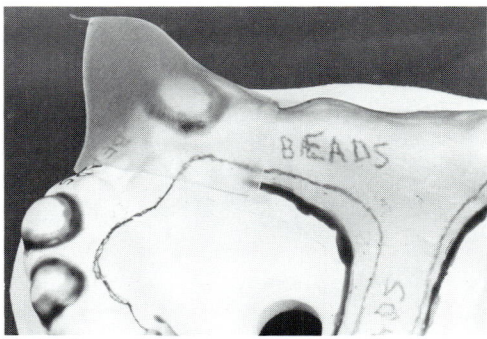

Fig. 14-13. Wax in place over abutment before adaptation.

first, wax is adapted carefully around the lingual surface, next over the incisal surface, and down the facial surface. The wax puckers or bunches up on the facial surface as the adaptation proceeds. At this point a wedge-shaped piece of wax is removed from the facial aspect (Fig. 14-14) to permit complete adaptation without strain and undue thinning of the wax. Another cut can be made in the wax if it is needed to relieve any strain (Fig. 14-15). The wax is trimmed to meet adjacent sections, and all junctions and border areas are sealed well with blue pattern wax (Fig. 14-16). Using the uniformly gauged wax sheets over an abutment is superior to flowing wax onto the abutment, for it is difficult to "free flow" with uniformity.

Mandibular tissue-bearing areas are waxed similarly; however, knife edged mandibular ridges are not amenable to the adaptation of a single sheet of wax over the posterior ridge area. The wax tears and becomes excessively thin when adapted over the ridge crest. Therefore two sections are used, one for the buccal slope adapted slightly over the ridge crest and one for completion of the lingual slope. The pieces are joined together with soft pattern wax immediately lingual to the ridge crest to assure more uniform thickness in this portion of the mandibular wax-up. If extra reinforcement is required, as in mandibular castings, one length of 12-gauge half-round wax is placed lingual to the ridge area; however, use of 22-gauge wax sheets usually makes this procedure unnecessary.

Although different gauges of wax can be used together in various portions of the same wax-up, sheets thicker than 22-gauge are too bulky, and those thinner than 24-gauge may not cast if well adapted because of thinned-out spots produced during adaptation.

In the event that open retention is desired in a portion of the wax-up, the technique is modified slightly by using the same procedure as for areas of open retention on conventional removable partial denture frameworks. When relief is also desired in areas of open retention, relief wax is applied to the master cast before duplication. In most instances, using open resin retention and cast-metal–bearing areas is of questionable merit, for a weaker, more complicated, and bulkier casting is inevitable.

The entire surface of the wax-up is flamed lightly with a torch to produce a smooth surface by sealing any surface defects and releasing stress in the wax. Care must be exercised to avoid overheating the wax during flaming, especially on convex surfaces, or undesired thinning can occur, especially at the tips of the abutments. Then the

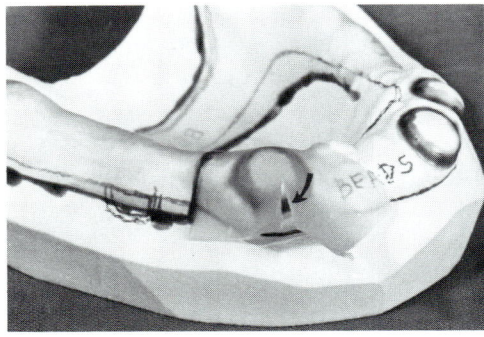

Fig. 14-14. Wedge shape cut in wax to facilitate adaptation to abutment.

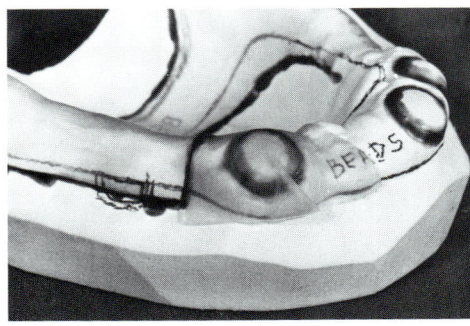

Fig. 14-15. Final adaptation of wax over abutment before trimming.

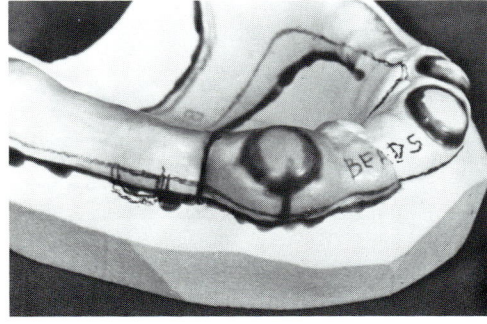

Fig. 14-16. Wax adapted and sealed on refractory cast.

wax-up is examined closely for defects under high illumination.

SPRUING

After completion of the wax-up, the case is sprued, and resin retention beads and jaw relation handles are added (Fig. 14-17). Inasmuch as ideas about spruing vary, the recommendations of manufacturers and the success factors of individual technicians deserve recognition. In other words, if a method gives good results for a technician, he or she should use it. As stated previously, the objective is to obtain an acceptable casting. Over-jet spruing is effective in casting chrome-cobalt alloys through the cast; however, it may be necessary to modify the method for other alloys.

Mandibular castings

For mandibular castings two 6-gauge, half-round sprues originate from the main sprue lead. They are attached lingually to the wax pattern and bilaterally in the cuspid and premolar area to provide an initial flow of metal to and around the abutments (Fig. 14-18). No additional sprues are required for posterior abutments.

Maxillary castings

Horseshoe design. In making maxillary castings of the horseshoe or other designs, except for the circular bar, two 6-gauge, half-round sprues from the main sprue lead are attached to the palatal aspect of the case and "aimed" toward the anterior abutments.

Circular bar design. For maxillary castings of the circular bar design, four 6-gauge half-round sprue leads are used, one to each corner of the pattern palatally (Fig. 14-17). These larger castings require the flow of more metal into a larger thin area. The four sprues also seem to have an effect of tying down the casting and allowing less distortion. Being more rigid, this configuration is less likely to distort during removal from the refractory material and the initial sandblasting of the casting.

Technical procedures

In spruing, a stainless steel sprue pin is always inserted in the sprue hole of the refractory cast and sealed to the cast with hard inlay wax. Use of the hard wax permits cleaner removal of the stainless pin before burnout procedures. The 6-gauge, half-round wax sprues from the main sprue lead to the wax-up are attached at both ends with soft blue pattern wax. The sprues also are sealed down well onto the cast to prevent refractory material from running under during investing.

The rather bulky wax sprue is attached to the thin wax-up by fanning out the point of attachment to avoid creating sharp corners, which impede the flow of metal. Fanning out the wax also reduces the high risk of dislodging refractory material in sharp corners at the time of casting. The dislodged material causes porosity in the completed casting.

Handles. If desired, jaw relation handles made

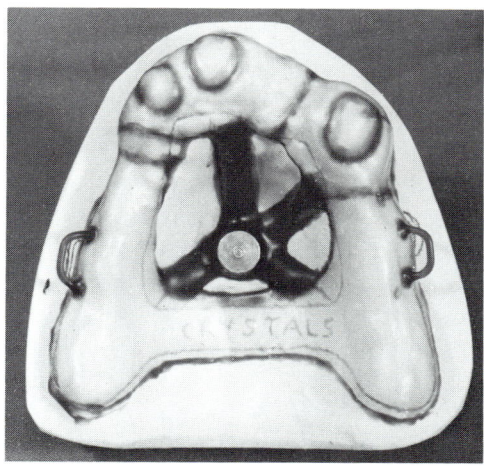

Fig. 14-17. Completed wax-up, sprued and ready for application of resin retention beads. Note position of sprue leads.

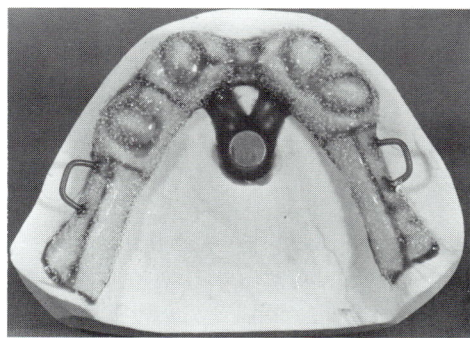

Fig. 14-18. Retention beads on completed wax-up. Note position of handles, raised and perpendicular to surface of cast.

of 18-gauge pattern wax are attached to the completed, sprued wax-up in the designated position perpendicular to the surface of the cast. They are sealed to the wax-up with soft pattern wax and flamed lightly. Placement of the handles is deferred until this time, for they can be deformed or displaced while handling the cast during spruing.

Resin retention. Resin is retained on the metal base by applying a tacky fluid adhesive to the surface of the wax-up and adding fine acrylic beads* or crystals (Fig. 14-18). This adhesive can be made by dissolving resin patterns in acetone; its consistency must be thin to avoid adding bulk to the wax-up. When the adhesive is thin and tacky, it is volatile and dries quickly. Therefore the adhesive and the beads are applied to only small sections of the wax-up at a time. A small sable brush

---

*Retention beads for crown and bridge, L. D. Caulk Co., Milford, Del.

is used to apply the adhesive, and the retention beads are sprinkled onto the adhesive immediately. A plastic squeeze bottle with a small orifice aids in placing the beads. The technician must exercise extreme care in applying the tacky adhesive and the beads to avoid excessive use and an undesirable thickening on the wax-up. Since valleys or depressed areas of the wax-up are especially sensitive to thickening, the beads are applied to the entire surface of the wax-up, a section at a time. Clumping of beads is to be avoided, especially over the abutments. A small brush dipped in acetone can be used to remove heavy concentrations of beads. An evenly applied, fine distribution of the retention beads gives the desired acrylic retention without undue thickening of the resulting casting. Now the completed wax-up is ready for investing (Fig. 14-19).

INVESTING WAX PATTERN

Investing procedures depend on the metal and the refractory material selected. A gypsum-bound investment usually requires the use of a surface paint-on layer of investment. It is mixed and measured according to the manufacturer's specifications and vacuum spatulated. The surface of the wax-up is treated with a surface tension reducing agent before application of the paint-on layer. A thin, uniform layer of the premixed refractory material is applied to the entire surface of the wax-up with a soft brush. It is essential that this paint-on layer of investment be uniform and thin. Success in making thin castings requires a rapid, uniform release of mold pressure at the time of casting. Experience indicates that a thin paint-on layer permits the desired effect and minimizes the number of miscasts.

The outer investment material is applied in the manner specified by the manufacturer. It must be air-laden to augment release of the mold pressures during casting.

BURNOUT

Burnout of the invested wax-up depends on the metal-refractory system selected. The procedure must not be speeded up, for complete burnout and adequate thermal expansion are essential in achieving thin, well-fitting castings. Adherence to the manufacturer's recommendations in burnout procedures materially contributes to success in

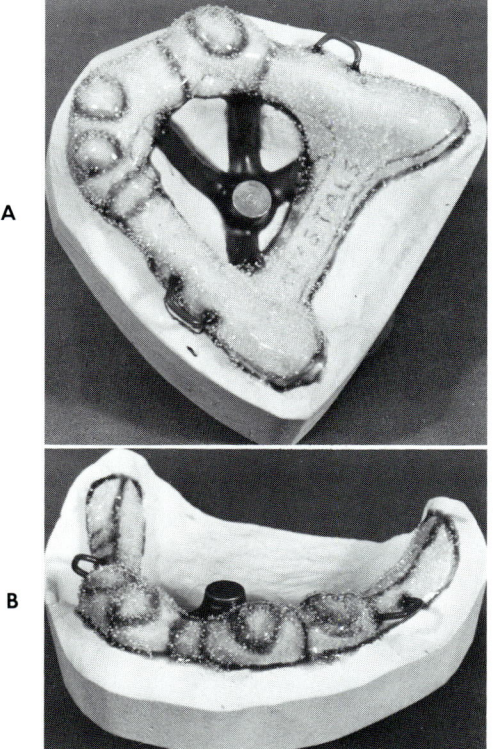

Fig. 14-19. **A**, Completed maxillary wax-up, sprued and ready for investing. **B**, Mandibular wax-up. Note handles in raised position.

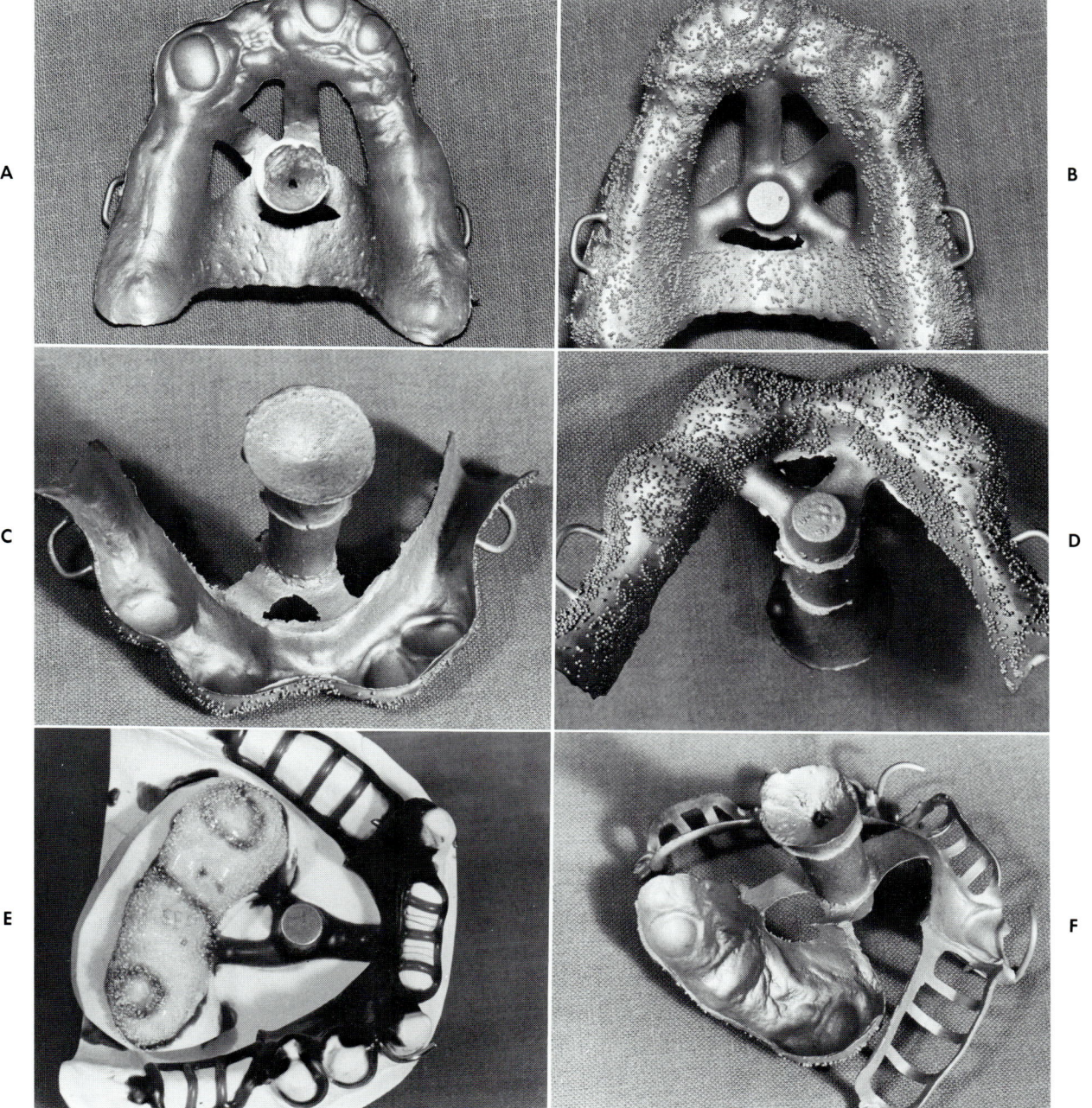

Fig. 14-20. **A**, Interior of maxillary casting prior to finishing. Note absence of nodules. **B**, Maxillary casting ready for finishing. **C**, Mandibular casting before removal of sprue. **D**, Superior surface of mandibular casting. Note position of handles, which are removed after recording jaw relationship. **E**, Small overdenture bases, frequently cast as "add-on" to conventional partial dentures. **F**, "Add-on" casting, which reduces laboratory costs.

casting. Burnout ovens must be calibrated periodically for accuracy, and the length of the burnout must be timed accurately. Setting expansion as well as hygroscopic and thermal expansion affect the final fit of the casting. Maximum thermal expansion, the most significant factor, must be attained. The technician must be thoroughly cognizant of all these factors for the material selected and must adhere closely to the time-temperature charts.

CASTING

Induction casting of the chrome series of alloys is an effective method. The casting equipment must be tuned periodically and calibrated exactly. Human error is minimized by using electronic equipment. Use of a torch for melting these alloys is possible, but to obtain consistent results it requires considerable skill on the part of the technician.

DEVESTING THE CASTING

The completed casting is allowed to cool, usually for 30 to 45 minutes, until the investment can be held comfortably in the hand. The method of cooling varies with the particular metal-investment system, and following the manufacturer's recommendations closely is essential. The casting is removed from the investment carefully, and the remaining investment is removed by sandblasting. Then the casting is examined carefully to determine its acceptability (Fig. 14-20).

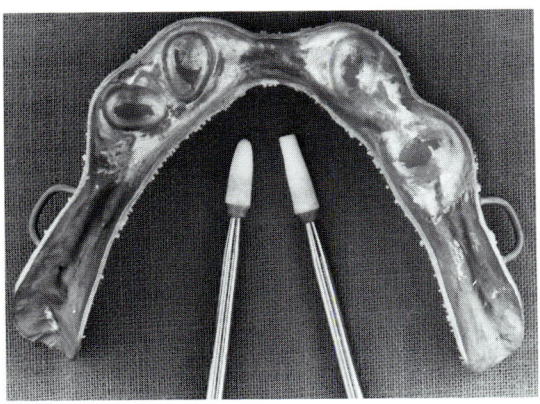

Fig. 14-21. Stones should be shaped like stone on left to facilitate finishing of abutment indentations.

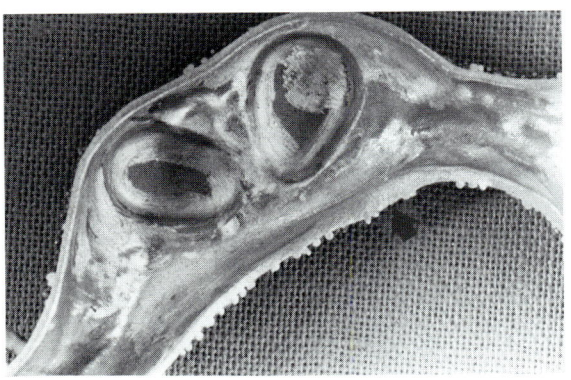

Fig. 14-22. First stage in finishing abutment indentations and adjacent surfaces. Arrow indicates thickened border where sprue was attached. Border is thinned with a Carborundum disk.

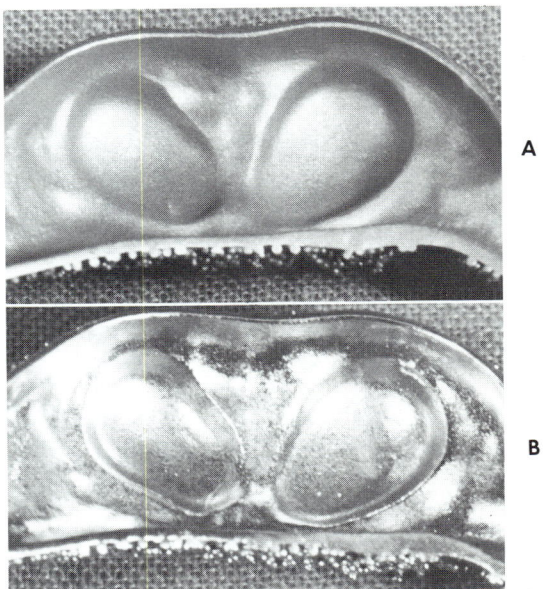

Fig. 14-23. A, Interior surface of casting after fine finishing and sandblasting. B, Interior surface of same casting after electropolishing.

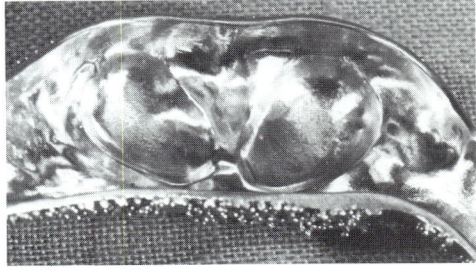

Fig. 14-24. Smooth semipolished casting after use of rubber point.

LABORATORY PROCEDURES FOR METAL BASES

FINISHING AND POLISHING

If the casting is acceptable, the sprues are removed with a thin carborundum disk on a high-speed chrome finishing lathe. Then the borders of the casting are adjusted to the desired extension and finished perpendicular to the cast surface. Bubbles and nodules on the interior surface are removed with fine finishing stones. Few defects are seen when vacuum-spatulated investment is used. Almost all finishing of the interior of the casting is confined to the area immediately adjacent to the abutments. The axial walls of the abutment indentations and the adjacent tissue surfaces of the casting are finished with a fine finishing stone (Fig. 14-21). Care is taken to avoid the bearing area in the depths of the abutment indentations (Fig. 14-22). A fine finishing stone is used to reduce the sharp edges by rounding slightly the borders contacting the tissue. Then the casting is sandblasted, inspected closely, and electro polished (Fig. 14-23). All surfaces previously finished with a stone are smoothed with a rubber point (Fig. 14-24). A mirrorlike finish is obtained in and around the

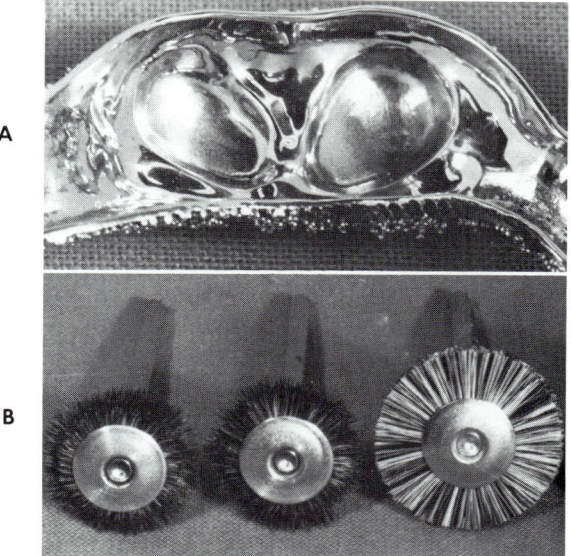

Fig. 14-25. **A,** Mirrorlike surface facilitates cleansing and contributes to abutment health. Thick border where sprue was attached has been reduced with Carborundum disk. **B,** Brushes used for final polishing. On left are two brushes of correct diameter for polishing of critical area immediately adjacent to abutments. Brushes of good quality are essential for polishing at high rotational speeds.

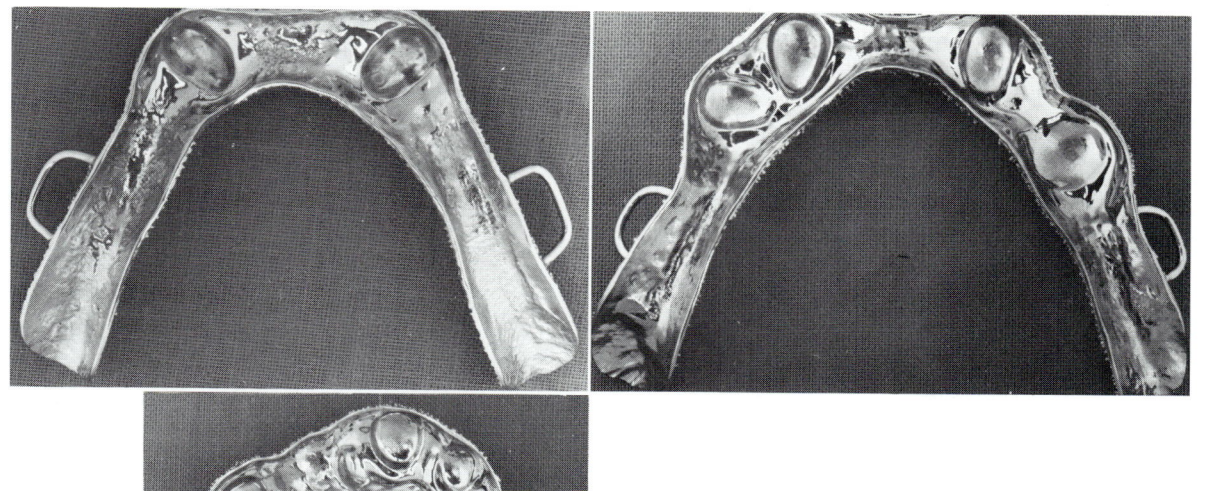

Fig. 14-26. **A,** Interior of polished mandibular casting. **B,** Interior of overdenture casting for four abutments. Note high polish in gingival margin area of abutment indentations. **C,** Maxillary overdenture casting for three abutments after polishing has been completed.

206 METHODS

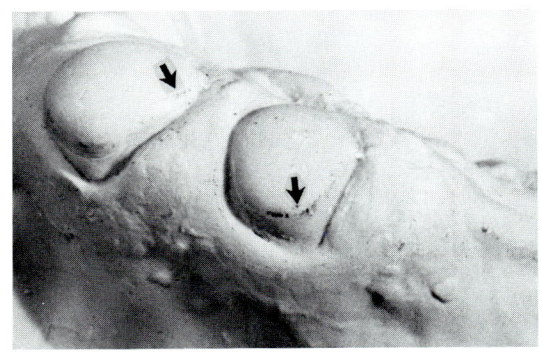

Fig. 14-27. Scuff marks on abutment, indicating need for adjustment of casting.

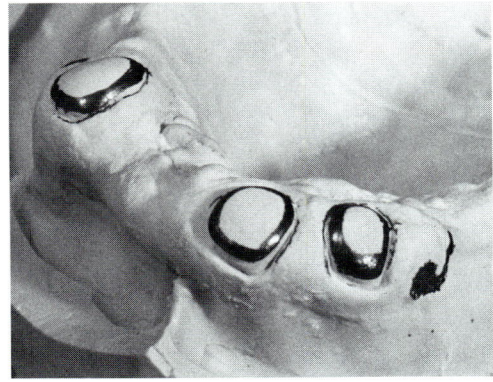

Fig. 14-28. Soft pencil is rubbed on cast as indicator.

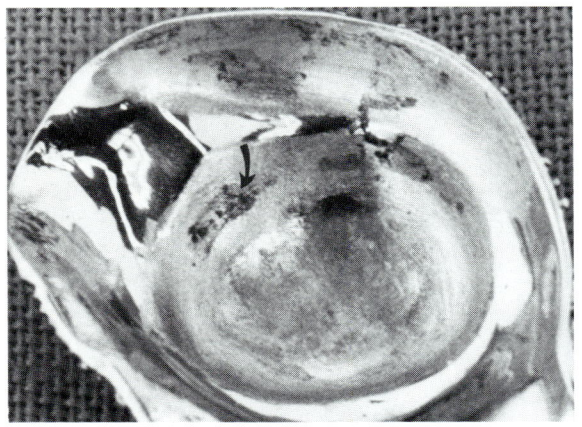

Fig. 14-29. Area requiring adjustment is indicated by carbon.

abutments with small soft bristle brushes* and polishing compounds (Fig. 14-25), and high illumination is required throughout this procedure. Tissue-bearing surfaces remote from the abutments are highlighted with polishing brushes and compounds; excessive polishing in these areas is to be avoided. Then the borders and handles are polished. Smooth, polished borders are essential for the comfort of the patient at the time of try-in and during jaw relation recording procedures. All traces of polishing compound are removed in an ultrasonic cleaner with suitable cleansing solutions. Then the polished casting is examined carefully (Fig. 14-26).

FITTING THE CASTING

The casting is checked for fit on the master cast. A duplicate master cast can be used for fitting if preferred. Occasionally some minor adjustment to the casting is needed for accurate adaptation to the cast. Such areas of impingement are primarily

---

*Brush, bristle dental, soft bristle, Buffalo Dental Manufacturing Co., Buffalo, N. Y.

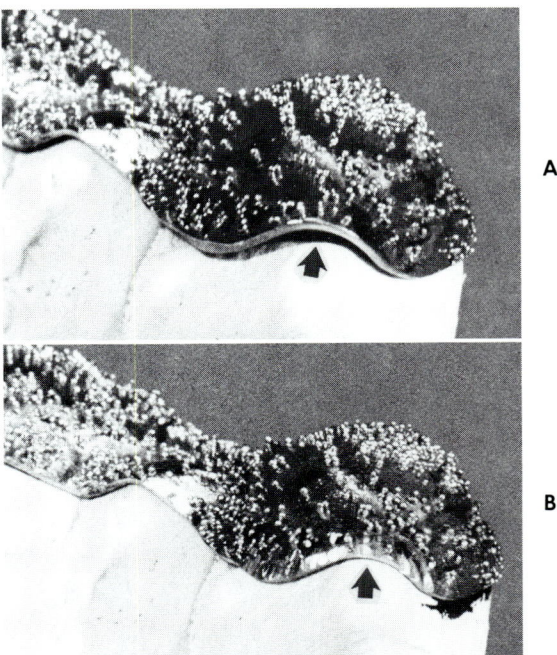

Fig. 14-30. A, Impingement, preventing accurate seating of casting. B, Adjusted casting that fits cast.

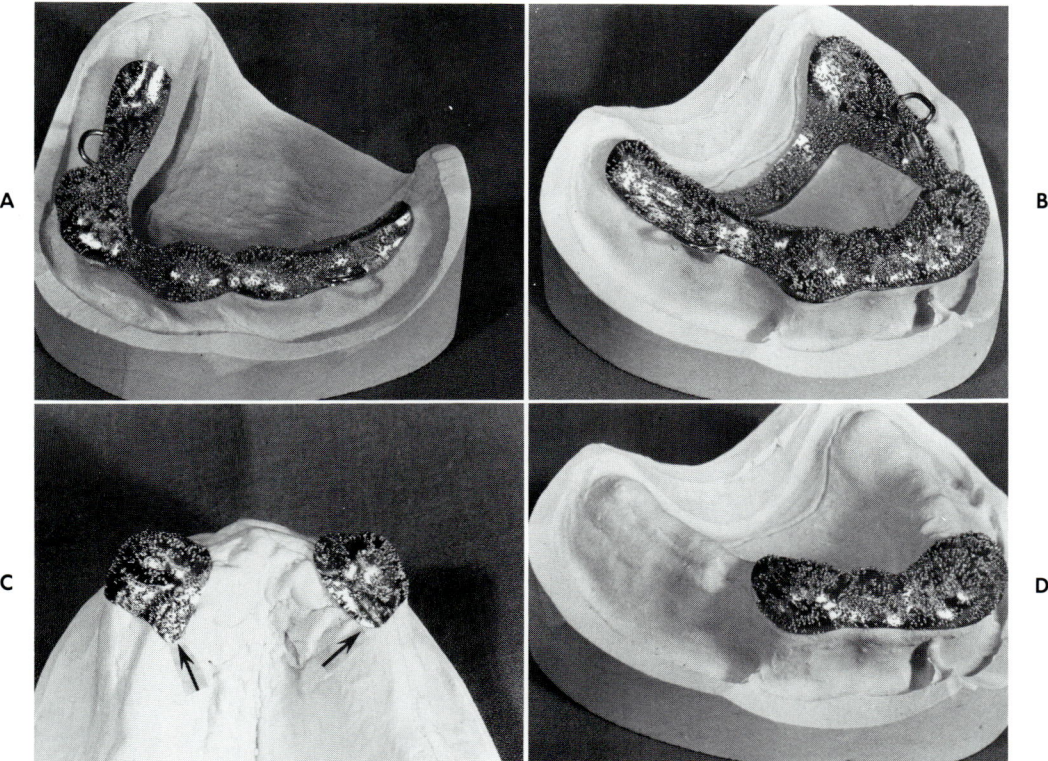

Fig. 14-31. A, Completed mandibular overdenture casting ready for return to dentist. **B,** Completed maxillary overdenture casting, circular bar design. **C,** Individual abutment castings on master cast. Design does not provide strength obtained with other designs. Note palatal extension to facilitate identification and orientation on cast. **D,** Maxillary "minibase" casting on master cast.

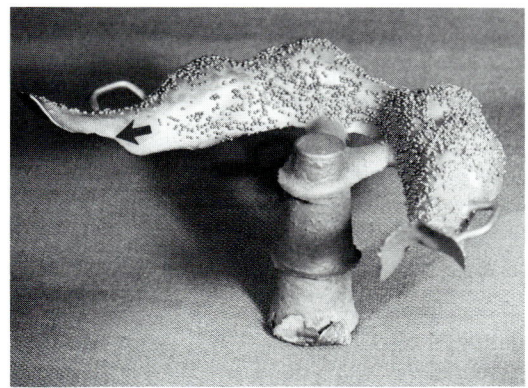

Fig. 14-32. Miscast. Note rounded edges, possibly as a result of incomplete burnout.

found on the abutments and are detected by close examination of the cast after removal of the casting. Small metalic scuff marks on the facial aspect of the abutment tooth generally indicate impingement (Fig. 14-27). Areas requiring adjustment can be identified readily by applying a soft No. 1 pencil to the appropriate area on the cast (Fig. 14-28). The casting is reseated on the cast and then removed; the areas of interference, now easily identified, are adjusted with an appropriate stone (Fig. 14-29) and repolished. In this manner, the casting is adapted accurately to the master cast (Fig. 14-30). Then the completed overdenture metal base castings are returned to the dentist for try-in (Fig. 14-31).

PROBLEMS

Among problems encountered in fabricating thin, light castings is the possibility of a casting failure. In making overdenture bases, miscasts can result from a variety of causes: (1) use of too thin a gauge of casting wax, (2) excessive thinning when adapting the wax to the refractory cast, (3) injudicious flaming of the pattern, contributing to thinning, particularly over abutment convexities, (4) a thick paint-on layer of investment material, restricting the release of mold pressure during casting, (5) inadequate burnout, (6) underheating of metal when making the casting, (7) defective spruing, (8) too few sprues, (9) too thin sprues, and (10) improperly placed sprues (Fig. 14-32). Careful attention to the multitude of technical details invariably results in better castings.

15

DUPLICATING OVERDENTURES

ROBERT M. MORROW

The principal advantage of making duplicate overdentures is having them readily available if the original ones need repair or modification. Several methods for duplicating dentures with heat-curing and autopolymerizing denture base resins have been reported (Geiger, 1955; Adam, 1958; Shaw, 1962; Manoli and Griffin, 1969; Zoeller and Beetar, 1970; Azarmehr and Azarmehr, 1970). A method that has proved to be effective in my practice depends on the use of an alginate irreversible hydrocolloid mold and an autopolymerizing pour-type resin. Both resin and metal base overdentures can be duplicated by this method. Generally the original overdenture is duplicated on its completion, and the duplicate is stored in water until it is needed.

MODIFYING FLASK

An upper denture flask is modified by removing a rectangular section from the back surface of the upper part (Fig. 15-1). This opening accommodates the utility wax sprues, approximately 15 mm. in diameter and 75 mm. in length, that are added to the overdenture. The sprues are attached to the lingual surface of the heels of the mandibular overdenture and to the palatal surface of the tuberosity area of the maxillary overdenture (Fig. 15-2). Before the mold is poured, the round plate from the lower part of the flask is inserted from the exterior, rather than from the interior in the usual manner (Fig. 15-3). This method of insertion prevents distortion of the alginate mold by inadvertent displacement of the plate when handling the flask. Application of an adhesive* to the interior of the flask also helps to keep the mold from being displaced, particularly when the flask halves are separated (Fig. 15-4).

FLASKING OVERDENTURE

Six scoops of alginate impression material are mixed with twice the recommended volume of water. Regular-set alginate is preferred to give extra working time, and the mixing water can be

---
*Hold, William Goetz Dental Products, Chicago.

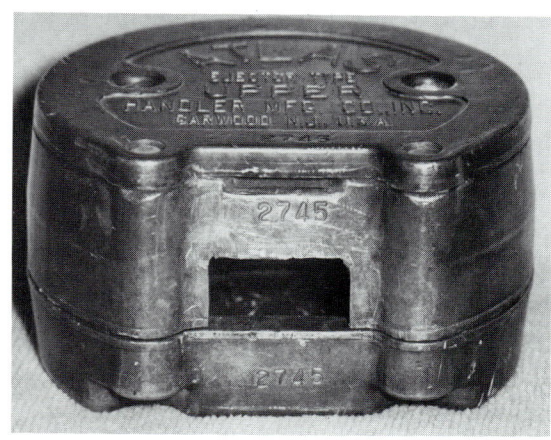

Fig. 15-1. Rectangular section removed from upper half "cope" of denture flask.

cooled to gain even more time if necessary. Although hand spatulation can be used, generally better results are obtained if the alginate is mixed in a mechanical spatulator* under reduced atmospheric pressure. After mixing, the alginate is placed in the interior of the denture with a finger or brush to minimize voids (Fig. 15-5). The remainder of the mix is placed in the lower part of the flask, and the denture is settled into the mix as in routine flasking procedures. The wax sprues are pressed into the back of the flask to support

*Combination Vac-U-Vestor and power mixer, Whip-Mix Corp., Louisville, Ky.

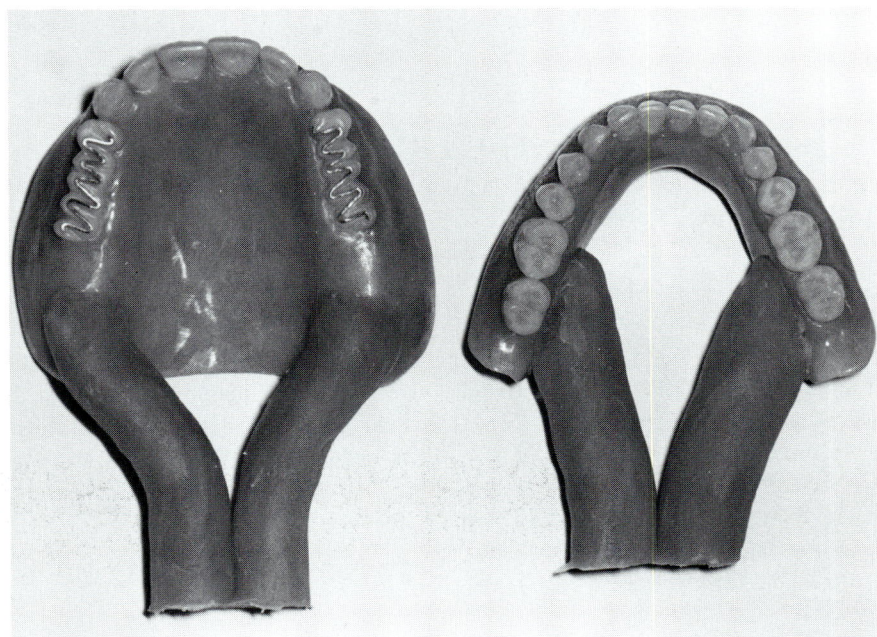

Fig. 15-2. Utility wax sprues attached to maxillary and mandibular overdentures.

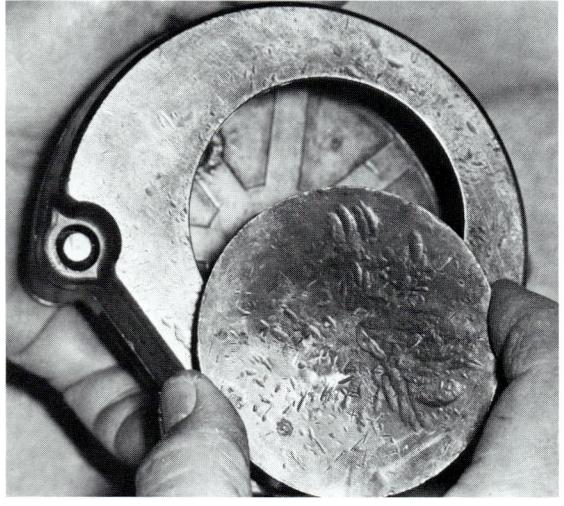

Fig. 15-3. Bottom plate is inserted from exterior rather than from interior of flask. This prevents displacement of alginate mold during handling of flask.

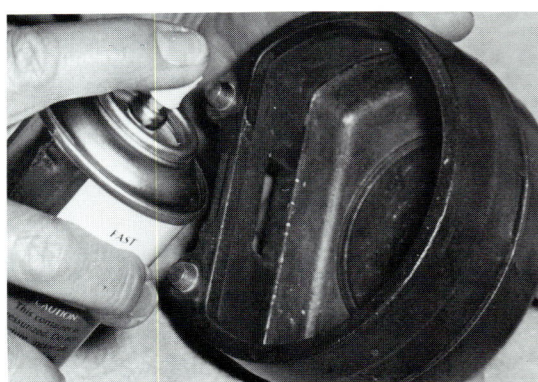

Fig. 15-4. Interior of flask is coated with adhesive to aid in retaining alginate during opening of flask.

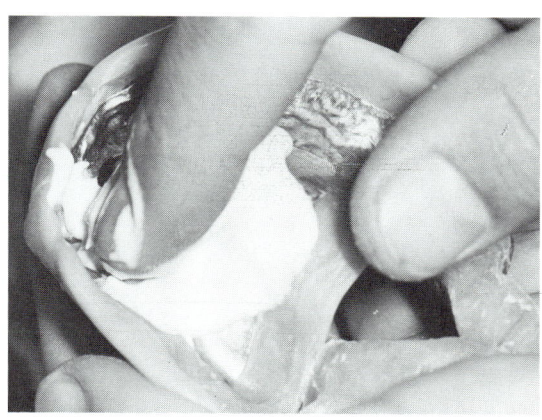

Fig. 15-5. Alginate is placed into interior of overdenture to minimize voids in mold.

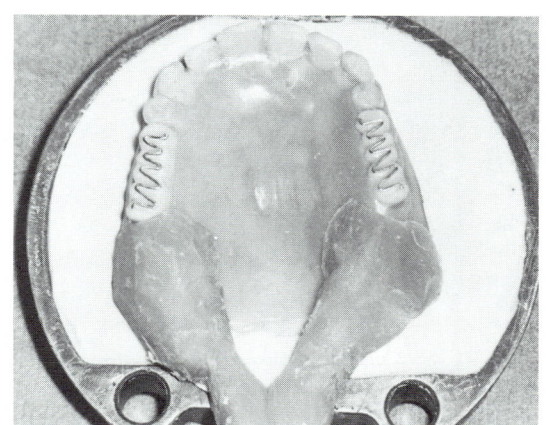

Fig. 15-6. Wax sprues are pressed onto flask to prevent settling of overdenture into alginate impression material.

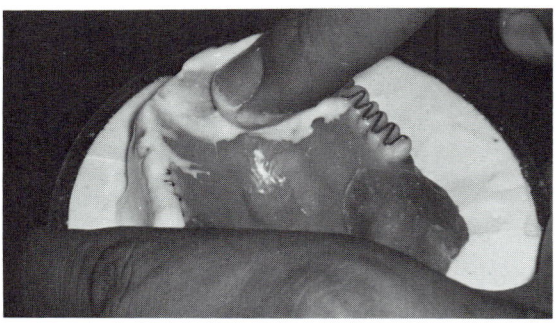

Fig. 15-7. Alginate is placed on overdenture with finger or brush to minimize voids.

the denture and keep it from settling too deep into the alginate (Fig. 15-6). After the setting of the alginate, the excess is removed from the edges of the flask, the upper part of the flask is assembled, and the rear opening is sealed with wax. Six scoops of alginate are mixed with three times the recommended volume of water to make a pourable consistency. Flasking is completed by pouring the alginate into the flask and using a brush or finger to place the alginate on the denture (Fig. 15-7). The top is placed and the alginate is allowed to set, usually approximately 15 minutes, and then the flask is opened. The denture and the sprues are removed from the flask.

MAKING TEETH

The tooth indentations in the alginate mold are dried gently with an air syringe. Autopolymerizing resin* of the appropriate shade is sifted

---

*Neopar, Miner Dental Products, Emeryville, Calif.

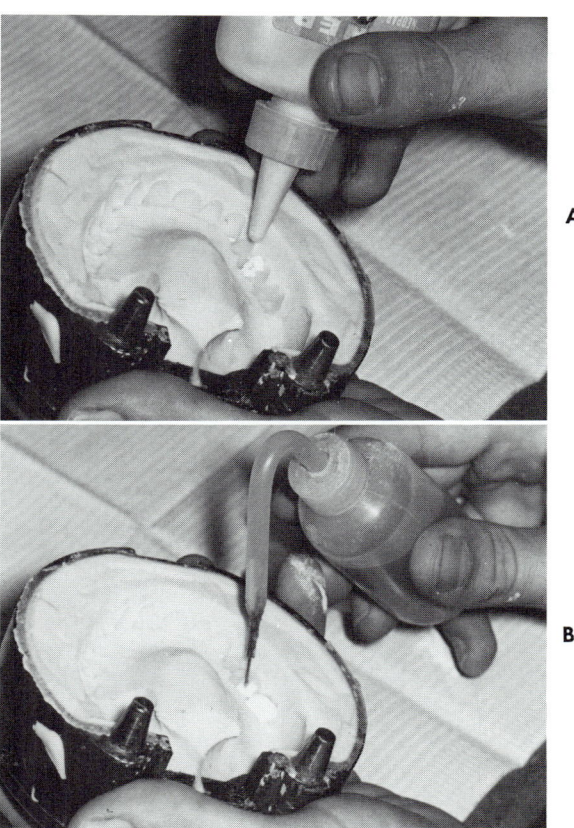

Fig. 15-8. A, Autopolymerizing resin of proper shade is sifted into tooth indentations. B, Resin saturated with monomer.

into the tooth indentations and saturated with monomer. In this manner, sufficient resin is added to conform to the cervical contours of the tooth indentations (Fig. 15-8). Care with this procedure contributes materially to improve the esthetic effect of the duplicate denture. If desired, incisal shades, followed by body and gingival shaded resins, can be used to simulate the natural teeth better. The teeth in the flask are placed in a pressure container at 30 p.s.i. for 10 minutes, and the teeth are left in the mold after curing.

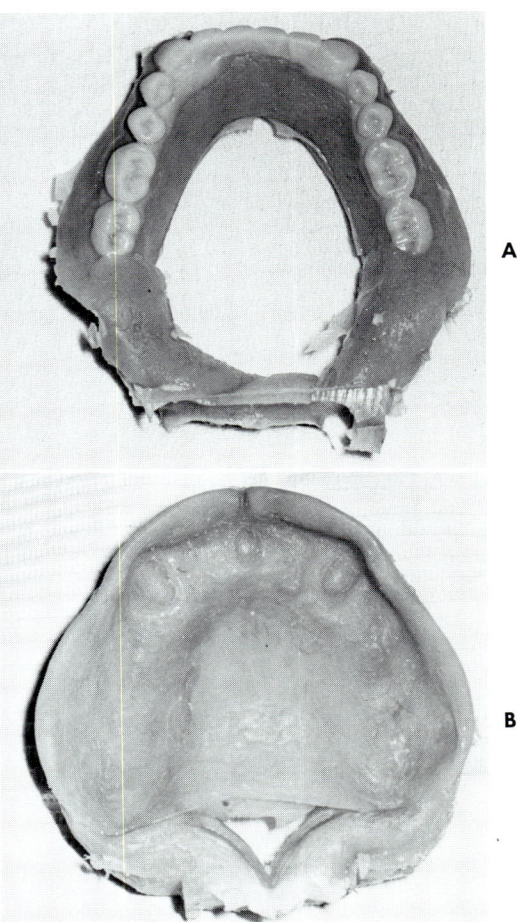

Fig. 15-10. A, Cured mandibular overdenture duplicate after removal from flask. B, Cured maxillary overdenture duplicate after removal from flask.

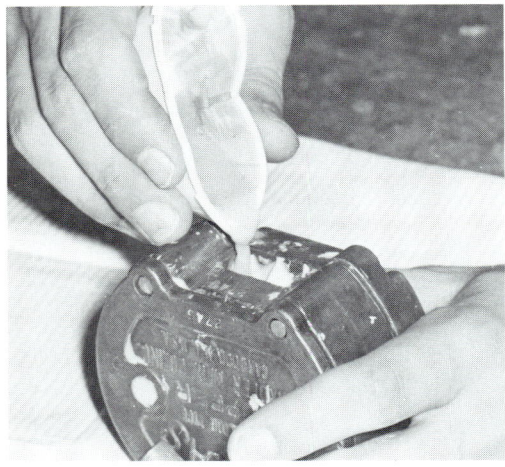

Fig. 15-9. "Pour-type" autopolymerizing resin is mixed and poured into mold through one sprue. Flask can be rocked gently to assure complete filling.

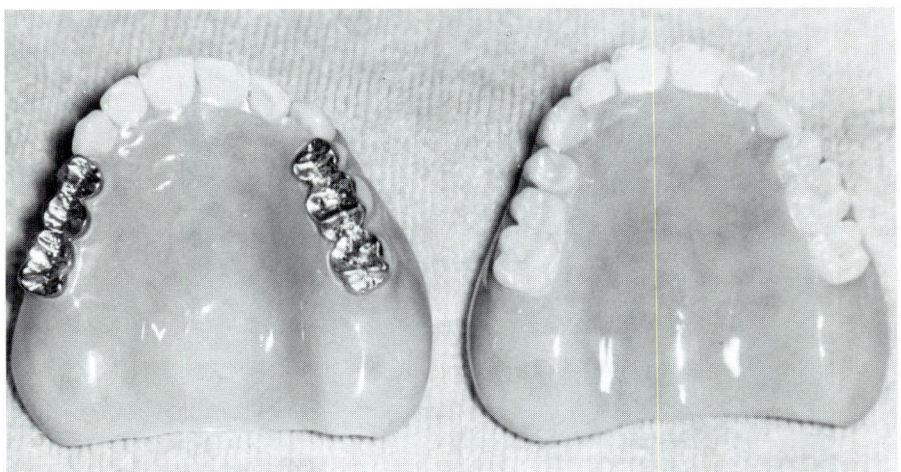

Fig. 15-11. Original overdenture and completed duplicate overdenture.

POURING THE BASE

Pour-type resin* is mixed according to the manufacturer's directions and poured into one sprue hole of the assembled flask (Fig. 15-9). The flask is held together with clamps or large rubber bands. Resin is poured until it rises to the surface in the other sprue, which acts as a vent. The flask can be rocked gently during pouring to minimize voids in the duplicate denture. When the pouring is completed, the flask is placed, with sprues upright, in a pressure container and cured at 30 p.s.i. for 30 minutes. Then the duplicate overdenture is removed and examined for bubbles or voids (Fig. 15-10). The finishing and polishing time is minimal as a result of the smooth surface imprinted by the alginate mold.

INSERTING THE DUPLICATE OVERDENTURE

Duplicate overdentures made from pour-type resins in hydrocolloid molds seem to demonstrate more dimensional change during curing than those made in plaster or stone molds. This can be observed readily when the overdenture is adapted with pressure-indicating paste. Usually more pressure areas are noted in the duplicate overdenture than in the original. Therefore, more "fitting" usually is necessary and, in my experience, the overdenture-supporting tissue adaptation is acceptable only after fitting. Relining of the duplicate overdenture can also be used to improve denture-tissue adaptation. The duplicate overdenture should be reserved for emergency use only and should not be used routinely. However, the duplicate constructed from the readily available materials and equipment does permit the dentist to furnish the patient at a reasonable cost with a spare or backup overdenture that has acceptable accuracy and esthetics (Fig. 15-11).

REFERENCES

Adam, C. E.: Technique for duplicating an acrylic resin denture, J. Prosthet. Dent. **8:**406-410, 1958.

Azarmehr, P., and Azarmehr, H. Y.: Duplicate dentures, J. Prosthet. Dent. **24:**339-345, 1970.

Geiger, E. C. K.: Duplication of the esthetics of an existing immediate denture, J. Prosthet. Dent. **5:**179-185, 1955.

Manoli, S. G., and Griffin, T. P.: Duplicate denture technique, J. Prosthet. Dent. **21:**104-107, 1969.

Shaw, D. R.: Duplicate immediate dentures, J. Prosthet. Dent. **12:**47-57, 1962.

Zoeller, G. N., and Beetar, R. F.: Duplicating dentures, J. Prosthet. Dent. **23:**346-353, 1970.

---

*Pour-N-Cure, Coe Laboratories, Chicago, or Pronto II, Vernon-Benshoff Co., Inc., Albany, N. Y.

16

CENTRIC CHECK-POINT PROCEDURE FOR DETERMINING THE ACCURACY OF JAW RELATION RECORDS

ROBERT M. MORROW

Centric check points are an effective method for verifying the accuracy of jaw relation records for overdentures (Brewer, 1963). Successful application of the technique is predicated on stable, well-adapted baseplates. Accurate records are difficult to obtain if record bases do not demonstrate adequate stability and retention in the mouth. It is also impossible to accurately transfer the recorded relationship if the record bases are not stable on the casts. The centric check-point technique is ideally suited for overdentures due to the inherent stability of the record bases supported by abutments. Record bases may be of cast metal as in the case of metal base overdentures, or they may be made from heat-curing or autopolymerizing resin. Baseplates can be constructed from thermoplastic material such as shellac or gutta percha, although these are not commonly used. However, if used, frequent readaptation is necessary to maintain fit. As previously stated, bases of chrome cobalt alloys or gold that are to become a part of the completed overdenture are excellent.

PROCEDURE

1. The casts are mounted on an articulator in centric relation at the desired vertical dimension of occlusion. Artificial stone accelerated with slurry water is an excellent medium for mounting casts. The method used to record the initial jaw relation is a matter of the dentist's preference.

2. The baseplates are prepared for attaching the centric check points by removing all traces of occlusion rim wax, recording medium, or other materials used to obtain the initial jaw record.

3. The centric check points are assembled for use. A set of centric check points* consists of three

---

*Centric check points, Hanau Engineering Co., Inc., Buffalo, N. Y.

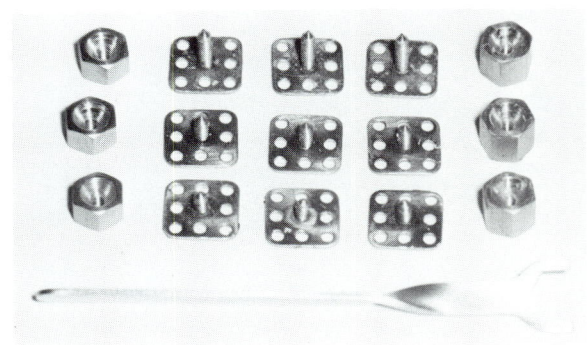

Fig. 16-1. Centric check-point set: long points at top, medium points in center, short points at bottom. Short cups on left are used with medium on mandibular when relationship record is to be reaccomplished.

short points, three medium points, three long points, three short cups, three long cups, and a wrench (Fig. 16-1). The centric check points are assembled by screwing the long cup onto the short point, hollow end first. The long point is then screwed into the flat end of the long cup until the points touch (Fig. 16-2). The medium point is substituted for the long point if the interarch space is inadequate. Three short and three long points are thus joined by the long cups (Fig. 16-3).

4. The assembled points and cups are attached to the baseplates on the mounted casts. One is placed in the anterior midline region and one on each side in the first molar area. They are slanted slightly forward at the top so that the points are in line with the arc of closure. The bases of the long points are attached to the mandibular baseplate with impression compound or artificial stone whose setting time has been accelerated with slurry water (Fig. 16-4). If stone is used, seal the set stone to the baseplate with sticky wax as a safety measure to prevent separation. With the articulator closed and the bases firmly seated on the casts, attach the bases of the short points to the maxillary baseplates in the same manner (Fig. 16-5). The point and cup assemblies should be firmly attached to the baseplates. With the wrench, each cup is then rotated clockwise until the short point is freed (Fig. 16-6). Now the articulator bow may be opened, and each cup may be rotated off its respective long point. When the articulator is closed, the points must be positioned tip to tip as in Fig. 16-7.

5. The baseplates with attached points are removed from the articulator and inserted into the mouth. The baseplates are seated and the patient is coached into centric relation. The lips are gently retracted and the position of the tips of the points is observed.

If the initial record was accurately registered and accurately transferred to the articulator, the tips of the points should coincide exactly (Fig. 16-

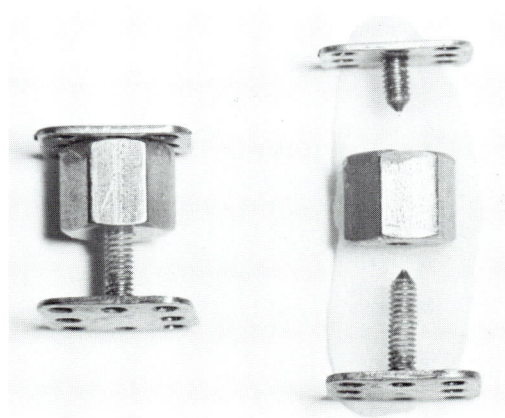

Fig. 16-2. Assembled points and cup on left. Base of long point is attached to mandibular record base.

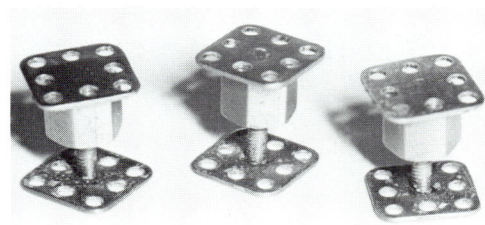

Fig. 16-3. Assembled points ready for attachment to baseplates.

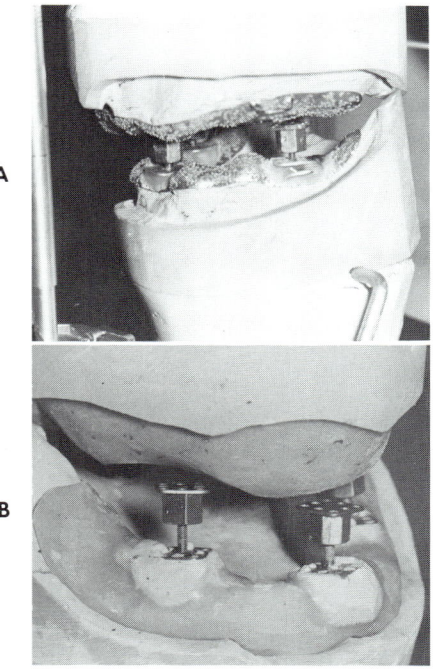

Fig. 16-4. **A,** Bases of long points are attached to mandibular record base, in this instance a metal base. **B,** bases of long points are attached to resin baseplates.

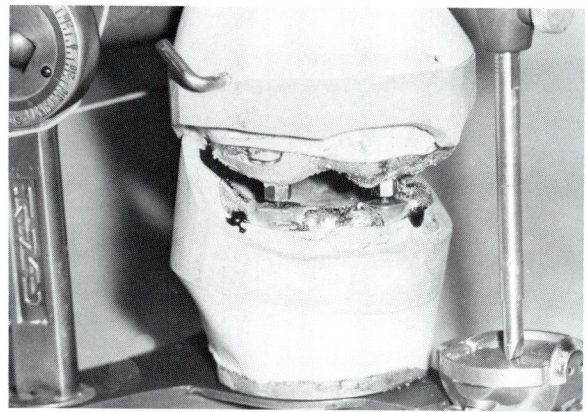

Fig. 16-5. Points are attached to maxillary and mandibular metal overdenture bases.

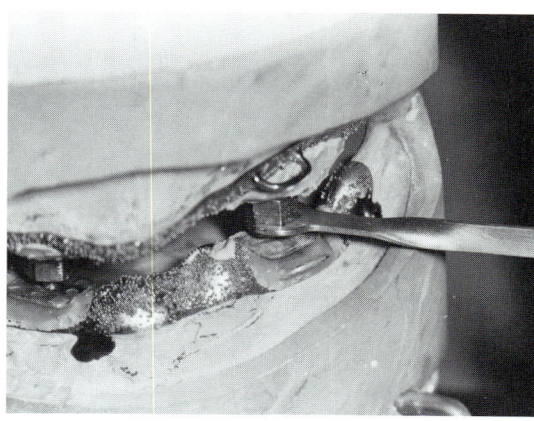

Fig. 16-6. Cup is backed off with wrench, freeing short point.

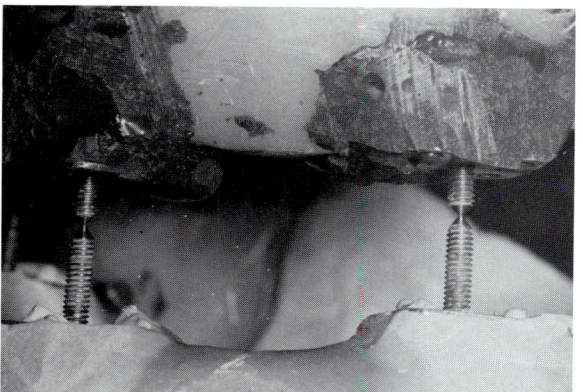

Fig. 16-7. Point tips should align on articulator.

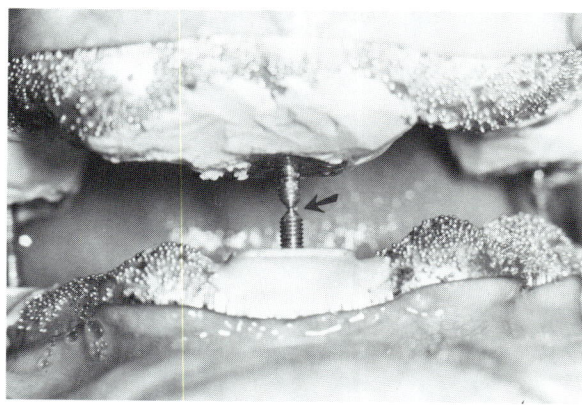

Fig. 16-8. Point tips contact properly in mouth indicating accurate mounting (arrow). Each point must contact at the same time.

8). If they do not coincide, and if you are certain that the patient's mandible is indeed in centric relation, an error is indicated either in the original jaw relation record or in its transfer to the articulator and possibly in both (Fig. 16-9). When centric check points are used to verify the accuracy of one's favorite method for making jaw relation records, it will be found that errors occur rather frequently as manifested by the failure of the points to coincide. This rather startling disclosure is due to the fact that centric check points are capable of indicating minute errors, and the contact between the two bases is reduced to such small areas that the error is much more easily observed.

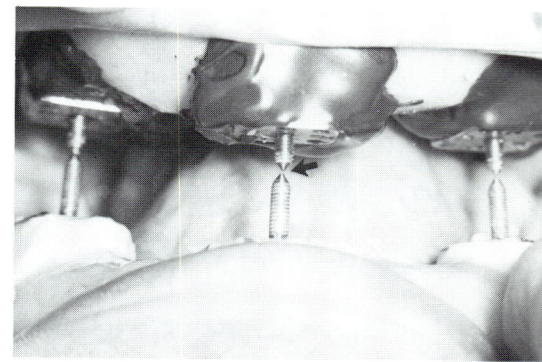

Fig. 16-9. Anterior points do not contact properly (arrow), indicating error.

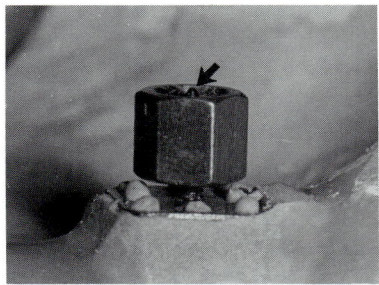

Fig. 16-10. Long cup is screwed down on long point (arrow) until point is level with cup rim.

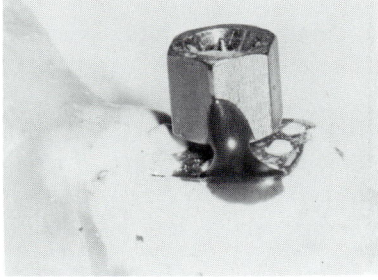

Fig. 16-11. Sticky wax prevents further rotation of cup on point. Note level of point.

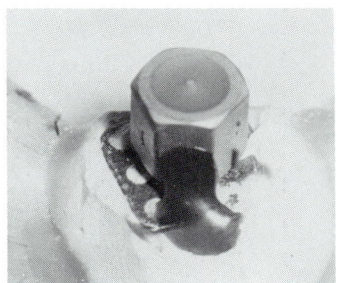

Fig. 16-12. Cup concavity is filled with baseplate wax and leveled to rim.

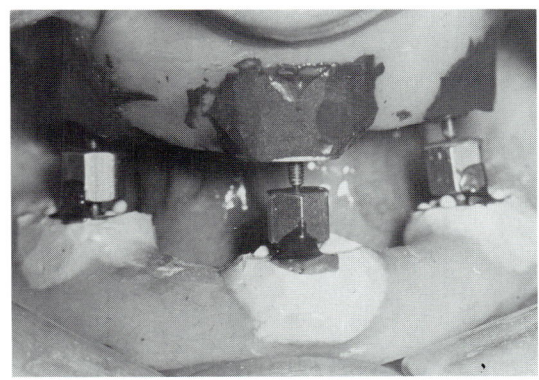

Fig. 16-13. Patient closes, indenting wax.

ERROR CORRECTION

When the tips of the points do not coincide, the centric relation record must be reaccomplished, and a remount is necessary. The long cups are screwed, flat end first, onto the long points on the mandibular baseplates until the tips of the points are flush with the top of the cups (Fig. 16-10). This serves as a check for maintenance of the vertical dimension. If the medium points were used on the mandibular base, the short cup is used when reaccomplishing the record. Sticky wax is used to fix the cups to the baseplate, preventing further rotation of the cups on the points (Fig. 16-11). The hollow portions of the cups are then filled with hard baseplate wax, which is leveled to the borders of the cups (Fig. 16-12). The short points on the maxillary baseplate are not changed. The baseplates with points and cups are then returned to the mouth, and the patient closes in the retruded position. The points should just penetrate the wax, creating small indentations. Deeper penetrations of the wax may alter the vertical dimension of occlusion.

1. To correct small horizontal errors the above procedure is adequate.

2. Should the error be in the vertical plane, it may be necessary to build up the level of the wax in the cup opposite the pin failing to make contact.

3. In those instances in which the error is of such magnitude that the points on the maxillary baseplate will not contact the surface of the cups, a new centric relation record must be made by conventional means, and points must be assembled and attached as previously described.

The patient should close lightly in centric relation several times. The accuracy of this new record should be demonstrated by the patient being able to close repeatedly into the same wax indentations (Fig. 16-13). With the patient's jaws closed in this newly registered position, the baseplates may be luted together intraorally with accelerated artificial stone. Some prefer to remove the baseplates from the mouth, position them correctly by hand, and lute them together with wax or accelerated stone (Fig. 16-14). The mandibular cast is removed from the articulator and remounted to the new relationship.

The short points are removed from the maxillary baseplate, cleaned, and reassembled as described for the initial verification. The long cups are returned, hollow end first, to the short points and are then screwed onto the long points, taking care that they are inserted only until point touches point. Forcing the points together will tend to flatten and bur the tips, thus reducing their effectiveness.

After the points and cups are assembled on the mandibular baseplate, the bases of the short points are reattached to the maxillary baseplate with impression compound or stone as described earlier. The long cups are backed off the short points with the wrench and rotated off the long points. The tips of upper and lower points are again in correct alignment (Fig. 16-15). The baseplates with points are returned to the mouth, and the accuracy of the new mounting is evaluated. The points of the pins should coincide (Fig. 16-16). If they do not, the corrective procedure must be repeated. When the articulator mounting has been proved correct, the procedures incident to completion of the overdenture are accomplished.

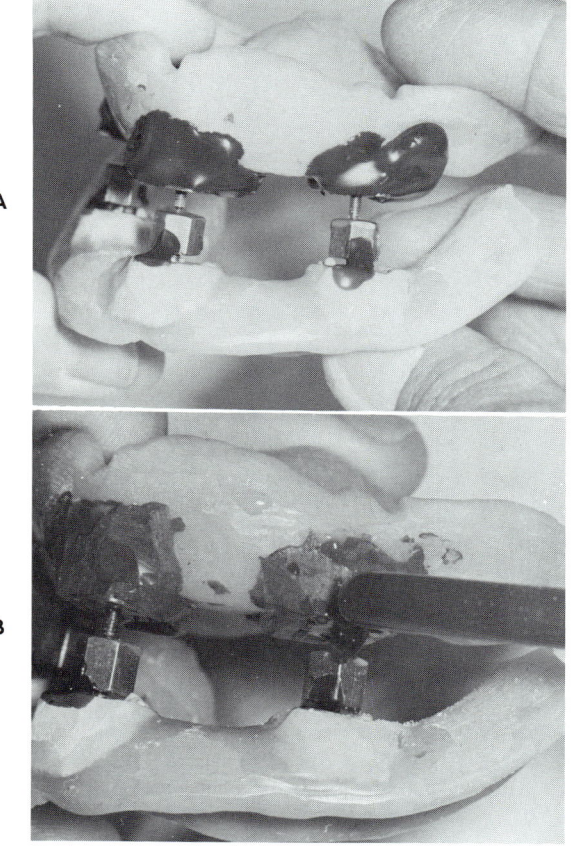

Fig. 16-14. **A,** Baseplates are assembled with points in wax indentations. Care is taken to not force points further into wax. **B,** Baseplates are assembled and luted together with sticky wax.

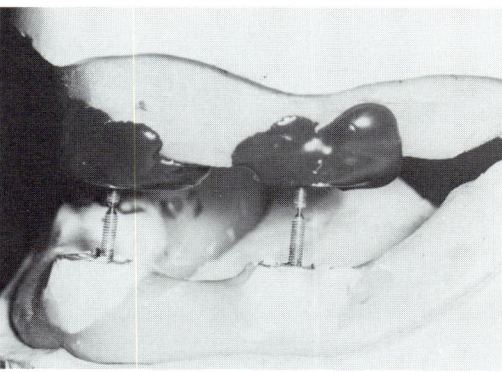

Fig. 16-15. Maxillary and mandibular check points are realigned in articulator.

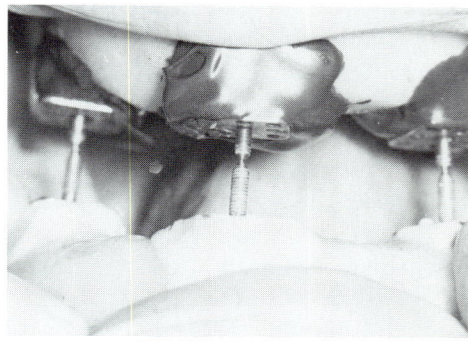

Fig. 16-16. Points are properly contacting in mouth, indicating accurate record and transfer.

CENTRIC CHECK POINTS AND THE SINGLE OVERDENTURE

Centric check points can also be used to verify the accuracy of jaw relation records for overdentures opposed by natural dentitions. After the casts are mounted in an articulator, points of proper length are mounted on the overdenture baseplate so as to contact selected cusps of the opposing dentition. The baseplate is then removed from the cast and inserted, and the contact of the points and cusps is verified. Errors are readily apparent and are corrected by reaccomplishing the jaw relation recording procedure.

REFERENCE

Brewer, A.: Prosthodontic research in progress at the school of aerospace medicine, J. Prosthet. Dent. 13:49-69, 1963.

17

METAL OCCLUSAL SURFACES FOR OVERDENTURES

ROBERT M. MORROW

INDICATIONS

Metal occlusal surfaces are indicated (1) when an overdenture is constructed to oppose a natural dentition or a reconstructed dental arch with metal occlusal surfaces, (2) where wear-resistant occlusal surfaces of maximum durability are desired when using an overdenture to oppose an overdenture, (3) where considerable modification of the denture teeth is needed to achieve their adaptation to the core when using a functionally generated path technique to construct an overdenture, and (4) when special wax-to-wax carving techniques are used to develop a functional occlusion.

A technique that I have found effective in constructing denture teeth with metal occlusal surface is described by Koehne and Morrow (1970). The technique, a modification of one reported by Wallace (1964), uses gold for the occlusal surfaces; however, chrome-cobalt alloys can be used after appropriate technical alterations.

METAL OCCLUSAL SURFACES FROM CARVED WAX PATTERNS

The occlusal surfaces to be duplicated in metal can be carved in wax to function with opposing tooth surfaces or a stone core, as in functionally generated path concepts, or the metal duplicates can be made from the occlusal surfaces of monoplane or anatomic posterior denture teeth.

After the jaw relation records are made and the casts are mounted on an articulator, resin denture teeth of the appropriate mold are positioned and waxed for the try-in (Fig. 17-1). Usually the anterior teeth are selected and positioned by the dentist before setting the posterior teeth. The buccolingual position of the posterior teeth, the occlusal curve or plane, and the length of the posterior segment of the arch are evaluated carefully to assure compliance with physiologic requirements. The dentist should make these and other pertinent evaluations at the time of the wax try-in.

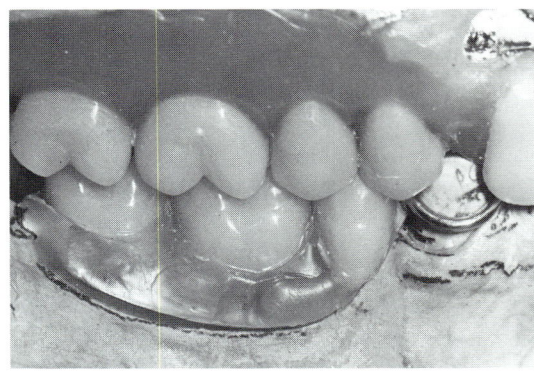

Fig. 17-1. Resin denture teeth are positioned for try-in. In this case both overdenture and removable partial denture are to receive gold occlusal units.

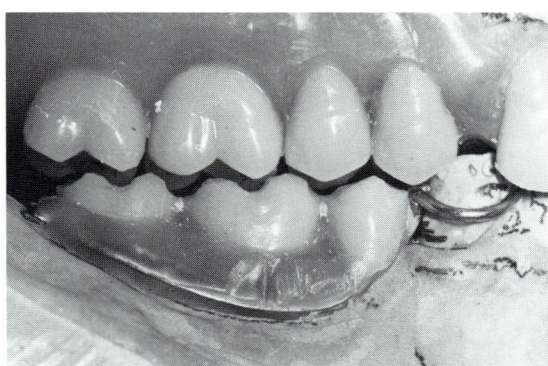

Fig. 17-2. The resin denture teeth are reduced by grinding to provide space for carving wax.

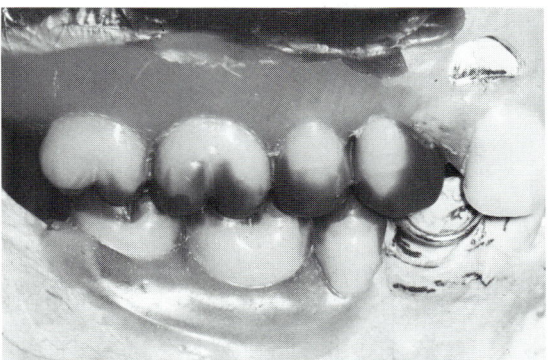

Fig. 17-3. Carving wax is added and contoured to develop cusp heights and sulci depths. For this patient, maxillary and mandibular occlusal anatomy were developed simultaneously.

Laboratory procedures

If the occlusion is developed by waxing techniques rather than by duplication of the existing occlusal surfaces of the denture teeth, the occlusal surfaces of the resin denture teeth are reduced by grinding to provide space for the carving wax and, subsequently, for the gold (Fig. 17-2).

Carving wax occlusal surfaces. The opposing denture teeth, cast, or core is lubricated to prevent the carving wax from sticking when occluded. The carving wax is added to the prepared denture teeth, and the articulator is closed to record the cusp height and sulci depths while the wax is soft (Fig. 17-3). Several closures may be needed to reestablish the recorded vertical dimension of occlusion. Attempts to close the articulator after the carving wax has hardened result in either fracture of the wax or displacement of the denture teeth on the baseplate. The articulator is moved to the various eccentric positions, the occlusal surfaces are contoured, and the secondary anatomic details are carved (Fig. 17-4). A disclosing powder dusted onto the wax occlusal surfaces facilitates making necessary adjustments in the pattern. Although only posterior teeth usually receive gold occlusal surfaces, cuspids can be included, particularly when they are the abutment teeth for the overdenture and it has been necessary to incorporate a pronounced vertical overlap in the anterior setup. Use of gold on the cuspids makes the replacement stronger and reduces the possibility of breakage. The wax occlusal surfaces are cleaned by washing gently with green soap and rinsing in cool water. Excess water is removed with an air syringe.

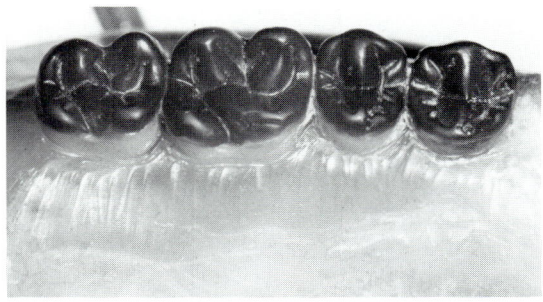

Fig. 17-4. Secondary anatomic details are carved, and wax-up is completed.

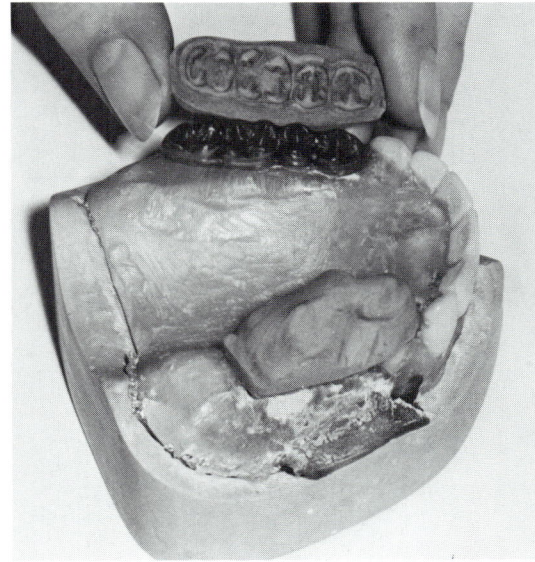

Fig. 17-5. Investment is removed from wax occlusal units in one piece and examined for defects.

222 METHODS

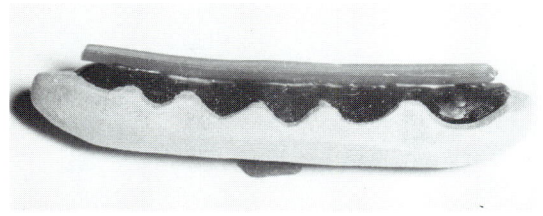

Fig. 17-6. Investment mold is reduced occlusogingivally to create desired thickness for gold occlusal units. Reduction is accomplished in such a manner as to make gold of same thickness over occlusobuccal line angle. This makes better esthetics by minimizing gold display.

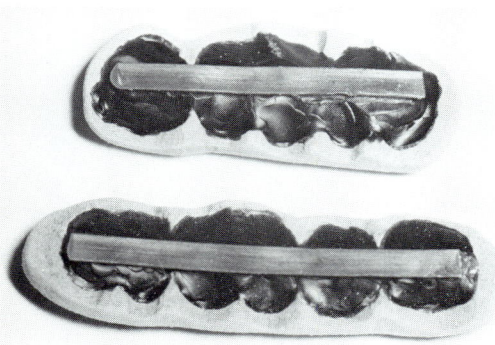

Fig. 17-7. Casting wax is flowed into mold and reinforced with a strip of 12-gauge half-round casting wax. Small beads or crystals can also be added if desired for additional retention.

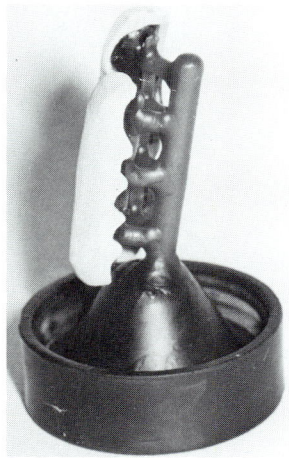

Fig. 17-8. Pattern is sprued and ready for investing.

Investment core. An investment that is compatible with the alloy to be used is mixed and placed over the wax occlusal surfaces. Care is taken to paint the investment thoroughly in the grooves of the wax-up to avoid trapping air and to assure faithful reproduction of the carved surfaces. The investment placed over the wax patterns should be approximately 4 or 5 mm. thick and should extend approximately 2 mm. onto the facial and lingual surfaces of the resin teeth. After setting, the investment is removed carefully from the wax-up and examined for defects (Fig. 17-5). The investment procedure can be redone if it is necessary to correct defects or to construct duplicate occlusal surfaces.

Making wax pattern. The thickness of the investment mold is reduced occlusogingivally to make the gold castings of the thickness desired. This reduction is accomplished in such a manner as to make the gold of the same thickness over the entire occlusobuccal line angle (Fig. 17-6). Casting wax is flowed into the mold, and 12-gauge half-round casting wax is sealed onto the interior surface of the wax pattern to provide rigidity and retention for the resin that is added later (Fig. 17-7).

Investing the pattern. The pattern in the investment is sprued and placed in a casting ring (Fig. 17-8). The ring is filled with cool water to soak thoroughly the investment covering the wax patterns; this procedure contributes to a smooth juncture with the refractory investment to be added. After the soaking, the water is poured from

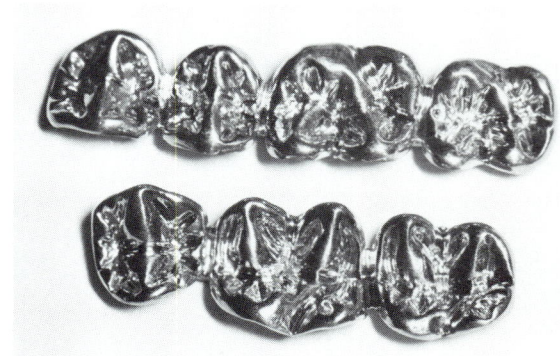

Fig. 17-9. Polished gold castings.

METAL OCCLUSAL SURFACES FOR OVERDENTURES 223

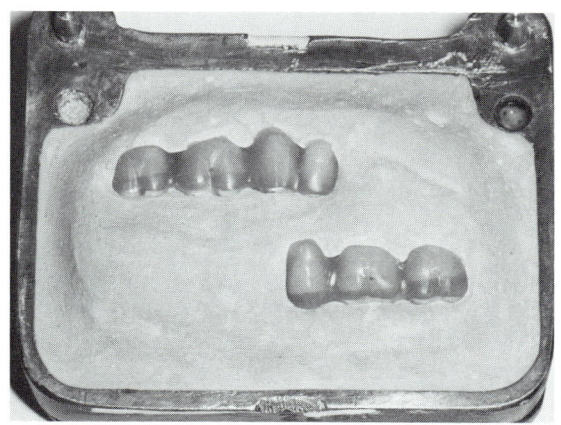

Fig. 17-10. Waxed occlusal units are flasked in a conventional manner.

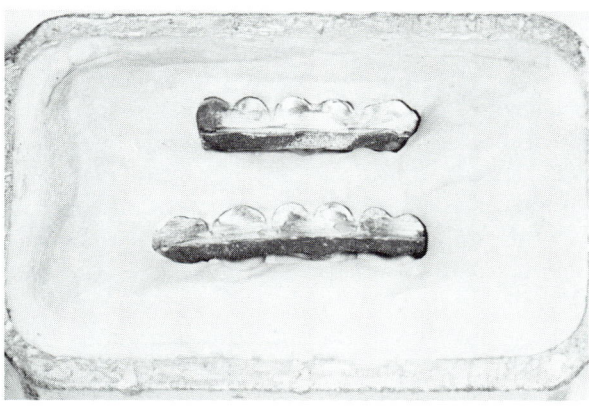

Fig. 17-11. Wax is eliminated with clean boiling water. Opaquing can be accomplished at this stage.

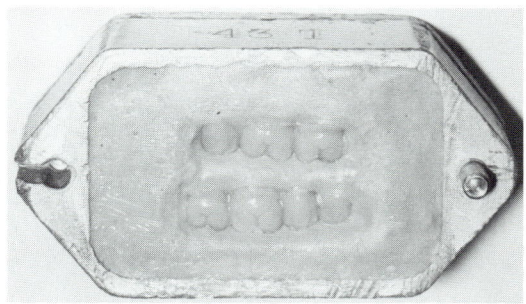

Fig. 17-12. Cross-linked heat-curing resin of appropriate shade is packed into mold. Characterization such as simulated cracks and restorations can be placed if desired.

the ring, and the excess is removed by shaking gently. The outer refractory investment is mixed, and the ring is filled.

Casting metal occlusal surfaces. Burnout and casting are accomplished by a technique compatible with the type of metal alloy and investment used. The completed casting is cleaned and examined; any nodules or bubbles are removed. The sprues are removed and the castings checked for accuracy by positioning them against the opposing occlusal surfaces used during the carving procedures. It may be necessary to reduce the resin teeth further to accommodate the 12-gauge half-round retentive bar. The gold occlusal surfaces are then polished (Fig. 17-9), placed in the proper position on the opposing cast, and sealed with a sticky wax.

Waxing occlusal units. The articulator is closed, and ivory casting wax is flowed between the gold occlusal surfaces and the resin denture teeth. The sticky wax is chipped away, and the articulator is opened to permit the addition of ivory wax to areas otherwise inaccessible. The buccal and lingual surface anatomy can be modified at this time if desired.

Flasking occlusal units. The teeth with the gold occlusal surfaces are removed in a block. Flasking is accomplished in the usual manner; however, the buccal surfaces are depressed in the mold slightly toward the occlusal surface (Fig. 17-10). This procedure facilitates positive retention of the cast occlusal surfaces in the mold and permits removal of the resin teeth after boilout. Boilout procedures are completed, and the resin teeth are retrieved from the mold (Fig. 17-11). The teeth can be retained to make metal occlusal surfaces on other overdentures at a later time. All stone surfaces are coated with a tinfoil substitute.

Packing the resin. A cross-linked heat-curing resin of the proper shade is mixed and packed into the mold in the same manner as for veneer crowns (Fig. 17-12). Characterization can be added if desired.

Completing the denture. At the end of the recommended curing cycle, the teeth are removed from the flask and polished. Then they are replaced on the baseplates, the occlusion is verified and tried in, and the denture is completed in the usual manner (Fig. 17-13).

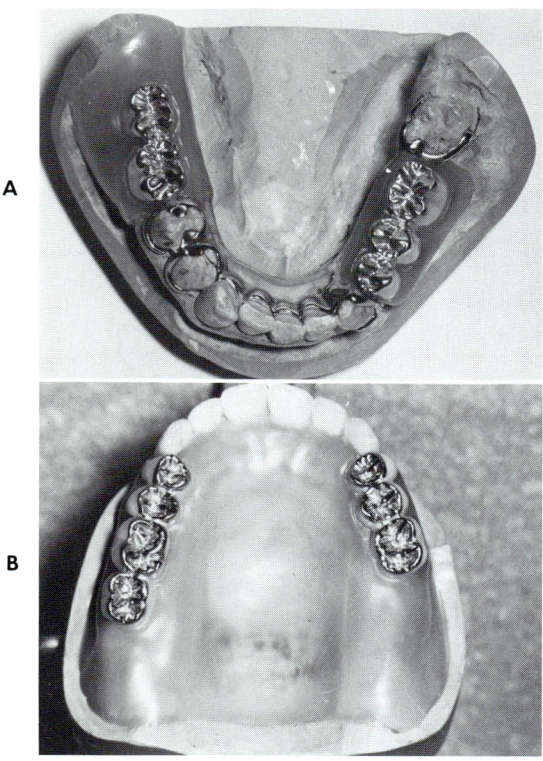

Fig. 17-13. **A**, Gold occlusal units are repositioned on cast for mandibular removable partial denture. **B**, Gold occlusal units are repositioned on maxillary overdenture.

METAL OCCLUSAL SURFACES FROM DENTURE TEETH

If the occlusal surfaces of unmodified denture teeth instead of carved wax surfaces are to be duplicated, the investment is placed on the occlusal surfaces of these teeth. A reusable mold of artificial stone can be made for monoplane posterior teeth. The stone mold is lubricated, and casting wax is flowed into the mold; the pattern is sprued, removed from the mold, invested, and cast. In this manner, monoplane occlusal units can be made in advance.

METAL OCCLUSAL SURFACES FOR EXISTING DENTURES

Metal occlusal surfaces to duplicate the occlusal surfaces of an existing denture can be constructed readily if the teeth are of resin. In this instance, the denture is mounted in a relining jig, and an occlusal core is made to preserve the occlusal relationships. After setting, the denture is separated from the core, and the investment is placed on the occlusal surfaces by the same procedure as for duplicating occlusal surfaces of denture teeth. The wax pattern is made as described previously, invested, cast, and polished. The teeth on the denture are reduced to allow space for the castings. The castings are seated into the stone core, and the relining jig is assembled to determine whether reduction of the denture teeth is adequate. Auto-

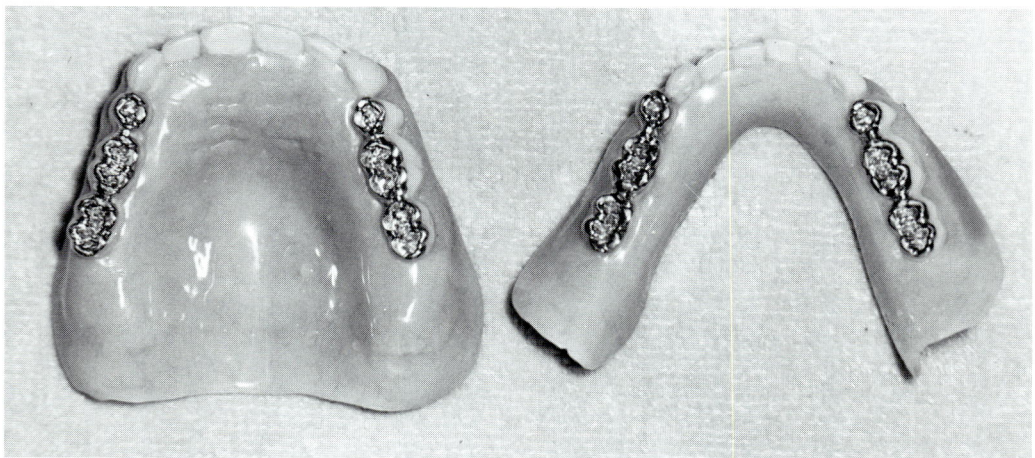

Fig. 17-14. Gold occlusal units for a maxillary and mandibular overdenture. In this case a monoplane occlusion was used.

polymerizing resin of the correct shade is mixed and used to attach the metal occlusal surfaces to the denture teeth. The jig with the denture is placed in a pressure pot for 30 minutes at 30 p.s.i. for curing, and, after removal, the teeth are trimmed and polished. Modification of dentures with porcelain teeth is more difficult, for these teeth often fracture during reduction to make space for the metal. In addition, porcelain teeth require retentive grooves or pin holes for cementing the metal occlusal surfaces.

Often the use of gold occlusal surfaces on denture teeth contributes to the clinical success of an overdenture (Fig. 17-14). The advantages are the inherent physical properties of the metal, the adaptability to unusual opposing occlusion problems, and a definite, albeit subjective, psychologic advantage. In many instances, patients who have overdentures with gold occlusal surfaces are better motivated and more interested in improved oral hygiene with a resultant increased service life of the remaining dentition. The disadvantages are higher cost and possible impairment of esthetics.

REFERENCES

Koehne, C. L., and Morrow, R. M.: Construction of denture teeth with gold occlusal surfaces, J. Prosthet. Dent. 23:449-455, 1970.

Wallace, D. H.: The use of gold occlusal surfaces in complete and partial dentures, J. Prosthet. Dent. 14:326-333, 1964.

18
RELINING, REBASING, AND SOFT LINERS

ALLEN A. BREWER

At some time the majority of dentures need refitting to compensate for changes in the tissue that occur after insertion and use of a denture. This requirement applies to overdentures as well as to other types of dentures.

IMPRESSION PROCEDURES

A variety of materials such as irreversible hydrocolloids, zinc oxide–eugenol impression pastes, silicones, and thiokols can be used to make the impression. However, a tissue conditioning material, such as Hydrocast tissue conditioner* or Coe Comfort† is preferable, for it not only aids in restoring abused tissues to a healthier state, but also makes possible a check of the fit of the denture and the maxillomandibular relativity.

When supporting tissues have been abused, application of the tissue conditioner is repeated at 3-day intervals until the desired comfort and adaptation are obtained. At the last sitting, before taking the denture from the patient for relining and rebasing, all tissue conditioning material is removed again and replaced with fresh material. The denture is returned to the patient's mouth; after 30 minutes the maxillomandibular relativity is checked visually and, if it is incorrect, a new record is obtained.

---

*Kay See Dental Manufacturing Co., Kansas City, Mo.
†Coe Laboratories, Chicago.

CENTRIC JAW RELATION RECORD

Centric jaw relation is a three-dimensional relationship that is registered most accurately in two steps. The armamentarium used consists of a small plaster bowl, a small quantity of quick-setting bite

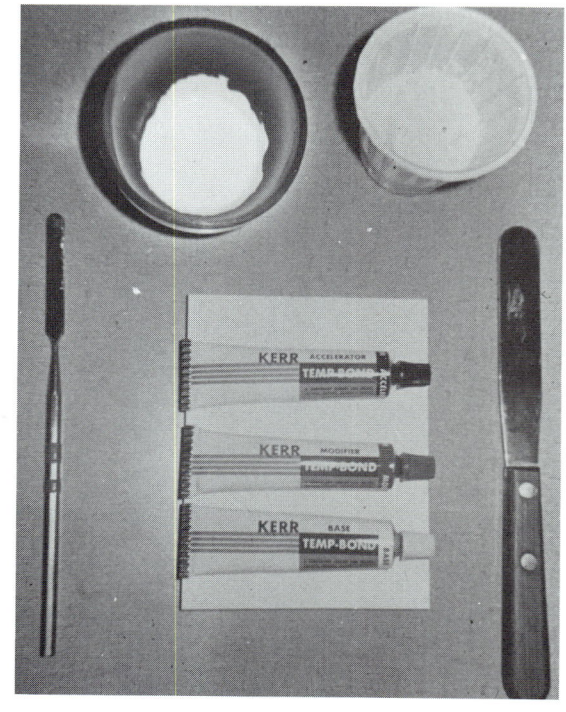

Fig. 18-1. Armamentarium for centric jaw relation record.

RELINING, REBASING, AND SOFT LINERS 227

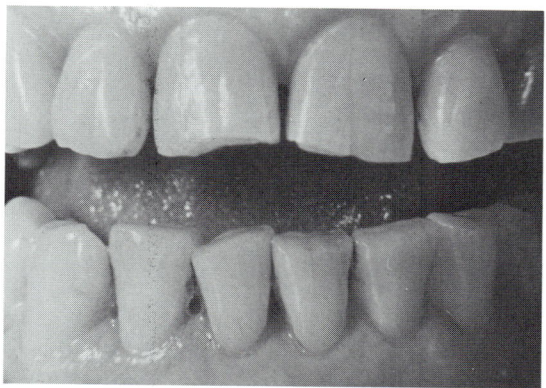

Fig. 18-2. Mouth opened to receive stone placed over mandibular anteriors.

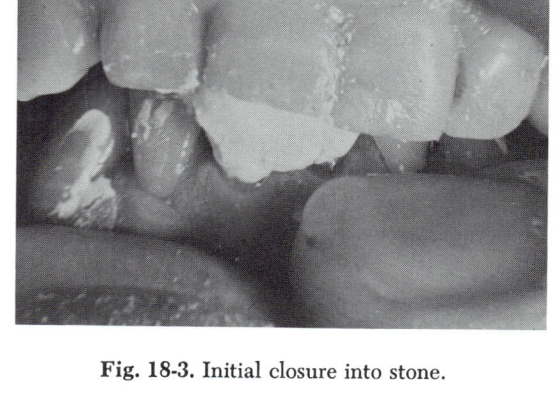

Fig. 18-3. Initial closure into stone.

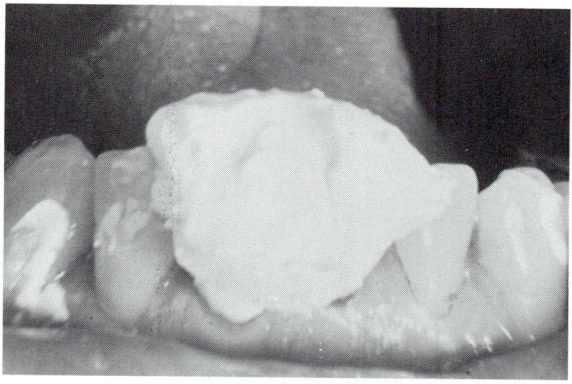

Fig. 18-4. Stone index on mandibular incisors.

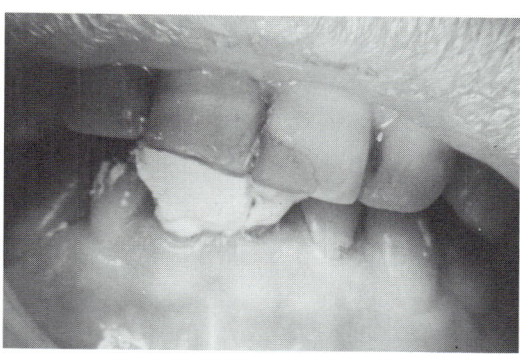

Fig. 18-5. Reclosure in centric jaw relation shows incorrect record.

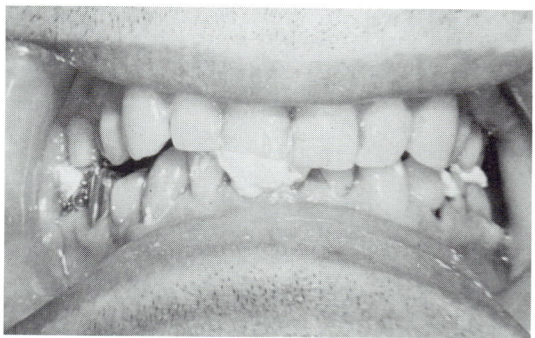

Fig. 18-6. Reaccomplishment in correct centric jaw relation.

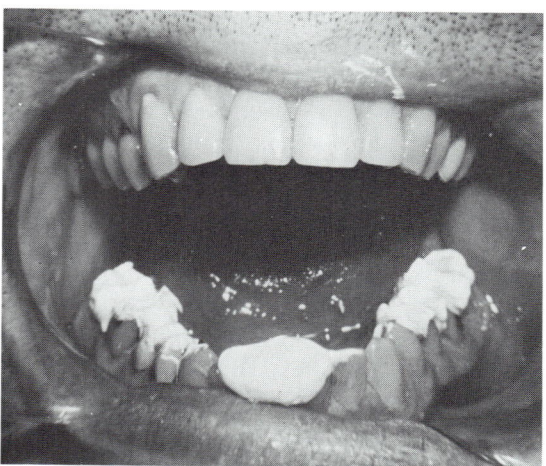

Fig. 18-7. Record of vertical component of centric jaw relation when properly related to horizontal and lateral components.

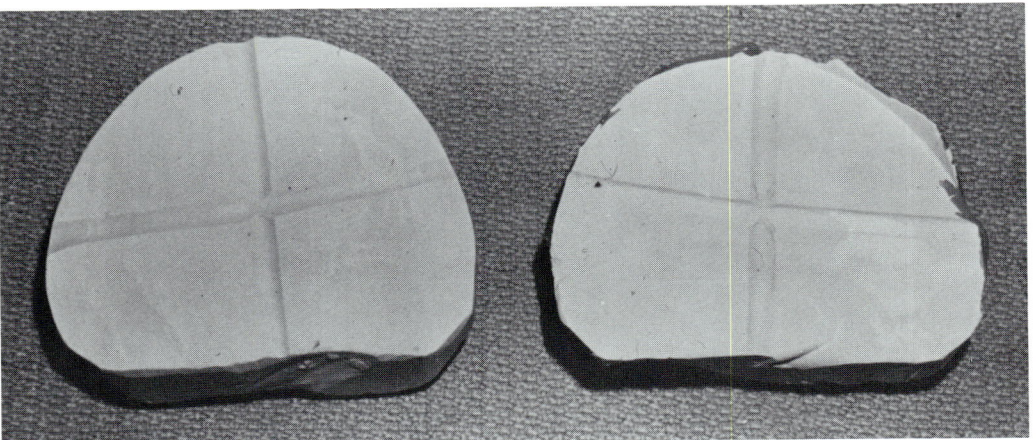

Fig. 18-8. Indexed casts (grooves).

stone, distilled water, a plaster spatula, Temp-bond,* and a cement spatula (Fig. 18-1). The patient is asked to open the mouth (Fig. 18-2), and a small quantity of quick-setting stone is mixed and placed over the mandibular incisors with the cement spatula. Then the patient is guided to the centric jaw relation position, and the mouth is closed to near-tooth contact (Fig. 18-3). After it has been held in this position until the stone sets, the patient is asked to snap the jaw open (Fig. 18-4). Any lingual incline impression of the tooth on the stone is cut away carefully with a sharp knife, so that only the cutting edge of the maxillary incisor contacts the stone on closing. The patient is guided to the centric jaw relation position again. After the mouth is closed, any error in determining the horizontal and lateral components of the centric jaw relation is readily apparent (Fig. 18-5). In the event of an error, the stone is removed and the procedure is repeated until a positive seating is obtained on subsequent closures. Then a small quantity of Temp-bond* is mixed and placed over both sides of the posterior teeth with a cement spatula. Once more the patient's mandible is guided to the centric jaw relation position as indicated by the anterior stone guide (Fig. 18-6). This procedure also establishes a record of the vertical component of the centric jaw relation, *not* the mean vertical dimension. The patient is asked to snap open the jaw again (Fig. 18-7), and the denture is removed from the mouth.

*Kerr Manufacturing Co., Romulus, Mich.

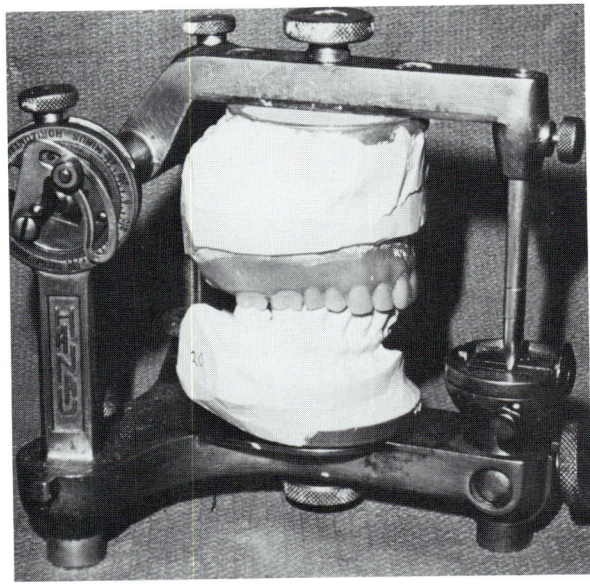

Fig. 18-9. Maxillary cast of denture with relining impression mounted on articulator to opposing cast of natural teeth.

LABORATORY PROCEDURES

Preparation of cast and mounting on articulator. A cast is poured in the denture to be relined (Fig. 18-8); it is indexed, and, after an application of petrolatum, the cast is mounted on the instrument of choice (Fig. 18-9). Inasmuch as the mounting casts on all dentures should be retained, neither a face-bow transfer nor a new opposing cast is required when relining only one denture.

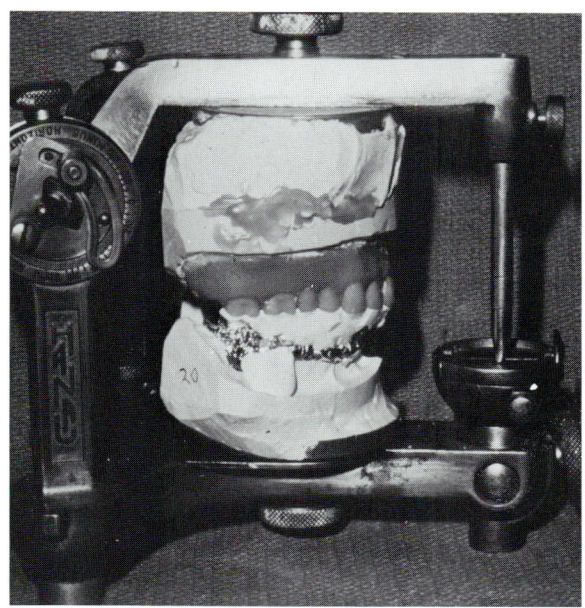

Fig. 18-10. Mandibular cast covered with tinfoil with stone painted over it and articulator closed to form matrix for teeth.

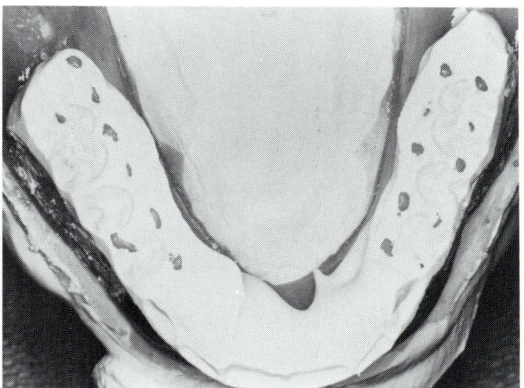

Fig. 18-11. Stone matrix showing seating of denture teeth.

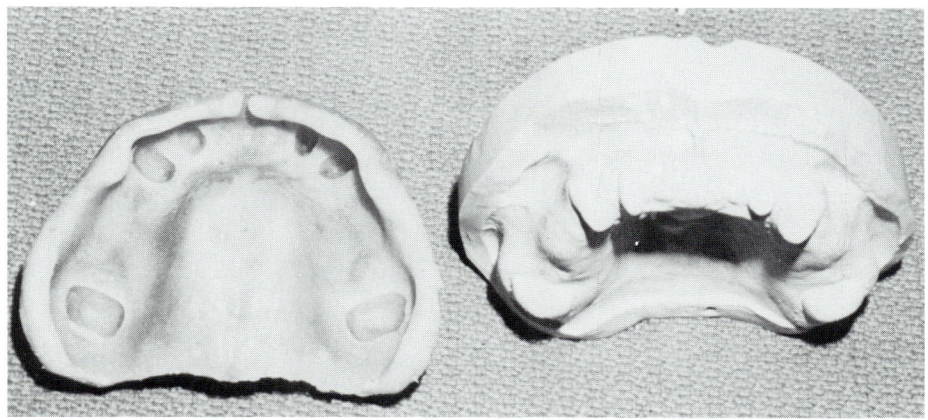

Fig. 18-12. On left is denture after removal from cast; on right is maxillary cast after removal from articulator.

However, a new face-bow transfer is essential to reline both dentures at the same time.

Preparation of opposing cast as matrix. When a maxillary overdenture opposed by a natural dentition is relined, the teeth on the stone cast of the natural teeth are covered with tinfoil. Then a thin mix of quick-setting stone is painted over the foil, and the denture is closed into the stone (Fig. 18-10). It is essential that the incisal guide pin be in contact with the incisal table. After the stone is set, the articulator is opened (Fig. 18-11) and closed to assure proper seating of the denture into the matrix.

Preparation of denture on articulator. After the maxillary cast is removed from the articulator and placed in warm water, the denture is removed from the cast (Fig. 18-12). The palate is cut out, and the peripheral borders and posterior edge are

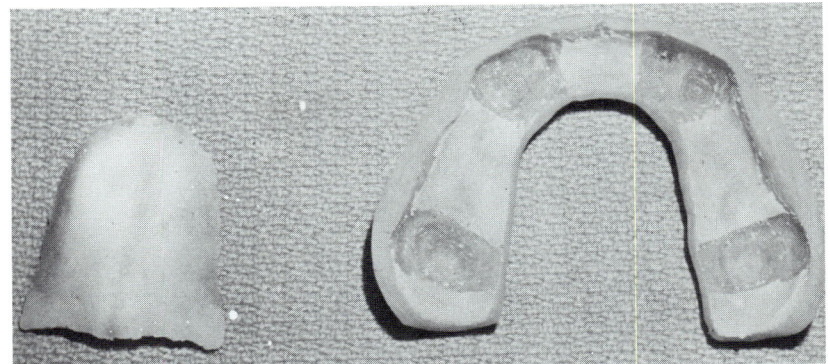

Fig. 18-13. Denture prepared for relating to cast and opposing stone matrix.

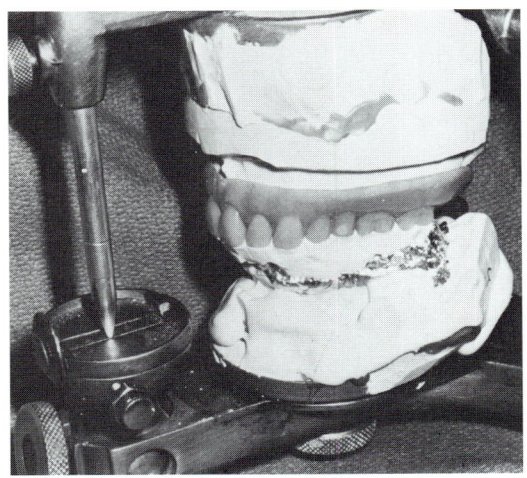

Fig. 18-14. Prepared denture with cast re-related to articulator and matrix guides.

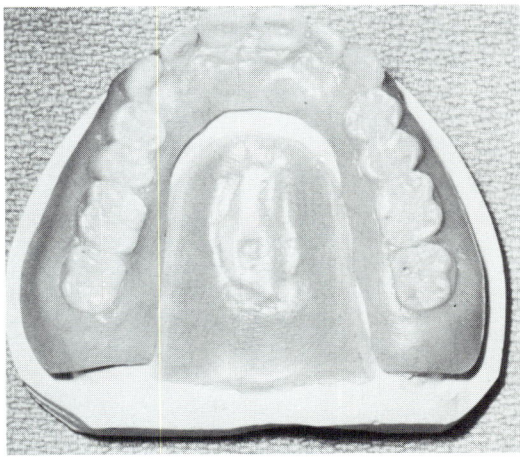

Fig. 18-15. Sectioned palatal portion of denture returned to cast for repositioning.

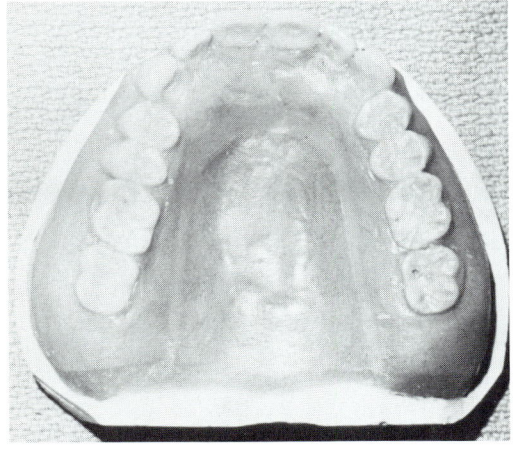

Fig. 18-16. New palatal section waxed.

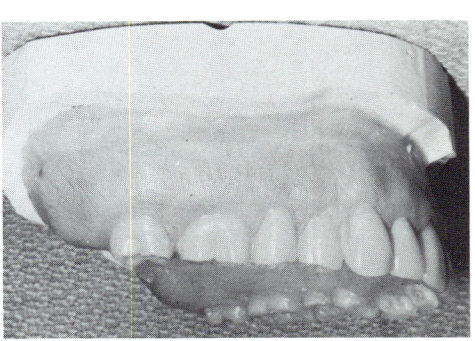

Fig. 18-17. Denture waxed for processing.

RELINING, REBASING, AND SOFT LINERS 231

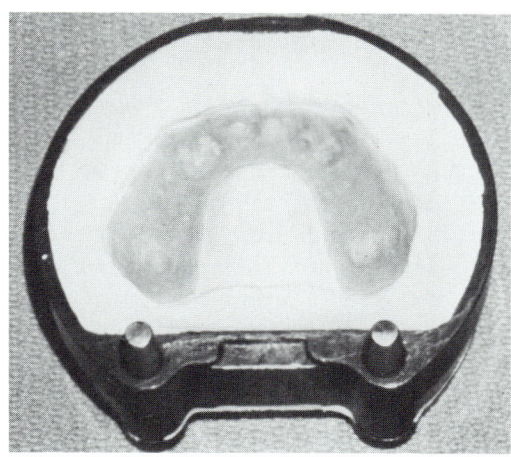

Fig. 18-18. Denture after flasking, opening, and removal of wax and palatal section. Intaglio surface was reduced to assure adequate thickness of new material.

reduced by ⅛ inch. The hydrocast is removed from the intaglio surface of the denture except in several "step" areas (Fig. 18-13). The denture is reseated on the cast, which is returned to the articulator and closed to assure proper seating on the stone matrix (Fig. 18-14). Then the denture is waxed to position on the cast; at this time it is imperative that the relationship to the matrix be maintained. The articulator is opened, and the palatal section is finished by waxing it only in the part cut out (Fig. 18-15) or by rewaxing the entire section (Fig. 18-16). After completion of the waxing (Fig. 18-17), the denture is returned to the articulator to verify the seating in the matrix.

Preparation of denture in flask. After flasking and opening of the flask, the wax is boiled out, the palatal section and the balance of the hydrocast are removed, and the entire intaglio surface is reduced to assure adequate thickness of the new material (Fig. 18-18). However, when a soft liner, such as Molloplast-b,* is used, the palate is not cut out.

Rechecking on articulator after processing. After being packed and processed, the cast with the denture is returned to the articulator and

---

*K. G. Köstner & Co., 6370 Oberursel/Taunus, PostFach 271, West Germany.

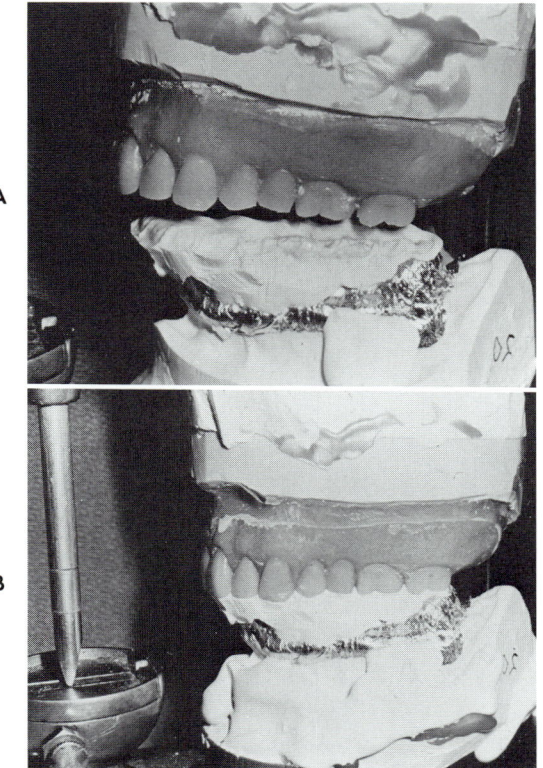

Fig. 18-19. A, Relined denture and cast returned to articulator. B, Relined denture seated into opposing stone matrix showing proper positioning and no pin opening.

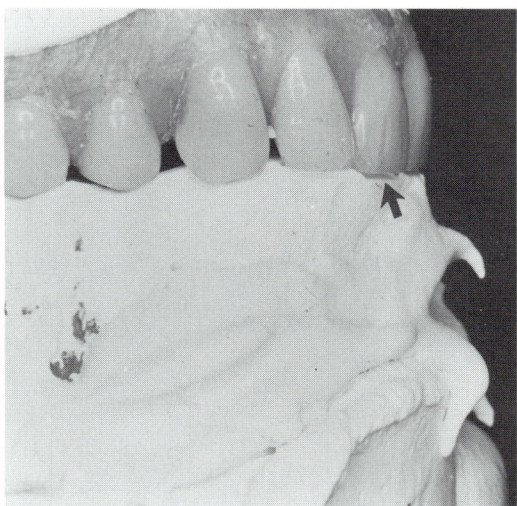

Fig. 18-20. Error (arrow) caused by change during processing.

closure into the matrix is verified (Fig. 18-19). If a processing change is found (Fig. 18-20), the stone matrix and foil are removed from the opposing cast, and the errors in occlusion resulting from the change are corrected by selective grinding. This method assures the correct maxillomandibular relativity of the denture when placed in the mouth. Relining of the mandibular denture is accomplished in the same manner.

Relining opposing dentures. If both dentures are taken from the patient for relining at the same time, they are mounted on the articulator as described previously. In this instance, one denture reline is completed and returned to the articulator for checking and correcting, if necessary, before instituting the procedures on the opposing denture. In this manner the relationship can be maintained.

Rebasing procedures. The procedures for rebasing differ in only the following respects:

1. Although the denture is removed from the cast after articulating, neither reduction of the peripheral borders nor cutting out of the palate are required. It is essential that enough of the hydrocast be removed to avoid fracturing the tooth prominences on the cast when separating the flask.

2. The porcelain teeth can be separated from the denture by heating them with an alcohol

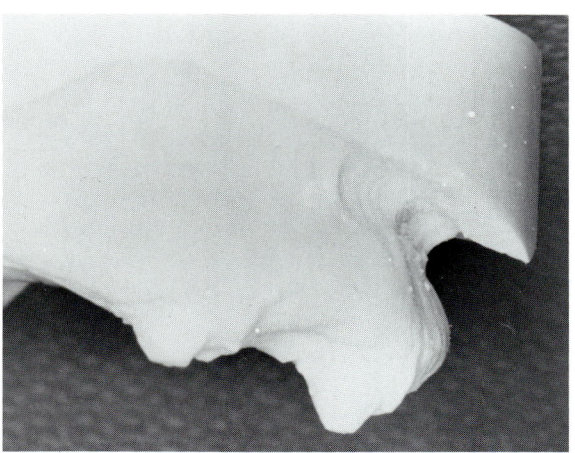

Fig. 18-21. Cast with severe undercuts, which can be obturated with a soft liner.

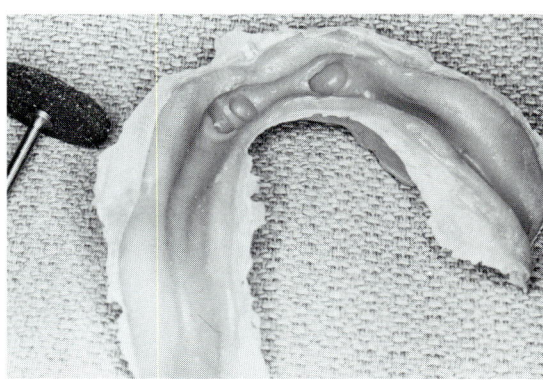

Fig. 18-22. Overdenture with soft liner before trimming.

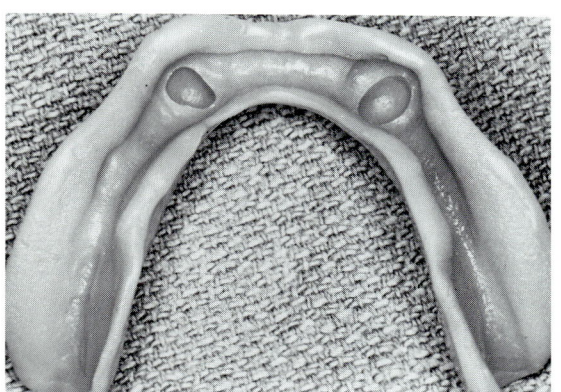

Fig. 18-23. Overdenture with entire tissue surface in soft liner.

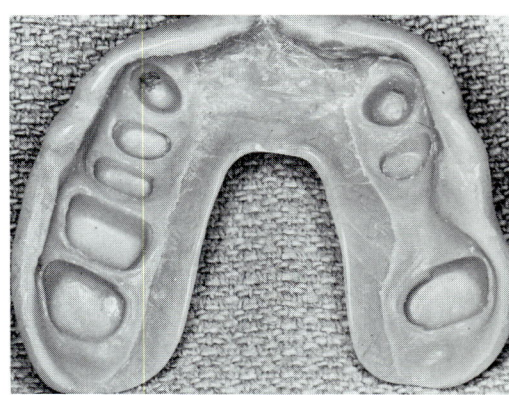

Fig. 18-24. Overdenture with multiple abutments. In this instance soft liner around teeth greatly improved retention.

torch. The acrylic extending into the diatorics is cut away, and the teeth are reseated in their respective "sockets" in the denture base.

3. The resin teeth can be cut off individually or as a unit and repositioned to the denture base with the opposing stone matrix.

4. After separation of the flask, all of the old acrylic is removed and replaced.

The subsequent procedures are the same as described previously.

SOFT LINERS

In many situations bony or soft tissue protuberances (Fig. 18-21) require that the overdenture be relieved over these areas to avoid "scuffing" of the tissue and to permit seating. Invariably this breaks the peripheral seal and reduces the retention of the denture. I have found that these spaces or undercut areas may be filled with a soft liner. This enhances the retention in two ways. The peripheral seal is maintained, and the material may be adapted closely to the retained teeth and even into the gingival crevice. The tissues appear to respond favorably to this close adaptation. The entire denture may be so lined (Figs. 18-22 and 18-23), or the material may be placed only in these undercut areas or additionally around the teeth (Fig. 18-24). This may be accomplished at the time of denture fabrication or subsequent to the initial insertion.

At the present my material of choice as a soft liner is Molloplast-b.* The manufacturer claims that the material will not undergo a gradual hardening process, nor will it absorb saliva. I do, however, explain to the patient that the material has a limited life and may have to be replaced at any time from 6 months to 2 years. I recommend that the manufacturers' instructions be followed in using this material.

---

*K. G. Köstner & Co., 6370 Oberursel/Taunus, PostFach 271, West Germany.

PART FOUR
SPECIAL CONSIDERATIONS

protective to dentin surfaces. It is impossible to make a direct extrapolation of all enamel protection data to dentin, for the chemical composition of these two tissues differs so markedly.

At pH 3.5 the order was reversed, with enamel more soluble than dentin and dentin more soluble than bone. At all pH values, after removal of the organic matter, bone dissolved faster than dentin,

Based on the previous work reviewed and the current research presented in this chapter, some recommendations can be made for the chemical protection of dentin surfaces exposed to oral fluids when preparing patients for overdentures. Dentin surfaces are highly susceptible to protective reactions that follow treatment with either APF or SnF_2 used singly. Combination treatments using APF and SnF_2 give significantly more protection than the single treatments. The performance of APF followed by SnF_2 is outstanding in this respect.

The following treatment procedure is particularly appropriate in managing the overdenture patient. At each office visit, the dentin surfaces are given a 2-minute topical application of APF first. The research reported here indicates that the concentration of fluoride in this APF can be reduced from the conventional 1.23% to 0.5% without loss of efficacy. The APF treatment is followed immediately by a 2-minute treatment with 0.4% SnF_2. The latter treatment solution can be prepared quickly and easily from a glycerin-based SnF_2 concentrate shown in Fig. 19-5.

Although professionally administered treatment can be expected to be highly effective, the inescapable fact is that after the patient has been given dentures, visits to the dentist become less frequent. Therefore it is essential that patients with overdentures receive a chemical preventive program that they can apply themselves in a home-care, oral hygiene regimen.

This requirement is met readily by the use of a water-free, completely and indefinitely stable 0.4% SnF_2 gel developed in this laboratory and distributed for clinical use throughout the 168 hospitals of the Veterans Administration. It is recommended that the overdenture patient use this gel in a daily program of chemical preventive dentistry.

The ability of fresh stannous fluoride solutions to protect dental enamel is unquestioned. Advocates of other forms of topical treatment frequently criticize stannous fluoride by the following statements: (1) deleterious chemical changes ensue when stannous fluoride is placed in aqueous solution; (2) this characteristic prohibits treatment with stannous fluoride in a gel vehicle, one of the currently popular methods used for topical treatment with other compounds; (3) pigmentation or staining frequently results from stannous fluoride treatment; (4) some concentrations of stannous fluoride induce untoward soft tissue reactions, par-

Table 19-5. Effect of solvent and age on stannous tin concentration of SnF_2 solutions

Age of solution (months)	Stannous tin (mg./100 ml.)					
	Aqueous solutions			In solution in glycerin		
	1% SnF_2	0.4% SnF_2	0.1% SnF_2	1% SnF_2	0.4% SnF_2	0.1% SnF_2
Fresh	740.0	298.6	74.7	743.1	297.2	74.3
1	601.6	262.3	60.1	737.2	282.2	73.3
2	577.5	254.3	60.8	758.2	276.2	70.5
3	499.3	241.1	44.3	756.5	274.3	67.9
4	535.4	240.0	42.1	743.1	285.1	69.0
5	469.2	243.4	39.3	732.4	282.4	67.2
6	403.1	208.3	39.8	725.1	277.6	70.9
7	439.2	180.5	33.7	731.2	276.9	65.2
8	427.1	171.5	27.6	755.3	284.1	67.2
9	435.2	171.5	24.1	749.1	286.4	67.7
10	391.0	159.4	23.2	733.1	288.6	72.3
11	379.0	138.6	19.3	741.2	298.4	68.1
12	337.1	97.8	19.9	758.6	273.7	66.9
13	334.6	92.5	20.1	736.4	281.1	65.3
14	330.9	88.6	20.3	755.2	285.8	70.8
15	264.7	84.2	19.7	746.3	288.9	70.4

ticularly in areas of preexisting inflammation; and (5) taste characteristics are far from ideal.

In an attempt to obviate these criticisms of aqueous solutions of SnF_2, a method of forcing SnF_2 into solution in glycerin was developed (Shannon and co-workers, 1968). It was suggested that preparation of this solution would prevent the hydrolysis and oxidation of stannous tin that occurred after SnF_2 was dissolved in water and that it might extend the shelf life indefinitely.

Both aqueous and glycerin-based solutions of SnF_2 in concentrations of 1.0%, 0.4%, and 0.1% were prepared and analyzed throughout a 15-month ing period. This deleterious effect of water on the stannous tin concentration of these solutions and the completeness with which dissolution in glycerin protects this ion are apparent in Table 19-5 (Shannon, 1969).

The effect of the 15-month aging period on the fluoride concentration of the SnF_2 solutions is seen in Table 19-6. As with stannous tin, there was a significant loss of fluoride in the aqueous solutions as they aged, but there was no indication of fluoride decrease in the glycerin-based solutions.

An important evaluation of the 0.4% SnF_2 gel was completed recently; the patients were 209 children receiving orthodontic treatment over an 18- to 24-month period (Stratemann, 1973). The controls were 110 patients managed routinely by graduate orthodontic students under the direction of faculty members. Ninety-nine other children were treated in the same manner as the controls except that they received a daily treatment with the 0.4% SnF_2 gel. After the evening brushing of the teeth, each gel user rinsed his mouth thoroughly and then applied the gel with a toothbrush. He was told not to rinse or remove the gel from his teeth, not to consume any water, other beverage, or food of any type after gel treatment, but merely to expectorate without rinsing.

The incidence of decalcification in the 110 control patients was 58%, whereas in the 99 patients given the gel, it was only 27%. The incidence of decalcification was reduced more than 50%.

However, the relationship between the incidence of decalcification and the frequency with which patients used the gel was more important. Of the 99 patients using the gel, 29 used it infrequently (once a week or less), and the incidence of decalcification in this group was 66%. Of the 19 patients who used the gel two or three times a week, 26% had areas of decalcification. The ob-

Table 19-6. Effect of solvent and age on fluoride concentration of SnF_2 solutions

	Fluoride (mg./100 ml.)					
	Aqueous solutions			In solution in glycerin		
Age of solution (months)	1% SnF_2	0.4% SnF_2	0.1% SnF_2	1% SnF_2	0.4% SnF_2	0.1% SnF_2
Fresh	239	95.6	23.8	237.6	95.1	23.8
1	213	83.2	21.8	233.4	95.1	23.8
2	206	80.8	20.3	241.5	93.6	23.8
3	203	78.4	18.9	243.7	95.1	23.7
4	198	78.4	19.7	241.5	95.6	23.8
5	197	78.4	19.9	249.6	95.1	23.8
6	196	78.4	19.6	250.4	93.6	23.8
7	196	78.4	20.8	250.7	93.6	23.8
8	198	78.4	18.0	248.7	95.6	23.9
9	183	78.4	18.1	245.3	96.1	23.9
10	198	76.8	19.1	241.8	95.6	23.6
11	200	69.2	18.8	238.5	96.6	23.8
12	192	73.2	18.9	241.6	95.1	23.5
13	189	72.0	19.0	249.7	93.6	23.5
14	193	72.0	19.0	230.7	95.1	23.8
15	179	75.6	19.2	228.6	93.6	23.7

servation to be emphasized was that of the 51 patients who used the gel daily as directed, only 2% showed any evidence of decalcification. Therefore it was concluded that frequent use of the 0.4% SnF_2 gel as directed in this study would be a helpful adjunct in an orthodontic practice for the prevention of active caries as well as the unsightly and highly undesirable decalcification of enamel seen so frequently in this type of practice.

SUMMARY

On the basis of the evidence presented, it is recommended that management of the overdenture patient include a vigorous program of chemical preventive dentistry. Nearly maximal protection can be provided for the exposed dentin surfaces in these patients by strict adherence to a program of recall appointments and home care.

Recall office appointments. Ideally, the overdenture patient is seen every 3 months. During these recall appointments, maintenance of the retained teeth and soft tissues is evaluated. Disclosing solutions are used on both the retained teeth and the overdenture to reveal plaque deposits. At each office visit the dentin and root surfaces exposed to the oral environment are cleaned with a zirconium fluoride paste and treated with a sequential 2-minute application of APF, followed by a 2-minute application of fresh SnF_2. The fluoride concentration of the APF can be reduced from the conventional 1.23% to 0.5% without appreciable loss of efficacy. The fresh 0.4% SnF_2 topical solution can be prepared quickly and easily from an indefinitely stable glycerin-based SnF_2 concentrate (5.33%) described earlier in the chapter.

Home care regimen. The portion of the program that is of major importance is the daily home care treatment by the patient. The primary purpose of overdenture therapy is the preservation of the remaining oral tissues; without efficient home care, this goal is negated. A daily home care regimen consisting of the following should be followed:

1. Both the oral cavity and the overdenture should be cleansed after each meal. This is accomplished by brushing, but if brushing is impossible, at least a thorough rinsing should be done.

2. In addition to the after-meal cleansing, one thorough cleansing is necessary each day, preferably at bedtime. Depending on the oral conditions and the manual dexterity of the patient many helpful hygiene devices can be used, such as dental floss, a tightly twisted nylon yarn, interdental stimulators, interproximal brushes, disposable mouth mirrors, gauze strips, water irrigators, and contra-angle toothpick holders. The use of disclosing solutions is recommended highly. Initially, these solutions should be used on the overdenture and in the oral cavity daily. After the patient demonstrates proficiency in oral hygiene, the disclosing solutions should be continued weekly. In addition to the thorough cleansing of the retained teeth, it is important to provide for the stimulation and hygiene of the soft oral tissues.

3. The patient is given a stable, water-free 0.4% SnF_2 gel for use after the vigorous bedtime cleansing. The gel can be applied to the dentin surfaces with a toothbrush or any other suitable means. After swishing the gel around the mouth for 30 seconds, the patient holds it in the mouth for 2 minutes and then expectorates but does not rinse, thereby completing the treatment. The patient retires and generally leaves the overdenture in a cleaning solution while he sleeps.

4. This program of oral hygiene should be continued on a permanent basis because of the increased risk of caries in areas of exposed dentin and root surfaces in the retained teeth that support the overdentures.

REFERENCES

Apostolopoulos, A. X., and Buonocore, M. G.: Comparative dissolution rates of enamel, dentin and bone. I. Effect of the organic matter, J. Dent. Res. 45:1093-1100, 1966.

Brudevold, F., and Chilton, N. W.: Comparative study of a fluoride dentifrice containing soluble phosphate and a calcium-free abrasive: second year report, J. Am. Dent. Assoc. 72:889-894, 1966.

Brudevold, F., and Soremark, R.: Chemistry of the mineral phase of enamel. In Miles, A. E. W., editor: Structural and chemical organization of teeth, New York, 1967, Academic Press, Inc.

Brudevold, F., Savory, A., Gardner, D. E., Spinelli, M., and Speirs, R.: A study of acidulated fluoride solutions. I. In vitro effects on enamel, Arch. Oral Biol. 8:167-177, 1963.

Buonocore, M. G.: Dissolution rates of enamel and dentin in acid buffers, J. Dent. Res. 40:561-570, 1961.

DeShazer, D. O., and Swartz, C. J.: The formation of CaF_2 on the surface of hydroxyapatite after treatment with acidic fluoride-phosphate solution, Arch. Oral Biol. 1:1071-1075, 1967.

Frazier, P. D., and Engen, D. W.: X-ray diffraction study of the reaction of acidulated fluoride with powdered enamel, J. Dent. Res. **45**:1144-1148, 1966.

Gehl, D. H.: Overlay of tooth supported dentures, J. Wis. State Dent. Soc. **47**:362-363, 1971.

Goldman, B. M., and Shannon, I. L.: Application of fluorides to dentin surfaces, J. Ga. Dent. Assoc. **46**:17-22, 1973.

Kalista, W. T., Jr: Tooth supported complete dentures, Dent. Stud. **49**:38, 58, 63, 1971.

Loiselle, R. J., Crum, R. J., Rooney, G. E., and Stuever, C. H.: The physiologic basis for the overlay denture, J. Prosthet. Dent. **28**:4-12, 1972.

Miller, P. A.: Complete dentures supported by natural teeth, Texas Dent. J. **83**:4-8, 1965.

Sandoval, E., and Shannon, I. L.: Stannous fluoride and dentin solubility, Tex. Rep. Biol. Med. **27**:111-116, 1969.

Shannon, I. L.: Water-free solutions of stannous fluoride and their incorporation into a gel for topical application, Caries Res. **3**:393-347, 1969.

Shannon, I. L.: Dual application of fluorides, N. M. Dent. J. **21**:12, 32, 36, 1970a.

Shannon, I. L.: Enamel solubility reduction by topical applications of fluoride compounds, J. Oral Med. **25**:12-17, 1970b.

Shannon, I. L.: In vitro enamel solubility reduction through sequential applications of acidulated phosphofluoride and stannous fluoride, J. Can. Dent. Assoc. **36**:308-310, 1970c.

Shannon, I. L.: Antisolubility effects of acidulated phosphofluoride and stannous fluoride in the treatment of crown and root surfaces, Aust. Dent. J. **16**:240-242, 1971.

Shannon, I. L., Cook, J. M., III, Henson, W. T., and Moore, R. E.: Reduction of enamel solubility by stannous fluoride, J. Houston Dist. Dent. Soc. **40**:7-10, 1968.

Shannon, I. L., Edmonds, E. J., and Madsen, K. O.: Single, double and sequential methods for fluoride applications, J. Dent. Child. **41**:35-38, 1974.

Shannon, I. L., and Gibson, W. A.: Laboratory effectiveness of a two percent stannous fluoride prophylaxis paste, J. Can. Dent. Assoc. **29**:457-461, 1963.

Shannon, I. L., Uribe, T. R., and Wightman, J. R.: Topical treatment of prepared cavities, Tex. Dent. J. **91**:6-8, 1973.

Shannon, I. L., and Wightman, J. R.: Treatment of root surfaces with a combination of acidulated phosphofluoride and stannous fluoride, J. La. Dent. Assoc. **28**:14-17, 1970.

Stratemann, M. W.: Clinical effect of 0.4% stannous gel on orthodontic patients, M.S. thesis, Houston, Texas, 1973, University of Texas Dental Branch.

Wei, S. H. Y., and Forbes, W. C.: X-ray diffraction analyses of the reactions between intact and powdered enamel and several fluoride solutions, J. Dent. Res. **47**:471-477, 1968.

250 SPECIAL CONSIDERATIONS

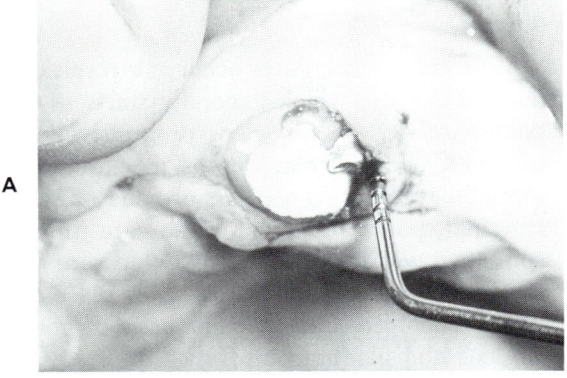

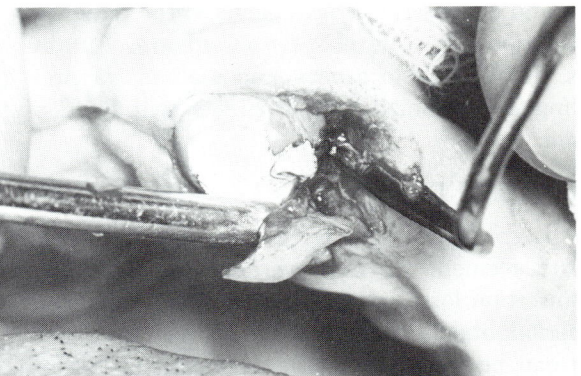

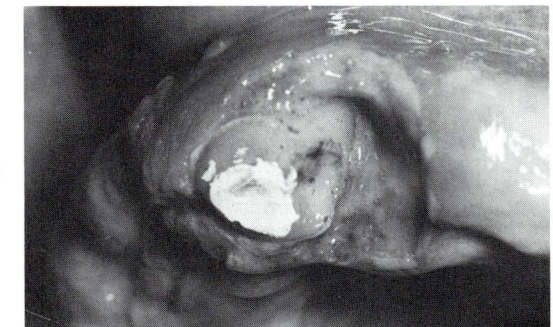

Fig. 20-3. **A,** Deep pocket on distal aspect of cuspid abutment. **B,** Pocket being eliminated by periodontal surgery. **C,** Surgical site after removal of pack.

abutment teeth with a silicophosphate cement* has seemed to improve their resistance to caries. Although evidence on effectiveness of fluorides in inhibiting caries in dentin or on root surfaces is limited, their use does not seem to be contraindicated. This subject is discussed in Chapter 19.

Other abutment losses

Loss of abutment teeth associated with the failure of endodontic therapy has been rare in our experience. However, the performance of endodontically treated abutment teeth without coping reinforcement over an extended service period of 15 to 20 years remains problematical. Abutment loss as a result of an accident involving facial injuries can be singularly catastrophic for the overdenture patient.

CLINICAL PROBLEMS

Providing acceptable overdentures does not require unusual skill or competence of the dentist.

---

*Fluoro-thin silicophosphate cement, S. S. White Dental Manufacturing Co., Philadelphia.

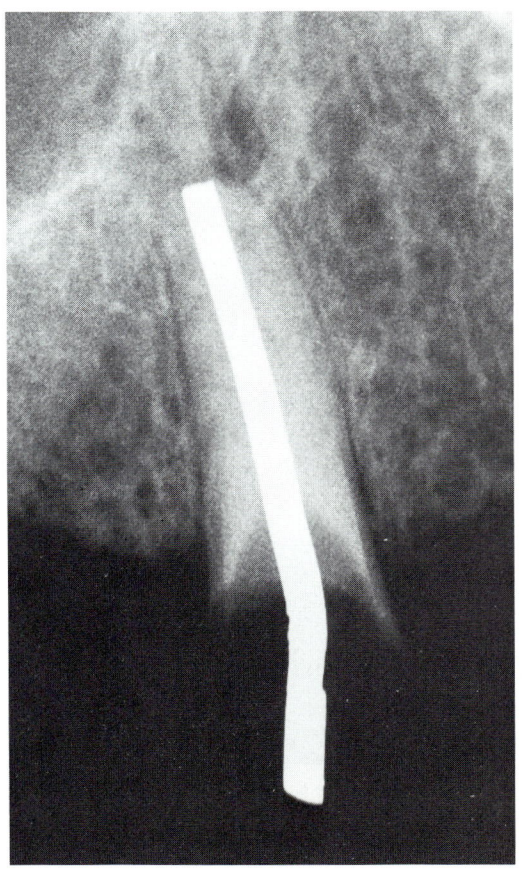

Fig. 20-4. Failure of abutments as a result of caries is possible with or without copings.

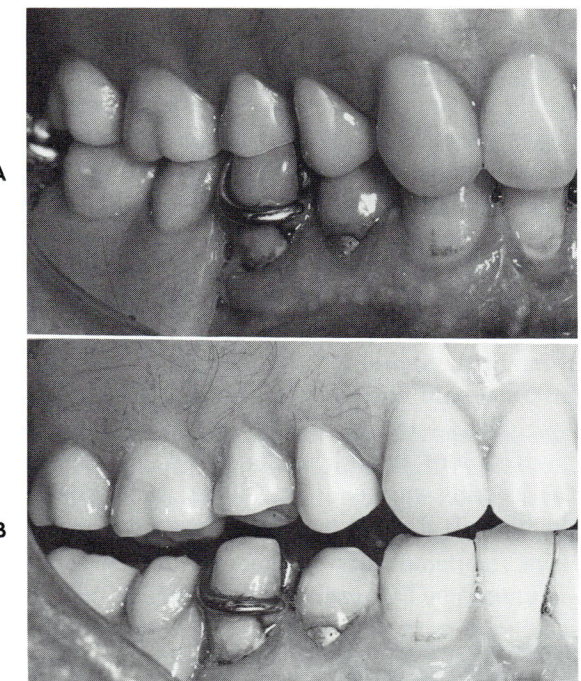

However improperly extended and contoured impressions, inaccurate jaw relation records, poorly prepared abutment teeth, and nonesthetic tooth arrangements contribute to overdenture problems. Impressions should be extended and contoured properly; overextended impressions produce overextended denture bases that often cause discomfort and inadequate retention of the overdenture. Adequate occlusal harmony can be developed only if accurate jaw relation records are accurately transferred to the articulator (Fig. 20-5).

Inadequate abutment reduction

In our early overdenture attempts, we thought that if more tooth structure was left above the

Fig. 20-5. A, Patient with maxillary overdenture in seemingly good occlusion. **B,** Same patient with deflective contacts preventing closure in retruded position. This was corrected after remounting.

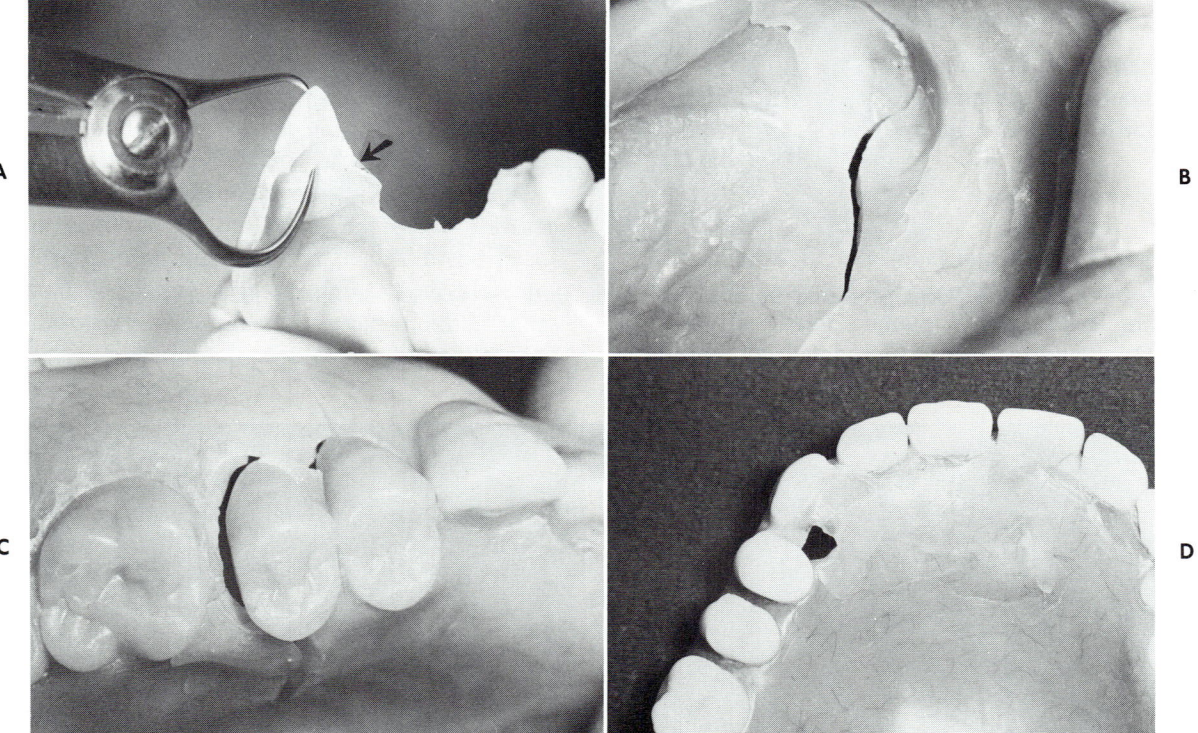

Fig. 20-6. A, Resin overdenture fracture through abutment tooth. Note thin lingual resin. **B,** Another resin overdenture fractured through abutment indentation. **C,** Overdenture fractured adjacent to abutment. Note again that resin was exceptionally thin. **D,** Abutment tooth was reduced inadequately and perforated base.

maxillary telescoping dentures after extensive preparatory procedures, Quintessence Int. 1:37-41, April, 1970.

Böttger, H., and Engelhardt, J. P.: The telescopic system in dental practice: prosthetic rehabilitation with a fixed maxillary bridge with telescoping elements and a unilateral free end denture in the mandible, Quintessence Int. 1:19-24, May, 1970.

Böttger, H., and Engelhardt, J. P.: The telescopic system in the dental practice: prosthetic restoration with a splint sence Int. 1:29-32, Dec., 1970.

Böttger, H., and Engelhardt, J. P.: The telescopic system in the dental practice: prosthetic treatment wtih telescopic prosthesis in the nearly edentulous mouth, Quintessence Int. 2:31-34, Jan., 1971.

Böttger, H., and Engelhardt, J. P.: The telescopic system in the dental practice: prosthetic treatment with a removable partial denture, Quintessence Int. 2:19-22, Feb., 1971.

Böttger, H., and Engelhardt, J. P.: The telescopic system

Flange, 80, 89
Flap
    mucoperiosteal; *see* Mucoperiosteal flap
    surgery, 49
Flasking, 106-108
    duplicate overdentures, 209-211
    immediate overdentures, 106-108
    metal base overdentures, 148-152
Flour of pumice, 111
Fluoride
    acidulated phosphate, and dentin solubility reduction, 240
    agents
        single, research on, 239-240
        topical, 238-246
    combinations, topical treatment with, 240-242
        current research on, 242-246
    dentin solubility reduction by different treatments, 243
    enamel solubility reduction by, 241
    gel, 116
        stannous, 86
    root surface solubility and, 242
        flowing tap water and, 242
    stannous
        concentration of, effect of solvent and age on, 245
        dentin solubility
            multiple applications, 238
            single application, 238
            various concentrations, 240
        mouthwash concentrate, 243
        stannous tin concentration of, effect of solvent and age on, 244
        topical treatment with, 238-239
Forces; *see* Occlusal forces
Fracture of resin overdenture through abutment tooth, 251
Future of overdentures, 256

G

Gauge, EM, 171
Gauze roller bandage for cleansing overdenture, 50
Gerber attachment, 157, 177-179
    nonresilient, 177-178
    resilient, 178-179
Gingivectomy, 49
Ginta attachment, 181-182
Gloves, plastic, for packing, 109
Grooves, retention, 107

H

Hader bar joint, 170, 187-188
Handles and sprung, 201-202
Heat-curing resin, 109
History, 24-26
    dental, 24
    medical, 24
Home care regimen for chemical protection of tooth surfaces, 246
Hydrocolloid impressions, reversible, 82

Hygiene
    oral
        instructions, 116
        overdentures, metal base, 153, 154
        poor, after periodontal therapy, 51
    overdenture
        immediate, 116
        metal base, 153
Hypertension and endodontic therapy, 55

I

Implants, endodontic, 58-61
    cementing, 61
    contraindications for, 58-59
    endosseous, 253
    fitting, 61
    instruments for, 59
    preparation of, 60
    technique, 59-61
Impression(s)
    alginate, 100
        irreversible hydrocolloid, with partial denture, 88
    hydrocolloid, reversible, 82
    for immediate overdentures, 100-105
        pouring of cast, 102-105
    with modeling plastic, 101
    paste, zinc oxide, 104
    procedures
        for rebasing, 226
        for relining, 226
    rubber base material, 100
    tray, stock rim lock, 101
Incisor, lateral, as abutment, 35
Indicator paste, 113
Instruments
    blockout, 193
    for endodontic implants, 59
    for mucoperiosteal flap
        one-handed control of, 70
        two-handed control of, 70
Interoceptors, 4
Introfix, 179
Ipso-Clip, 189-190
Irritation from overdenture, 86

J

Jaw relation records
    centric, 226-228
        armamentarium for, 226
    centric check-points, 214-219
        error correction, 217-218
        metal base overdentures, 216
        procedure, 214-216
        set of, 214
        single overdenture, 219
    for immediate overdentures, 105
    for metal base overdentures, 137-147
        centric check-points, 216

Jaw relation records—cont'd
  for metal base overdenture opposed by complete denture, 137-139
    centric jaw relation record, 139
      verification of, 139
    establishing occlusal plane, 138
    face-bow transfer, 138
    vertical dimension of occlusion, 138
  for metal base overdenture opposed by natural or restored dentition, 141-147
    conventional procedure, 141
    path technique; see Path technique
  for metal base overdenture opposed by overdenture, 139-141
    pretreatment measurements, 139-140

K

Kerr Endoposts, 168
Kurer screw, 168

L

Lathe-mounted arbor band, 111
Liners, soft, 13, 233
  problems with, 254

M

Mandible
  dentulous
    appearance of, 64
    comparison with edentulous mandible, 64
    intact, appearance of, 64
  development, four stages of, 39
  edentulous
    after death, 64
    before death, 64
    comparison with dentulous mandible, 64
  prognathic, 79
  surgery and; see Surgery, mandible and
Maxilla
  dentulous, appearance of, 65
  surgery and, 63-66
Maxillary antrum, pneumatization into posterior alveolar ridge, 72-73
Maxillary cast
  face-bow transfer to articulator, 83
  mandibular cast related to, on articulator, 83
Measurements, 13, 99
Mechanoreceptor, definition, 4
Medical history, 24
Metal bases; see also Overdentures, metal base
  blockout procedures for; see Blockout procedures for metal bases
  burnout, 202-204
  casting, 204
    devesting, 204
    fitting of, 206-207
  design
    considerations, 130-136, 191-192
    modifications, 133-134

Metal bases—cont'd
  diagnostic cast, designing procedures, 135-136
  duplicating casts, 196-198
    pouring refractory cast, 196
    preparation for, 195-196
    removal of master cast from duplicating material, 196-197
    trimming refractory cast, 197-198
  examining casts, 192-193
  finishing, 205-206
  investing wax pattern, 202
  laboratory procedures for, 191-208
  mandibular
    design considerations, 130-133
    extension of metal base, 130-132
    finishing, 133
    polishing, 133
    relief for copings, 132
    resin retention, 133
    thickness of base, 132-133
  maxillary, design considerations, 133
  opaquing of, 150-152
  polishing, 205-206
  problems with, 207-208
  spruing; see Spruing
  survey, general considerations, 191-192
  try-in, 136-137
  typical, illustration, 192
  wax-up, 198-201
    armamentarium for, 198
    general considerations, 198
    technical considerations, 198-201
Metal dowels, prefabricated, 165-166
Metal occlusal surfaces, 220-225
  from carved wax patterns, 220-224
    carving procedures, 221-222
    casting, 223
    completing denture, 223-224
    flasking occlusal units, 223
    investing pattern, 222-223
    investment core, 222
    laboratory procedures, 221-224
    making wax pattern, 222
    packing resin, 223
    waxing occlusal units, 223
  from denture teeth, 224
  from existing dentures, 224-225
  indications for, 220
Millimeter ruler, 99
Mini Zest, 183
Mini-Presso-matic, 189
Mixer, power, 102
Modeling plastic, 101
  cotton fibers embedded in, 101
  trimming, 101
Molars
  as abutments, 53-55
  mandibular, first, two separate distal roots, 54
Mooser dowel, 166
M.P. channels, 185-186

Mucoperiosteal flap, 69-71
    one-handed control of instrumentation, 70
    two-handed control of instrumentation, 70
Muscle changes after natural tooth contacts, 7-8

N

Neuromuscular function and sensory input, 3-6
Nutritional guidance, inadequate, 254

O

Obturation, 57-58
Occlusal forces
    in conventional dentures, 9
    in overdentures, 9
Occlusal surfaces; *see* Metal occlusal surfaces
Occlusion
    check with transitional overdentures, 89
    ideal, with overdentures, 13
    rims, 103
Oligodontia, 78
    complete mouth radiographs, 80
    diagnostic casts, 81
Opaquing of metal base, 150-152
Oral hygiene; *see* Hygiene, oral
Overdentures
    for acquired defects, 77-87
        indications for, 77
        procedures, 77-87
    advantages of, 12-14
    alveolar bone preservation in, 9-10
    anatomic basis for, 39-40
    attachments for; *see* Attachments
    breakage of, 254-255
    care, follow-up, inadequate, 253-254
    cleansing; *see* Cleansing
    for congenital defects, 77-87
        indications for, 77
        procedures, 77-87
    construction simplicity, 12
    contraindications for, 14
    conversion to complete denture, 13
    cured, remounted in articulator, 110
    disadvantages of, 13-14
    duplicate, 209-213
        flasking overdenture, 209-211
        insertion of, 213
        making teeth, 211-212
        modifying flask, 209
        pouring base, 213
    effectiveness of, 12
    esthetic excellence of, 12
    fitted to mouth with disclosing wax, 85
    flange, short, 80
    future of, 256
    immediate, 29-30, 98-118
        adapting to abutments, 115-116
        advantages of, 98
        care
            follow-up, 117-118
            postinsertion, 115-118

Overdentures—cont'd
    immediate—cont'd
        clinical procedures, 99-105
        construction of, 105, 106-111
        diagnosis, 99
        disadvantages of, 99
        examination, 99
        finishing of, 109-111
        flasking of, 106-108
        hygiene, 116
        impressions for, 100-105
            pouring of cast, 102-105
        jaw relation records, 105
        packing, 107, 108-109
        placing of, 111-115
            abutment preparation, 111-112
            surgical procedures, 112-115
        polishing of, 109-111
            rubber cup and flour of pumice used, 111
        positioning teeth, 106
        pretreatment records, 99
        relining, 116-117
        selecting teeth, 106
        stippled surface, 111
        treatment planning, 99-100
        trimming with lathe-mounted arbor band, 111
        waxing of, 106-108
    indications for, 14
    maintenance of
        ease of, 12
        patient-dentist relationship and, 20-21
    metal base, 119-155; *see also* Metal bases
        abutment copings for; *see* Copings
        adaptation, verification of, 152-153
        advantages of, 119-120
        breakage of, 254
        bubble gum massage, 153
        contraindications for, 120
        disadvantages of, 120
        failures, 154
        finishing of, 152
        flasking of, 148-152
        hygiene, 153
            oral, 153, 154
        impression for, 128-130
            duplicate cast, 130
            pouring master cast, 129-130
        indications for, 120
        jaw relation records; *see* Jaw relation records for metal base overdentures
        maintenance of, 153-154
        packing of, 152
        placing overdenture, 152-154
        polishing of, 152
        positioning teeth, 148
        postinsertion instructions, 153-154
        processing, 148-152
            minimizing error, 148-149
        recall appointments, 153
        selection of teeth, 148

Overdentures—cont'd
  metal base—cont'd
    wax elimination, 149-150
  occlusal forces in, 9
  periodontal basis for, 38-39
  periodontics and; see Periodontics and overdenture patient
  problems with, 248-255
    clinical, 250-254
  procedures, familiar, 13
  refitting due to resorption, 253
  remote, 30, 119-155
    construction of, 30
    metal base; see Overdentures, metal base
  removable partial, 156-161
    abraded teeth retained for, 158
    eroded teeth retained for, 158
    existing, alteration of, 157-161
    Gerber attachments for, 157
    initial fabrication, 156-157, 158-159
  resin
    breakage, 254
    fracture through abutment tooth, 251
  retention of, 12
  retention of teeth for, rationale for, 3-11
  single, centric check-points for jaw relation records, 219
  stability of, 12
  successful, 162-163
  superiority of, 12
  transitional, 30, 88-97
    advantages of, 88
    completed
      after insertion, 95
      after polishing, 94, 97
    conversion using denture teeth, 89-91
      intermediate modifications, 89
      modifications, 90, 91
      removable partial denture, 88
    disadvantages of, 88-89
    postinsertion care, 97
    using patient's teeth, 91-97
      removable partial denture not present, 91-94
      removable partial denture present, 94-97
  types of, 29-30
  unilateral, 161

P

Packing of overdentures
  immediate, 107, 108-109
  metal base, 152
Pain after one-appointment endodontics, 58
Palate, open, 12-13
Parkel CI kit, 168
Paste
  impression, zinc oxide, 104
  indicator, 113
Path technique for jaw relation records, 141-147
  adapting denture teeth to core, 146-147
  baseplate fabrication, 142-143
  making compound rim, 143

Path technique for jaw relation records—cont'd
  positioning teeth, 143
  pouring path, 146
  pretreatment records, 143-145
  recording cuspal path, 146
  tentative record, 141-142
  wax try-in, 145
Patient
  acceptance, 13
  conference, 29
  -dentist relationship, 17-23
    appointments and, 20
    establishing relationship, 19-20
    fees and; see Fees
    human relations vs. practice management, 19
    maintaining relationship, 20
    overdenture maintenance and, 20-21
    treatment options, 17-18
  psychologic problems of, 18-19
  special factors related to, 18-19
Pawl connectors, 188-190
  Ipso-Clip, 189-190
  Mini-Presso-matic, 189
  Presso-matic, 188-189
Perception
  decrease in older people, 8
  definition, 3
  dimensional, 6-7
  of nonvital teeth, 8
  of teeth with reduced alveolar support, 8
Periodontal
  abscess, 51
  basis for overdentures, 38-39
  curettes, curved, 43
  disease, and abutment loss, 248, 249, 250
  examination, 27-28, 41
  ligament space, 40
  pathology, 40
  probes, double-ended Williams, 43
  probing, 42-43
  receptors, sensory input from, 6-8
  status of abutments, 31
Periodontics and overdenture patient, 37-51
  complications, 50-51
  diagnosis, 43-44
  evaluation, 40-43
  examination
    oral, 41
    radiographic, 41-42
  maintenance of overdenture, 49-50
  medical history, 40-41
  prognosis, 44
  treatment planning, 44-49
    construction of overdenture, 49
    endodontics, 47
    extraction of hopeless teeth, 47
    intermediate overdentures, 47
    periodontal therapy, 47-49
    tooth selection, 44-47
    transitional overdentures, 47

Periodontium, 40
Pins for overdenture copings, 123
    plastic, 123
Pivot
    Schenker step, 167
    Stutz, 166-167
Plastic
    gloves for packing, 109
    modeling; see Modeling plastic
Pneumatization of maxillary antrum into posterior alveolar ridge, 72-73
Polishing
    metal bases, 205-206
        mandibular, 133
    of overdentures
        immediate, 109-111
            rubber cup and flour of pumice used, 111
        metal base, 152
Power mixer, 102
Premolar, maxillary first, with three roots, 54
Presso-matic, 188-189
Pressoreceptors, definition, 4
Pressure button; see Studs
Probe, periodontal, double-ended Williams, 43
Probing, periodontal, 42-43
Prognosis, 36
Proprioception
    definition, 4
    salivary secretion and, 8
Proprioceptive sensibility, definition of, 3-4
Proprioceptors, definition of, 4
Prosthodontic patient; see Patient
Psychologic problems of patient, 18-19
Pumice, flour of, 111

Q
Quinlivan Snapper, 170, 182

R
Radiography
    in endodontic evaluation of abutments, 52-55
        examination, 28
            periodontal patient, 41-42
        in oligodontia, 80
Rebasing, 226-233
    impression procedures, 226
    procedures, 232-233
Receptors
    definition of, 4
    periodontal, sensory input from, 6-8
Records, 24-26
    jaw relation; see Jaw relation records
    pretreatment, 24-26
        for immediate overdentures, 99
        photographic, 26
Refitting due to resorption, 253
Relining
    immediate overdentures, 116-117
    impression procedures, 226
    jig, 117

Relining—cont'd
    laboratory procedures, 228-232
    opposing dentures, 232
    preparation of cast and mounting on articulator, 228-229
    preparation of denture
        on articulator, 229-231
        in flask, 231
    preparation of opposing cast as matrix, 229
    rechecking on articulator after processing, 231-232
Remote overdentures; see Overdentures, remote
Resin
    autopolymerizing
        saturated with monomer, 89
        sifted into abutment indentations, 89
    dowels, prefabricated, 165
    "flash," excess, removal of, 115
    heat-curing, 109
    overdentures; see Overdentures, resin
    packing for metal occlusal surfaces from carved wax pattern, 223
    retention
        for mandibular metal bases, 113
        in spruing, 202
    tray, 100
Resorption necessitating refitting of overdenture, 253
Restorations, amalgam, 112
Retention
    grooves, 107
    of overdentures, 12
Reversibility of overdentures, 13
Rheumatic fever and endodontic therapy, 55
Ridge
    alveolar; see Alveolar ridge
    laps and tinfoil substitute, 108
Rim(s)
    lock impression tray, 101
    occlusion, 103
Roentgenology; see Radiography
Root
    canals
        of bicuspid, maxillary second, files in, 53
        bifid, 54
        sealing of, 112
        split, 54
    surface solubility and fluoride, 242
        flowing tap water and, 242
Rothermann attachment, 179-180, 181
    nonresilient, 180
    resilient, 180
Rubber base impression material, 100
Ruler, millimeter, 99

S
Salivary secretion and proprioception, 8
Schenker step pivot, 167
Schubiger screw block, 180-181
Screws, 188
    block, Schubiger, 180-181
    Kurer, 168
    VK, 167-168

Sensation, definition, 3
Sensibility, proprioceptive, definition, 3-4
Sensitivity
   of anterior teeth, 6
   directional, 7
Sensory input
   neuromuscular function and, 3-6
   from periodontal receptors, 6-8
Snap grip, Baer, 174-175
SnF_2; see Fluoride, stannous
Soft liners, 13, 233
   problems with, 254
Soft tissues 5 years after overdenture insertion, 86
Spreaders for lateral condensation, 57
Sprinkle method, 97
Spruing, 201-202
   cast preparation for, 195
   handles and, 201-202
   mandibular castings, 201
   maxillary castings, 201
      circular bar design, 201
      horseshoe design, 201
   resin retention and, 202
   technical procedures, 201-202
Stabilization of existing structures, 13
Stannous fluoride; see Fluoride, stannous
Studs, 173
   comparison to bars, 169-170
   nonresilient, 173
   presentation of, 173-183
   resilient, 173
Stutz pivot, 166-167
Surgery, 62-73
   criteria for, 69
   future of, 73
   goal of, 68-69
   history of, 62
   limiting factors, 69
   as logical solution, 67-68
   mandible and, 63
      stability of field, 71
      two-handed use of instrumentation, 71, 72
   maxilla and, 63-66
   minimal, 68-73
   prescription, 66-68
   procedures, 69-73
Surveying procedure, 81

T

Teeth; see also Dental examination; Dental history
   abutments; see Abutment(s)
   anterior, sensitivity of, 6
   natural tooth contacts, muscle changes after, 7-8
   nonvital, perception of, 8
   with reduced alveolar support, perception of, 8
   retention for overdentures, rationale for, 3-11

Teeth—cont'd
   surfaces, chemical protection of; see Chemical protection of tooth surfaces
Tinfoil substitute and ridge laps, 108
Tissue
   blockout for metal bases, 194-195
   hard, 5 years after overdenture insertion, 86
   response to existing prostheses, 26
   soft, 5 years after overdenture insertion, 86
   supporting, less trauma with overdentures, 13
Tools; see Instruments
Toothbrush, soft multitufted nylon, 50
Toothpick for cleansing, 50
Training denture, 13
Trauma to supporting tissues, 13
Tray
   impression, rim lock, 101
   resin, 100
Treatment
   planning, 28-36
   prerequisite, 36
   sequence, 35
Trimming
   immediate overdenture with lathe-mounted arbor band, 111
   refractory cast, 197-198

V

Vac-U-Vestor, 102
Visual examination, 26-27
VK screw, 167-168

W

Water, tap, root surface solubility and fluoride treatments, 242
Wax
   baseplate, 100
   carved wax patterns, metal occlusal surfaces from; see Metal occlusal surfaces from carved wax patterns
   disclosing, 114
      overdentures fitted to mouth with, 85
   registration, mandibular cast related to maxillary cast on articulator by, 83
Waxing of immediate overdentures, 106-108
Wax-up; see Metal bases, wax-up
Whaledent Parapost, 168
Williams periodontal probe, 43

X

X-ray; see Radiography

Z

Zest anchor, 182-183
   mini, 183
Zinc oxide impression paste, 104